Epidemic Encounters, Communities, and Practices in the Colonial World

Epidemic Encounters, Communities, and Practices in the Colonial World

Edited by
Poonam Bala and Russel Viljoen

LEXINGTON BOOKS
Lanham • Boulder • New York • London

Published by Lexington Books
An imprint of The Rowman & Littlefield Publishing Group, Inc.
4501 Forbes Boulevard, Suite 200, Lanham, Maryland 20706
www.rowman.com

86-90 Paul Street, London EC2A 4NE

British Library Cataloguing in Publication Information Available

Library of Congress Cataloging-in-Publication Data Available

ISBN 9781793651228 (cloth) | ISBN 9781793651235 (ebook)

Dedicated to

Our late parents, who were remarkable individuals in their own right.

Sh Raghubir Narain and Smt. Sharda for their love and inspiration and for guiding me to the path of righteousness.

Ann and Brian Viljoen, who taught me the value of humility, faith and trust.

Contents

Acknowledgements

It is an extreme delight to see this book in print finally! The idea of a book project was conceived before the pandemic and completed during what would seem to be the back end of the pandemic, even though COVID-19 and the coronavirus will be with us for the rest of our lives. The book was envisioned to research the impact of colonization and disease on indigenous societies not knowing, of course, how an unknown disease disrupted and destroyed the lives and livelihoods of people from all walks of life in our present world. It, no doubt, provided researchers and academics a new and better understanding of disease and its impact on the lives of people past and present. With a long and tumultuous journey, occasionally halted by the pandemic that took a toll on humanity, globally, this book was not devoid of a roller coaster ride since its inception in 2019. Yet, this was no deterrent for this project and the journey continued!

Long-distance collaboration always poses a challenge when it comes to sharing the same academic platform of writing a volume jointly. Yet, the more than two-year journey of book writing has been immensely productive for which I thank my colleague and a friend I truly respect, Russel Viljoen, for his collegiality, commitment and cooperation in this long trek and I hope this will build up new collaborative academic ventures.

As co-editor of an important book on disease and colonial societies, my collaboration and association with Poonam Bala was equally rewarding and special, both personally and academically. As a senior scholar, her knowledge and expertise on the subject of disease studies, the social history of medicine and disease is exceptional and solid. Our friendship and collegial association spans well over a decade and this is our first collaboration as editors, for which I am very grateful.

The book is special and serves as a timely reminder of how destructive and lethal an outbreak of disease can be, especially when it transitioned into global pandemic. We, therefore, remember and mourn the many lives lost due to COVID-19 complications.

While we all worked under extremely difficult conditions when the libraries and institutions around the world witnessed lengthy closures during the recent pandemic, the academic zeal never faded and we are extremely thankful to all the chapter authors drawn from different continents and countries for their valuable contributions, their immense patience and cooperation in the making of this book. Without their support, this book would not have come to fruition. We also wish to thank the anonymous reviewers for their insightful comments.

To Wendy Recoegzi and Linda Francis, special thanks for their collegial support. Gillian, Hannah and Megan Viljoen deserve to be acknowledged for their support and patience.

Thanks also go to Lexington Books and the Publishing Editor, Eric Kuntzman, for his prompt responses and patience in awaiting the completion of this project. Thanks are also due to Rachel Kirkland for her editorial assistance and help in the finalization of the book. We would also like to express our gratitude to the Production Editors, Tricia Currie-Knight and Monica Sukumar for their assistance and input.

Thanks are also due to Nia Turner at the Heights Library (Cleveland) for her help in preparing the Index.

As always, I (Poonam Bala) owe a tribute to my (late) parents: I miss both of you dearly and your fond memories and countless blessings have become my fortune!

Poonam Bala, Cleveland, 2022
Russel Viljoen, Centurion, 2022

Introduction

Understanding Epidemics, Colonial Encounters and Communities

Poonam Bala and Russel Viljoen

Disease histories and the social history of disease, medicine, epidemics and pandemics have been researched, analysed and studied for decades by scholars drawn from the humanities to pure medical sciences.[1] Although their theoretical underpinnings and framework differed from discipline to discipline, in essence, the end result remains the same, namely, to provide plausible explanations on how infectious diseases disrupted humanity per se – over the centuries and in recent times, but also how humanity triumphed over numerous epidemiological disasters, as the human race. The Oxford-based archaeologist, Peter Mitchell, tracks the origins of disease to the very beginnings of human history. He argues that 'infectious disease has been part of human experience from the very origin of the hominid lineage, but the forms that it takes and effects exercised by different disease agents have altered enormously over time and space'.[2] Given the longevity in the 'coexistence' between humanity and infectious disease, as alluded to by Mitchell, it suggests that all diseases, like human beings, too have histories. At the very least, such histories often intersect at some point, or far worse, collide, leading to catastrophic consequences in the form of epidemics and pandemics translating into loss of life. Disease then, irrespective of when it occurred in the history of humanity throughout the ages, its impact was disruptive, devastating and brought into being a 'disbalance' in a structured world, as alluded to by William McNeill.[3] He identified a period, 'Transoceanic Exchanges 1500–1700', as a critical period of contact which witnessed the gradual introduction of diseases to the 'New World' societies to which many offered little or no resistance at all.

The 'discovery' of the 'Other World' during a period of exploration coined as the *Age of Discovery*[4] by scholars served as a precursor and catalyst to colonial conquest. These 'discoveries' not only sparked the remapping of geographical regions, renaming of conquered colonial territories and the introduction of new political agendas and ideologies, prompting new medical facilities, but soon spawned the introduction and dissemination of infectious diseases to newly acquired coastal colonies washed by the Indian and Pacific Oceans. The demonstration of colonial sea power followed by conquest of indigenous land systematically displaced and dismantled indigenous populations as many showed little or no resistance to the introduction of diseases to newly conquered territories. Soon, however, the previously isolated 'Other World' witnessed and experienced the emergence of a lethal and lasting liaison between 'discovery' and disease which, thus, forms a significant theme throughout the book. Indigenous societies, therefore, became a victim of both colonization and disease at the same time, during a period of commercial expansion accelerated by discoveries. It set forth a period and path whereby the gap of disease transmission between colonizer and colonized, country and country and continent and continent was significantly closed and the speed at which transmission and infection occurred. It paved the way for future endemics, epidemics and far worse, pandemics a distinct reality.

Disruptive colonial conquests and contradictions within disease situations and difficult health conditions made it well-nigh difficult for possible ameliorating efforts of the colonists. A 'disbalance' among infected and affected societies and people, and the rise and introduction of diseases, 'virgin spaces and landscapes',[5] thus continues to be a threat to indigenous people.

Historical studies and documented narratives, unlocking the histories of how epidemic and similar medical catastrophes shaped and continue to reshape the present and future of humanity, provide us with valuable lessons and coping mechanisms in dealing with current and future medical disasters. In defence of, and in recognition of, medical history and its current relevance in a modern world, Monica Green has written a powerful piece, entitled 'Emerging diseases, re-emerging histories'.[6] She takes on some issues with a report authored by a group of researchers at an American University for their blatant disregard of medical history and the 'comfortable erasure of the whole field of medical history', in their prediction of 'the world's next pandemic'.[7] While the researchers successfully predicted the futuristic scenario scientifically, it lacked historical input and knowledge of how past societies coped during times of medical crises. Similarly, David Arnold's reflection on the coronavirus using India as a test case is equally illuminating.[8] Using India as an example, he re-emphasized how knowledge of India's medical past in dealing with recurring medical disasters in the highly diseased-prone society proved vital in combating disease.[9]

A common and popular overarching theme that emerged in the study of disease within the humanities over the past few decades has been its analysis under the rubric of 'Epidemics and Society' or 'Disease and Society'. In their analysis, many scholars stressed how disease became a catalyst for social change as it came to be associated with disorder, disruption and ultimately, death. An excellent example of this theme is captured in the recent and mammoth study by Frank Snowden[10] titled *Epidemics and Society: From Black Death to the Present* and others that have preceded it.[11] Such studies sought and gave explanations how epidemics reshaped and reorganized the past and present world, but how its continuous presence in a modern and technologically advanced world still threatens the very existence of humanity. A major factor which brought about an equally disturbing 'disbalance' in conquered and newly colonized societies was the fact that the new colonizers emerged as the primary bearers of new diseases to settled indigenous societies of African, Indian and Australasian descent.

In his book *Contagion: How Commerce Has Spread Disease*,[12] Mark Harrison contends that the 'nineteenth century was a period of rapid change and saw an unprecedented redistribution of infections, but commerce had long shaped the epidemiological fate of humanity'.[13] His noteworthy mention of the affinity between commerce and contagion is a significant addition to our understanding of the spread of disease from Europe to indigenous communities with whom trade was carried on. Thus, the age of colonialism, furthered by European exploration and expansion, became a new catalyst for the introduction and transmission of infectious diseases and viruses to communities and societies that lived in isolation from Western societies. In this respect, the emergence of colonial powers and their quest to bring into being colonial societies visibly brought in a new dimension to 'disease and society' studies in later years.

It is now believed that colonial encounters and interactions between indigenous and Western medicine under colonial imperatives were often characterized by phases of contestation, negotiations and accommodation of knowledge and ideologies that eventually (re)defined both imperial and indigenous identities. In understanding the various processes in the context of transnational and transoceanic perspectives, it is certain that the various social and cultural interactions facilitated contacts between the communities; they also symbolized cultural and historical spaces within which were defined various social and cultural integrations. In this respect, the concomitant rise of empires exhibited a well-defined unity of land and sea wherein the maritime communities brought, for instance, 'Asia to the shores of Africa',[14] establishing new social and cultural fields. While this movement signified various aspects of social and cultural diversity[15] and the subsequent emergence of littoral communities around the Indian Ocean, for instance, it also offered new perspectives in maritime culture and in the unity of 'land and sea' environments.

The reclamation and restoration of the indigenous voice in a study by Sujit Sivasundaram entitled *Waves Across the South*[16] is yet another example of how globalized the world was during the eighteenth and nineteenth centuries. It masterfully combined studies produced in the past decade where the focus was either on *Oceanic Histories*,[17] detailing the interconnectedness between the oceans and the world's seas, or the *Pacific Worlds*[18] per se into one formidable historical account. It strengthened the magnitude of Ocean studies in the historiography of the global world, with special reference to the Indian and Pacific Oceans and the indigenous peoples whose lives past, present and future would have been profoundly shaped by it. While the Age of Revolutions across the Atlantic Ocean was held in high regard in the historiography of global studies, Sivasundaram has shifted academic attention to an equally significant part of the global world, namely, the Oceanic societies and island communities located in, bordered by or washed by the waters and waves of the Indian and Pacific Oceans. Conquest and colonization of the vast Indo-Pacific Oceanic region hardly suggests that it was a one-sided contest overshadowed by the expansion and consolidation of the empire, but sparked a period characterized by the rise of new revolutionary and political thought, political contestations, the emergence of rebel leaders culminating in the rise of resistance movements among a diverse group of indigenous societies.[19] As Sivasundaram puts it, 'the impact of the times as a phase of globalization is evident in how indigenous peoples saw their seas, their histories and their place on the globe'.[20]

More recently, scholars have analysed disease, medicine and health from a global perspective and began to link it to oceanic studies and oceanic histories. As such, the roots and the routes of contagion, colonial conquests and the introduction of disease were entrenched in the emergence and evolution of strategic sea routes expedited during the age of European colonial expansion and exploration. Strategic sea routes implied that explorers, navigators, sailors and ships sailed across three major oceans, notably, the Indian, Atlantic and Pacific to reach new societies. In their analysis, scholars established greater connections between Europe and the spread and introduction of new diseases to newly 'discovered' countries and societies bordered by the Atlantic, Indian and Pacific Oceans.[21] For instance, the existence of slavery in and around the Indian Ocean and its relation to colonial conquest is a noticeable theme in Winterbottom and Tesfaye's study that opens up new perspectives in understanding the interconnectedness between medicine, societies and colonialism across the seas.[22] A slightly different view is evident in Gómez's recent study. Based on the black Atlantic world, Gómez highlights the powerful contributions of black ritual healers and practitioners which engendered in great intensity in the scientific revolution, while also redefining the early modern world.[23] On a slightly different note, Campbell and Knoll portray an understanding of historical developments as a prelude to understanding the dynamic of disease in the Indian Ocean; their main focus is on the 'origin, dispersion and impact of disease in the Indian Ocean world societies.'[24] A significant impact was also seen in the transoceanic exchanges across the Atlantic when the exchange of plants and animals also meant exporting of several infectious diseases to the New World; this led to a 'mass destruction' of the indigenous peoples with more vulnerability to the new diseases.[25] So powerfully described as the 'Columbian Exchange',[26] Crosby takes the reader to a fascinating journey of understanding the diffusion of animals, plants and microbes and disease as a consequence of European colonization of the New World.[27]

Driven by commercial interests and having mastered navigating the Atlantic, Indian and Pacific Oceans, well-established seafaring nations, notably, the Dutch, British, French, Portuguese and Spanish fleets, began to pose a major threat to vulnerable coastal communities apart from colonial conquest. The founding of new communities and the frequency of person-to-person contact naturally coincided with the introduction of disease to unexposed communities. Disease studies obtained a new angle as scholars linked the frequent navigation of the three major oceans and the dissemination of disease. In his seminal work, David Arnold explains how the Indian Ocean,[28] as the lifeblood of trade and economic prosperity, actually triggered the dispersion of disease in the wide region. Trade, and later, colonial conquest soon transitioned into becoming medical conduits for the dissemination of disease.[29]

Colonial expansion, transcontinental trade and transoceanic sea travel exposed indigenous and local communities to new challenges of which face-to-face contact with Europeans was most significant. The transition from colonial contact to colonial conquest by powerful seafaring nations accelerated indigenous decline as many indigenous communities seemed incapable to resist colonial settlement and ultimately colonial conquest. Apart from the establishment of political control over indigenous societies, the introduction of disease by Europeans through person-to-person contact and subsequent exposure to an array of 'foreign' diseases to which indigenous communities had no immunity suggests that indigenous people suffered a 'double blow' of colonialism, namely, conquest of indigenous land as well as the body. Colonial contact and conquest proved catastrophic as many indigenous societies were incapable of handling outbreaks of infectious diseases, which invariably transitioned into lethal and lasting epidemics. The constant presence and introduction of unknown viruses, which resulted in high mortality and low recovery rates, destabilized not only their political structures of vulnerable indigenous communities, but systematically caused the erosion of their own social, economic, religious structures, including indigenous health structures. Written by a cohort of international scholars, the study seeks to uncover aspects relating to the social history of medicine, quarantine, epidemiology, disease, public health and epidemics in the geographically and oceanic defined regions of the Indian and Pacific Oceans. Based on archival material, case studies, historical narratives and travel accounts, expert contextualization, historical explanations and analysis are being provided by scholars in this volume. More specifically, the chapters in this volume unravel the trajectory of the introduction of disease brought about by the idea of a colonial project and an economic enterprise that favoured conquest. The idea and ideology subsequently transitioned into in-person physical contact and how this orchestrated the social, economic and political collapse of long-standing indigenous structures, institutions and peoples, facilitating further conquest.

The contributions propose a hybrid approach and seek to analyse the impact of global diseases on localized geographical regions and indigenous communities from the African continent, India and Australasia. Reclamation of such medical histories reveals how colonization and colonial conquest disrupted, dislocated and destroyed indigenous communities – from Africa, Australasia and India. This volume, therefore, demonstrates how global trends of conquest and colonization affected selected colonized regions and people since the early days of colonization in the eighteenth century to the present.

As the study concentrates on various outbreaks of disease, public health, race, politics of disease and quarantine, it tracks and traces how contagion aided by colonial contact accelerated colonial conquest and subjugation of the indigenous people. Besides, while the world finds itself in various waves of the current COVID-19 pandemic, the timely collection of chapters allows us a unique opportunity to rethink, reassess and reinvestigate the impact of disease on lesser-known micro-communities from new theoretical and historical perspectives. The editors have, therefore, succeeded in bringing together a group of scholars from different nationalities and continents to address how indigenous communities on the continents of Africa, Asia and Australia were infected and affected by a diversity of diseases and how they responded to the epidemics and sickness.

By the late eighteenth century, the British imperial power had expanded and had made inroads into world's seas and oceans, which also meant making way into and affecting the social, cultural and health environments of the colonized peoples. Noticeable especially with the onset of various epidemics, these changes also called for 'good governance'.[30] But what really triggered this call were the complexities in the relationship between trade, quarantine and public health – all of which were significant markers of power of the imperial regime. People's mobility through trade, the emergence of health issues, the enforcement of quarantine measures and the development of sanitary reforms changed the nature of colonial administrative policies. In particular, quarantine measures were seen as interfering with people's private spaces and any coercion met with serious opposition from them. The chapters in this volume reveal four overarching and interlinked major themes. One, the idea of imperial control, discipline and public health issues: Poonam Bala discusses imperial control and 'discipline' in relation to the impact of quarantine measures adopted by the colonial administration and their impact on the Indian peoples. And when these measures became mandatory, panic, resentment, and antagonism and hostility with the colonists surfaced; amidst all this, the role of the Epidemic Diseases Act of 1897 was equally significant in India as in Britain at the time. On a similar note, Apalak Das, in his discussion on the venereal disease, charts out the correlation between the much-discussed entanglements of health, 'discipline' and race with colonial investigations of this deadly affliction in the British troops in India. On a slightly different note, while labour history calls for a separate and detailed discussion, in this volume Amina Ameir Issa introduces the reader to a cogent relationship between bubonic plague, trade and mobility of goods and indentured labourers in the port cities of East Africa. Communities along the Pacific Island also were part of very important policies during the pandemic. While quarantine as a form of 'disciplining' and controlling public health issues seemed obvious here, it was deployed more for economic gains in the international community and hence of territorial expansion; in this context, the force of imperial diplomacy, as Harrison[31] remarks, seemed stronger than the force of 'scientific logic'.[32] Perhaps, this may have been true for the Pacific Islands where close contact with Australia and shorter sea voyages exposed the vulnerable indigenous peoples to infectious diseases.

The other theme that is drawn from the discussion in chapters here is the circulation of knowledge as a result of trade and travels. Both curiosities and discoveries through scientific travels were an integral part of imperial activities. Not surprisingly, they also became useful tools for imperial expansion alongside improvements in imperial economies and reforms. Besides, knowledge 'transfers', trade and travel posed a significant threat to the indigenous peoples. The history of the growth and expansion of the Dutch settlement at the Cape, for instance, is a case in point. As the Dutch settlement grew, so did the impoverishment of the Khoikhoi people who had, in most cases, no immunity to fight European diseases. Since 1713, a series of smallpox epidemics in the Cape had taken the lives of Khoikhoi, colonists and slaves. Russel Viljoen revisits the impact of three smallpox epidemics that ravaged the Cape colonial society in the eighteenth century. He emphasizes that the continuity of infection and transmission of communicable diseases among the Cape population, as a result, eventually threatened the autonomy of the Cape Khoikhoi people. This also extended into an era when transoceanic exchanges and colonial contacts also meant an introduction of new infections and diseases. Elizabeth van Heyningen discusses this trajectory in the context of measles in her chapter and how it impacted upon the indigenous populations. Unfavourable living conditions and a series of devastating epidemics induced labour exploitation, thereby enhancing their vulnerability to colonial control. But what was the main force behind these travels. While these disruptions and confusion in colonial societies were obvious, the need to undertake travels, nevertheless, is also an important issue. Matthew E. Franco in this volume throws light on the imperial desires to undertake scientific travels at a time when European travellers had limited knowledge of the colonized peoples and their social and cultural environment. More specifically, he focuses on the circulation of 'travel knowledge' in the Atlantic, Pacific and Indian Oceans. These travels also were part of colonial investigative modalities of knowing India better and what it represented. Sohini Das in her chapter discusses how colonial curiosities of India's medicinal herbs defined the manner in which useful information on local medicinal herbs was gathered, collated and compiled in the form of various books and travel documents; facilitated by travel, medical knowledge was exchanged and spread to other colonies, and in the process contributing to colonial expansion.

While imperial governance attempted to grapple with various health issues, it also created new health problems with a long-lasting impact on the populations they ruled. Coupled with the disease burden, colonial attempts at controlling health issues, thus, became increasingly difficult. Yet the significance of disease in the shaping of twentieth-century health policies cannot be dismissed. Few chapters in this volume come under this important theme. Jeff Ramsay discusses these aspects in Botswana in Southern Africa, projecting changes in the social order as a result of unfavourable administrative colonial policies; the decline in local livelihoods and subsequent resentment and resistance added to further social and economic problems. Saurav Kumar Rai's chapter adds a new dimension to the burden of disease and public health. His projection of disease as acquiring political, social and economic dimensions under colonial dictates in India is worth noting. Effects of the destruction of the social order as a result of colonialism have been detailed by Mark F. Briskey in his discussion on the First Nations peoples of Australia. Disruption of traditional livelihoods, disassociation of indigenous peoples from their lands and a subsequent destruction of culture all contributed to their overall social cultural decline; the introduction of diseases by the seaborne traders and invaders cannot be dismissed.

While trade, mobility and scientific travels strengthened imperial power prerogatives, new colonial establishments and infrastructures proved detrimental to colonial power. This theme runs in two chapters. Taking malaria as a case study, Arabinda Samanta, in this volume, portrays the creation of 'micro-environments' and habitats as a result of colonial interventions which became highly conducive to insanitary conditions such as water stagnation and hence of breeding of malaria-causing mosquitoes. Moving beyond this argument, certain structures proved inimical to maintaining sanitary and hygienic conditions. For instance, as Jacob Steere-Williams discusses in this volume, anti-plague measures in India and Cape Colony, which deployed several indigenous labourers to handle plague corpses, to disinfect and cleanse or destroy homes, were more crippling than effective in controlling the spread of plague; he discusses these specifically in the light of the racialized nature of colonial strategies in South Africa and India.

Deeper colonial engagements with the social and cultural environments in the colonies meant regulation of the latter from which emerged new forms of knowledge through the cultural and physical trial-and-error which they permitted; through the forms of governmentality and legality; and through the techniques of engagement with and regulation over hygiene, medicine and all kinds of disciplinary control of the body.[33]

Thus, in the early years of the twentieth century, as seen in the case of Asante society, there was a great deal of colonial anxiety and anguish about the local forms of religious beliefs and practices, seen as a result of the collision of 'discourse of power and knowledge of otherness'.[34] Knowledge of local customs of medicine and religious rites of healing then became the central focus of British efforts in 'bringing Africans to Christianity and in creating a civil society'.[35] Elsewhere in India, colonial engagements with science/medicine and religion witnessed the (re)invention of Indian medical system, Ayurveda, which eventually became the pivot of the national movement against British rule in Indian history.[36]

In contrast, various arguments on racial immunity against diseases dominated the British Indian medical discourse throughout most of the nineteenth century. Sahara Ahmed, in this volume, discusses colonial attempts at using various racial arguments and social construction of disease to explain immunity of the indigenous tribes in Bengal against epidemic diseases. This, Ahmed asserts, was done to defray any expenses otherwise needed for public health measures for the indigenous tribal populations.

Establishment of global trading networks which facilitated interconnectedness and colonial territorial expansion intensified the nature of tuberculosis from being local to becoming almost pandemic. While the Indian Ocean World was not devoid of tuberculosis, it was the rapid urbanization and industrialization which led to mass movement of people from villages and smaller towns to cities and port cities in search of employment. This further led to overcrowding and unhealthy environment. Suvankar Dey in this volume focuses on this movement of migrant labourers, and the changing urban environment, especially in South Africa and India, which aggravated the incidence of tuberculosis in cities. British imperial expansion, the series of epidemics and the creation of new disease environments as a result of colonial expansion decimated entire indigenous populations in her colonies.

The book will contribute to new understandings and insights into the 'forgotten' medical histories and narratives of indigenous communities, often ignored or subsumed by grand narratives of global histories. It has a strong focus on indigenous societies and shows how colonial discoveries, colonialism and disease affected such communities since the seventeenth century, often leading to their decline. It will also offer readers new insights into the medical narrative of many indigenous communities and their responses to disease and illness in different colonial contexts and geographical regions around the globe.

Humanity's long history of disease and disorders should ideally serve as sufficient warning that future outbreaks and far-reaching pandemics are inevitable. This also meant that all current diseases 'were once emerging diseases'.[37] The question we need to pose is one of recurrence? Since these diseases and epidemics demonstrated patterns of recurrence, new research, as well as fresh interpretations and analysis, is needed to possibly explain humanity's uncanny association with deadly viruses. This alone should serve as ample justification for further investigations into the medical pasts of colonial societies and regions affected and traumatized by colonial conquest and how it aided the introduction and dispersion of disease in the first place.

NOTES

1. See, for instance, J.N. Hays, *The Burdens of Disease: Epidemics and Human Response in Western History* (New Jersey: Rutgers University Press, 2009); Eric W. Banister, Allen Murray, Fadl Samia, Bhakthan Gordon, and Howard Dawn, eds., *Contemporary Health Issues* (Boston and London: Jones and Bartlett Publishers, 1988); C. Carroll and D. Miller, *Health: The Science of Human Adaptation* (Dubuque, IA: C Brown, 1986); Frank, Huisman and John Harley Warner, eds., *Locating Medical History: The Stories and Their Meaning* (Baltimore and London: The Johns Hopkins University Press, 2004); Cartwright Frederick Fox, *A Social History of Medicine* (London, New York: Longman, 1977); Eric J. Cassell, *The Place of the Humanities in Medicine* (New York: Hastings Centre, 1984); Ernst Waltraud and Harris Bernard, eds., *Race, Science and Medicine, 1700–1960* (London and New York: Routledge, 1999). Kenrad E. Nelson and Williams Carolyn, eds., *Infectious Disease Epidemiology: Theory and Practice* (Burlington, MA: Jones and Bartlett Learning, 2014).
2. Peter Mitchell, "The Archaeological Study of Epidemic and Infectious Disease", *World Archaeology*, vol. 35, no. 2 (2003):171–179.
3. William H McNeill, *Plagues and Peoples* (London: Penguin Books, reprint, 1994), 185.
4. Laurence Monnais and Pols Hans, "Health and disease in the colonies: Medicine in the Age of the Empire", in *The Routledge History of Western Empires,* eds.

Aldrich Robert and Kirsten McKenzie (London and New York, Routledge, 2014), see chapter 18; David Arnold, *The Age of Discovery 1400-1600* (London: Routledge, 2002); Walter M. Goldberg, *The Geography, Nature and History of the Tropical Pacific and Its Islands* (Cham: Springer, 2018), See especially "European Exploration of the Pacific during the Age of Discovery", 57–76.

5. H, Tilley, "Medicine, Empires and Ethics in Colonial Africa", *AMA Journal of Ethics*, vol. 18, no. 7, (2016):743–753. doi: 10.1001/journalofethics.2016.18,.7.mhstl -1607.

6. Monica H. Green, "Emerging Diseases, Re-Emerging Histories", *Centaurus: An International Journal of the History of Science and its Cultural Aspects*, vol. 62 (2020):234–247 (accessed on 20 June 2021).

7. Green, "Emerging Diseases, Re-Merging Histories", 235.

8. David Arnold, "Pandemic India: Coronavirus and the Uses of History", *The Journal of Asian Studies*, vol. 79, no. 3 (August 2020):569–577.

9. Arnold, "Pandemic India: Coronavirus and the Uses of History", 569–577.

10. Frank Snowden, *Epidemics and Society: From Black Death to the Present* (New Haven: Yale University Press, 2019).

11. Mack Arien, ed., *In time of Plague: This History and Social Consequences of Lethal Epidemic Disease* (New York: New York University Press, 1991); Jones Molly, *Epidemics and Society: AIDS* (Rosen Publish Group: 2010); D. Anne Herring and Alan C. Swedlund, eds., *Plagues and Epidemics: Infected Spaces Past and Present* (Oxford and New York: Berg, 2010). Watts Sheldon, *Epidemics and History: Disease, Power and Imperialism* (New Haven: Yale University Press, 1977); Charles Rosenberg, *Explaining Epidemics and Other Studies in the History of Medicine* (Cambridge: Cambridge University Press, 1992).

12. Mark Harrison, *Contagion: How Commerce Has Spread Disease* (New Haven: Yale University Press, 2012).

13. Harrison, *Contagion*, xii.

14. Abdul Sheriff, *Dhow Cultures of the Indian Ocean: Cosmopolitanism, Commerce and Islam* (London: Hurst & Co., 2010).

15. Sheriff, *Dhow Cultures of the Indian Ocean,* 1.

16. Sujit Sivasundaram, *Waves Across the South: A New History of the Revolution and Empire* (London: William Collins, 2020).

17. David Armitage, Alison Bashford and Sujit Sivasundaram, eds., *Oceanic Histories* (Cambridge: Cambridge University Press, 2018). This is an important and perhaps the first major comprehensive study on the history and historiographies of the oceans and world's seas and their connections.

18. David Armitage and Alison Bashford, eds., *Pacific Histories: Ocean, Land and People* (Basingstoke: Palgrave Macmillan, 2014); Matt Matsuda, *Pacific Worlds: A History of the Seas, People and Cultures* (Cambridge: Cambridge University Press, 2012).

19. Sivasundaram, *Waves Across the South*, 3–6.

20. Sivasundaram, *Waves Across the South*, 11.

21. Gwyn Campbell and Eva-Maria, Knoll, eds., *Disease Dispersion and Impact in the India Ocean World* (London: Palgrave Macmillan, 2020); Anna Winterbottom

and Facil Tesfaye, eds., *Histories of Medicine and Healing in the Indian Ocean World: The Modern Period* (London: Palgrave Macmillan, 2016).

22. Anna Winterbottom and Facil, Tesfaye, eds., *Histories of Medicine and Healing in the Ocean World: The Medieval and Early Modern Period* (Houndmills: Palgrave Macmillan, 2015).

23. Pablo, F Gómez, *The Experiential Caribbean: Creating Knowledge and Healing in Early Modern Atlantic* (Chapel Hill: University of North Carolina Press, 2017).

24. Campbell and Knoll, *Disease, Dispersion and Impact in the Indian Ocean World.*

25. Alfred W. Crosby, *The Columbian Exchange: Biological and Cultural Consequences of 1492* (Westport, CT: Greenwood Publishing Co., 1972).

26. Crosby, *The Columbian Exchange.*

27. Crosby, *The Columbian Exchange.*

28. David Arnold, "The Indian Ocean as a Disease Zone, 1500-1950", *South Asia: Journal of South Asian Studies*, vol. xiv, no. 2 (1991):1–21.

29. Monica Green and Jones Lori, "The Evolution and Spread of Major Human Diseases in the Indian Ocean World", in *Disease, Dispersion and Impact in the Indian Ocean World*, eds. Campbell Gwyn and Knoll Eva-Maria (Palgrave Macmillan, 2020, London), 25–57.

30. Harrison, *Contagion.*

31. Harrison, *Contagion.*

32. Cited from Rosner Lisa, "Policing Boundaries: Quarantine and Professional Identity in mid-nineteenth century Britain", in *Mediterranean Quarantines, 1750-1914: Space, Identity and Power*, eds. John Chircop and Francisco Javier-Martinez (Manchester: Manchester University Press, 2018), 125–144.

33. John L. Comaroff and Jean Comaroff, *Of Revelation and Revolution: Dialectics of Modernity on a South African Frontier, vol 2* (Chicago: The University of Chicago Press, 1997), 388. Cited from William C. Olsen, "The Empire Strikes Back: Colonial 'Discipline' and the Creation of Civil Society in Asante, 1906-1940", History in Africa, vol. 3 (2003):223–251, 228.

34. V.Y. Mudimbe, *The Invention of Africa: Gnosis, Philosophy and the Order of Knowledge* (Bloomington: Indiana University Press, 1988). Cited from Olsen, "The Empire Strikes Back", 230. In one of my earlier works, I have discussed Indian responses to colonial interventions and policies in terms of what I call, 'paradigms of defense'. For details, see Poonam, Bala, *Contesting Colonial Authority: Medicine and Indigenous Responses in Nineteenth- and Twentieth-Century India* (Lanham: Lexington Books, 2012; reprinted, Delhi: Primus Publications, 2015).

35. Olsen, "The Empire Strikes Back", 230.

36. For details, see Poonam, Bala, "Ayurveda (re) invented: Engagements with Science and Religion in Colonial India", in *The Routledge Handbook of Religion, Medicine and Health,* eds. Dorothea Lüddeckens and Philipp Hetmancyzk et al. (Abingdon: Routledge, 2021), 421–434.

37. Green, "Emerging Diseases, Re-merging Histories", 236.

BIBLIOGRAPHY

Arien, Mack, ed. *In time of Plague: This History and Social Consequences of Lethal Epidemic Disease*. New York: New York University Press, 1991.

Armitage, David, and Alison Bashford, eds. *Pacific Histories: Ocean, Land and People*. Basingstoke: Palgrave Macmillan, 2014.

Armitage, David, Alison Bashford, and Sujit Sivasundaram, eds. *Oceanic Histories*. Cambridge: Cambridge University Press, 2018.

Arnold, David. "The Indian Ocean as a Disease Zone, 1500–1950." *South Asia: Journal of South Asian Studies*, xiv, no. 2 (1991):1–21.

Arnold, David. *The Age of Discovery 1400–1600*. London: Routledge, 2002.

Arnold, David. "Pandemic India: Coronavirus and the Uses of History." *The Journal of Asian Studies*, 79, no. 3 (August 2020):569–577.

Bala, Poonam, ed. *Contesting Colonial Authority: Medicine and Indigenous Responses in Nineteenth- and Twentieth-Century India*. Lanham: Lexington Books, 2012; reprinted. New Delhi: Primus Publications, 2015.

Bala, Poonam. "Ayurveda (re) invented: Engagements with Science and Religion in Colonial India." In *The Routledge Handbook of Religion, Medicine and Health*, edited by Dorothea Lüddeckens and Philipp Hetmancyzk, et al., 421–434. Abingdon: Routledge, 2022.

Banister, Eric W., Murray Allen, Samia Fadl, Gordon Bhakthan, and Dawn Howard, eds. *Contemporary Health Issues*. Boston, MA and London: Jones and Bartlett Publishers, 1988.

Campbell, Gwyn, and Eva-Maria Knoll, eds. *Disease Dispersion and Impact in the India Ocean World*. London: Palgrave Macmillan, 2020.

Carroll, Charles R., and Dean F. Miller. *Health: The Science of Human Adaptation*. Dubuque, IA: William C Brown, 1986.

Cartwright, Frederick Fox. *A Social History of Medicine. London*, New York: Longman, 1977.

Cassell, Eric J. *The Place of the Humanities in Medicine*. New York: Hastings Centre, 1984.

Comaroff, John L., and Jean Comaroff. *Of Revelation and Revolution: Dialectics of Modernity on a South African Frontier, vol 2*. Chicago: The University of Chicago Press, 1997.

Crosby, Alfred W. *The Columbian Exchange: Biological and Cultural Consequences of 1492*. Westport, CT: Greenwood Publishing Co., 1972.

Goldberg, Walter M. *The Geography, Nature and History of the Tropical Pacific and Its Islands*. Cham: Springer, 2018.

Gómez, Pablo F. *The Experiential Caribbean: Creating Knowledge and Healing in Early Modern Atlantic*. Chapel Hill, NC: University of North Carolina Press, 2017.

Green, Monica H. "Emerging Diseases, Re-merging Histories." *Centaurus: An International Journal of the History of Science and its Cultural Aspects*, 62 (2020):234–247 (accessed on 20 June 2021).

Green, Monica H., and Lori Jones. "The Evolution and Spread of Major Human Diseases in the Indian Ocean World." In *Disease, Dispersion and Impact in the Indian Ocean World*, edited by Gwyn Campbell and Eva-Maria Knoll, 25–57. London: Palgrave Macmillan, 2020.

Harrison, Mark. *Contagion: How Commerce Has Spread Disease*. New Haven, CT: Yale University Press, 2012.

Hays, J.N. *The Burdens of Disease: Epidemics and Human Response in Western History*. New Jersey: Rutgers University Press, 2009.

Herring, D. Ann, and Alan C. Swedlund, eds. *Plagues and Epidemics: Infected Spaces Past and Present*. Oxford and New York: Berg, 2010.

Huisman, Frank, and John Harley Warner, eds. *Locating Medical History: The Stories and Their Meaning*. Baltimore, MD and London: The Johns Hopkins University Press, 2004.

Jones, Molly. *Epidemics and Society: AIDS*. New York: Rosen Publish Group, 2010.

Masuda, Matt. *Pacific Worlds: A History of the Seas, People and Cultures*. Cambridge: Cambridge University Press, 2012.

McNeil, William H. *Plagues and Peoples*. London: Penguin Books, reprint, 1994.

Mitchell, Peter, "The Archaeological Study of Epidemic and Infectious Disease." *World Archaeology*, 35, no. 2 (2003):171–179.

Monnais, Laurence, and Hans Pols. "Health and Disease in the Colonies: Medicine in the Age of the Empire." In *The Routledge History of Western Empires*, edited by Robert Aldrich and Kirsten McKenzie, 270–284. London and New York: Routledge, 2014.

Mudimbe, V.Y. *The Invention of Africa: Gnosis, Philosophy and the Order of Knowledge*. Bloomington, IN: Indiana University Press, 1988.

Nelson, Kenrad E., and Carolyn Masters Williams, eds. *Infectious Disease Epidemiology: Theory and Practice*. Burlington, MA: Jones and Bartlett Learning, 2014.

Olsen, William C. "The Empire Strikes Back: Colonial 'Discipline' and the Creation of Civil Society in Asante, 1906–1940." *History in Africa*, 3 (2003):223–251.

Rosenberg, Charles. *Explaining Epidemics and Other Studies in the History of Medicine*. Cambridge: Cambridge University Press, 1992.

Rosner, Lisa. "Policing Boundaries: Quarantine and Professional Identity in Mid-Nineteenth Century Britain." In *Mediterranean Quarantines, 1750–1914: Space, Identity and Power*, edited by John Chircop and Francisco Javier-Martinez, 125–144. Manchester: Manchester University Press, 2018.

Sheriff, Abdul. *Dhow Cultures of the Indian Ocean: Cosmopolitanism, Commerce and Islam*. London: Hurst & Co., 2010.

Sivasundaram, Sujit. *Waves Across the South: A New History of the Revolution and Empire*. London: William Collins, 2020.

Snowden, Frank. *Epidemics and Society: From Black Death to the Present*. New Haven, CT: Yale University Press, 2019.

Tilley, Helen. "Medicine, Empires and Ethics in Colonial Africa." *AMA Journal of Ethics*, 18, no. 7 (2016):743–753. doi: 10.1001/journalofethics.2016.18.7.mhstl-1607.

Waltraud, Ernst, and Harris Bernard, eds. *Race, Science and Medicine, 1700–1960*. London and New York: Routledge, 1999.

Watts, Sheldon. *Epidemics and History: Disease, Power and Imperialism*. New Haven, CT: Yale University Press, 1977.

Winterbottom, Anna, and Facil Tesafaye, eds. *Histories of Medicine and Healing in the Indian Ocean World: The Modern Period*. London: Palgrave Macmillan, 2016.

Chapter 1

Quarantine, Epidemics and Health

Framing Indigenous Engagements and Resistance in Colonial India

Poonam Bala

In the wake of the various epidemic situations, the nineteenth century presented opportunities for the colonial state in India to deal with public health issues in a manner that would disrupt the social and cultural fabric of Indian society. A lot of these public health policies were transferred from Britain where the professionalization of medicine owed allegiance to major advances in drug therapy. However, in India, these policies met with limited or partial success for various reasons: overemphasis on protection of trade and commerce which pushed health concerns for the Indian peoples into the background[1] and lack of sensitivity to India's social, cultural and religious conditions; the latter, Arnold[2] argues, limited colonial attempts at a successful implementation of health measures.

Among the various colonial strategies and plans to combat the epidemics, one that specifically proved consequential were the quarantine measures for fighting the plague epidemic. In this chapter, I argue that just as medicine and medical knowledge have existed as sites of contestation and various negotiations, quarantine, too, became a site that displayed colonial power and authority through which these negotiations could be formulated to exert authority and control of the people of India. I also argue that quarantine measures reinforced the emerging national identity, forging a new sense of medical and cultural nationhood as a result of its impact on the social, cultural and religious lives of the Indian people manifested through engagements with and resistance to colonial health policies. In the wake of these policies, practices and quarantine, social connotations of contamination and (im)purity in various discourses of disease and caste also came to the fore; varied experiences of epidemics based on caste, thus, provided new understandings of caste-epidemic situations in India.

POLICIES AND REFORMS

The turn of the twentieth century was a period of various social and political turmoils in India. These changes also influenced the manner in which public health measures were to be delivered and made accessible to the Indian peoples. The introduction of Montagu-Chelmsford Reforms (hereafter, Reforms) in 1919 was a welcome change in the political environment, especially when issues of patronage to Indian medicine were a cause of concern to Indian medical practitioners. By extending political power and autonomy to local self-governments, the Reforms established the dual system of control or *dyarchy*, also creating 'reserved' and 'transferred' categories. This also meant that matters pertaining to education and public health fell within the latter category and hence taken over by Indian ministers and local governments.[3] In 1935, the Government of India Act gave further impetus to engagements in matters of health by establishing the Central Advisory Board of Health in 1937 so that when 'new ideas of population problem dominated the thinking of public health officials in the interwar period', Indian intellectuals, patrons, economics, women social reformers and birth controllers were prompted to respond to the new 'concern'.[4] But what were the implications of the establishment of 'reserved' and 'transferred'? One, it provided grace to 'practitioners of Indian medicine'[5] so that medical practice, medical negotiations, matters of registration and other ordinances could be handled by Indians themselves. The Reforms were also 'instrumental in bringing about awareness of new negotiations'[6] between the people of India and British officials. Subsequently, with an increased Indian membership in the bureaucratic services, medical services too were categorized as 'transferred'. And the result: rapid Indianization of medical services.[7] Several Indian doctors participated in reaching the general public to persuade them to get inoculated or vaccinated. In some places, for instance, in Punjab, government schemes to deploy Indian practitioners (trained in Indian indigenous medicine, Ayurveda and Unani) to extend medical relief were successful in creating a demand for anti-plague vaccine where the disease was raging and a large vaccination scheme was underway.[8] Major Mercer, it is reported, introduced a scheme in Sealkote in Punjab[9] which aimed at establishing new village dispensaries managed by hakeems (practitioners of Unani medicine).[10]

The role of nationalists in connection with colonial policies is important here. Several influential elites and local magnates had begun to participate in India's national movement as a reaction to the consolidation of British rule and of Western ideologies in India. New social and cultural reform movements had already begun to take shape in this politically rife environment. The English-educated elites, the rich and influential Indians, sought employment under British administration, the elite Indian Civil Services, the legal services and education. In the late nineteenth century, several political organizations were founded by young leaders. The *Poona Sarvajanik Sabha* (Poona Public Society), for instance, was founded by Mahadev Govind Ranade in 1879, while other nationalists expressed their discontent against British rule through the press and writings. Bal Gangadhar Tilak, hailed as the leader of India's national movement, started a vernacular newspaper, *Kesari* (Lion) through which Tilak could voice his opinions and reach the Indian people. He was jailed in 1897 for his seditious writings and the two major religious festivals of Shivaji and Ganpati, through which he attempted to assert Hinduism, were subsequently banned in 1897 due to plague restrictions. Amidst all this, Indian medicine – Ayurveda and Unani – which in itself witnessed phases of competition and conflict with Western biomedicine, over the entire eighteenth century, received a fillip in 1919 with the establishment of the Montagu-Chelmsford Reforms.

PLAGUE, MEDICAL KNOWLEDGE AND PUBLIC HEALTH

'Plague was India's most feared and one of the deadliest maladies', writes Klein[11] claiming about 12 million lives, that brought great cities like Bombay and whole provinces, like the hard-hit Punjab, 'within compass of social disorganization and collapse'.[12] It was the outbreak of epidemics that forged new concerns and relationship between the colonial state and its subjects. The outbreak of the plague epidemic in 1896 in Bombay illustrates our point. Perhaps, this was the first time that 'the State acquired special legal and judicial powers for an apparently humanitarian cause to prevent the spread of the epidemic'.[13]

With the first case of Bombay Plague identified in September 1896, by one Dr Acacio Gabriel Viegas (Indian medical practitioner practicing Western medicine), the plague visitations which devastated parts of India nowhere else were comparably destructive.[14]

The onset of epidemics not only created fear and panic but also prompted 'insecurities and anxieties that disturbed the authoritative gaze'[15] of the British colonists. More significantly, it gave rise to a new and intricate culture of colonial medical correspondences and medical literature through which these anxieties could be communicated and which became a convenient tool for dissemination of medical ideas and information while also reinforcing colonial agendas.

They also 'shaped the acts of reporting, recording and recapitulating the epidemic'.[16] In Bengal, the case of the 'making' of Burdwan fever epidemic in Bengal offers insights into how colonial bureaucrats were able to repackage knowledge and information on malaria 'in accordance with the cosmopolitan codes of imperial correspondence', when 'knowledge of the locality and the epidemic converged to stereotype the Burdwan division as a malarial landscape',[17] often providing credibility to the projected stories of the epidemic.

Earlier notions of plague were replete with limited scientific knowledge of plague transmission. Contagionist view of plague still dominated the scientific thought. Although the plague bacillus had already been before the modern pandemic reached India, it continued to be seen as a 'disease of dirt', believed to be caused by insanitary and unhygienic living conditions; even the relationship between rat epizootics and the role of rat flea in human epidemics was not known well into the turn of the twentieth century. Although China and Indonesia followed closely, in India, plague mortality counted only 2% of the total mortality.[18] Since science, medicine and epidemics were closely intertwined, they inspired new social and political frameworks for understanding health and illness, thus modifying the knowledge and histories people brought with them; along with this, they gained a new understanding of their place in an expanding world. Travels and mobility across different oceans, thus, also opened up new movement of ideas of globalization and as these went along, they forged new alliances with indigenous populations, while also forging new concepts of racism, gender, and so on.[19]

Plague, as one of the most feared and deadliest epidemics in medical history, posed a mammoth challenge for the British premier ports of Calcutta and Bombay, both of which were flourishing administrative centres as well as important ports that maintained commercial relations with the world. Besides, plague challenged colonial commercial prosperity, as Bombay became the major centre connecting various commercial centres across India.[20] This entailed mobility and travel across places as a result of which it was believed that 'migrant labourers carried the epidemic with them as railway passengers, literally from town to town within days'[21] while travelling to India via the commercial steamships from Hong Kong. Commenting on the 'significance' of humans as 'carriers of infection,' Dr B. W. Brown, the then surgeon in the United States Public Health Service, wrote in one of his reports:

> The importance of Hong Kong as a shipping port, and the fact that vessels from all parts of the world call at this port, not only for cargo, but for repairs, this affording special opportunities for rat infestation, makes the history of plague in the colony of Hong Kong of interest and importance to health officers at every seaport. There is little doubt that certain of the plague epidemics of recent years in various ports of the world could be traced to rat infestation at Hong Kong.[22]

When it came to implementing public health measures, imperial medical practice combined both the contagionist and anti-contagionist views to handle the dreadful plague epidemic in India.

Although plague was accepted as an individual affliction instead of a group, medical knowledge at the time, despite its advances and gradual progress, continued to profess faith in the humoral theory of disease and health when Dr Richard Mead (1673–1754) emphasized the significance of balancing humors of the body in such a state so that they remain unaltered by any infection. This, he advocated, would protect one from all diseases.[23] Yet, anti-contagionist arguments firmly held that the 'disposition of the air than of human effluvia' was the chief cause and spread of plague.[24] Besides, various research committees were appointed to look into measures to deal with all matters of the plague epidemic, including assessment of the gravity of the situation and finding out means to prevent its spread. Camp hospitals and on-site field hospitals were set up to carry out research, experimentation and constant surveillance of the situation; detailed summaries of this research were later published in the various reports produced under the supervision of each committee.[25]

QUARANTINE: A BACKGROUND

While on the one hand, the onset of epidemics reinforced new medical policies, on the other, the same policy dictates were used to control the populations where epidemics occurred. One such effect of policies was the Epidemic Diseases Act (hereafter, the Act) passed in 1897. This also gave the British government added power to use segregation and isolation of patients as a means to control the cholera and smallpox epidemics. In some places, 'isolation huts' were established to segregate suspected men and women which caused a lot of resentment and suspicion in the minds of the people; they saw coercion and physical separation as interfering with their private lives and exclusion from their community; these restricted spaces and their rigid spatial partitioning were more like 'segmented, immobile, frozen spaces'.[26]

The Act not only invested authority in government officers to undertake compulsory inspection of corpses and reporting the number of deaths from plague. Local leading newspapers condemned the act for its mandates for flouting the social mores and intrusions into people's lives. Forceful entry into women's *zenanas*[27] was looked upon with suspicion and resentment for it interfered with ideas of seclusion and private space for women.

By the late nineteenth century, and more so 'from the 1870s, tropical medicine, its ideology European, its instrument the microscope, its epistemology the germ theory of disease, served the interests of dominant economic groups and obscured the relationship of disease to the social structure'.[28] The shifting social and political ideologies, thus, were central to new perceptions of disease.

The idea of quarantine which was based on contagion was, thus, deeply entrenched in the colonial minds as sine qua non for various assertions of scientific hegemony, to say the least, hence of colonial power and authority. British medical men in India saw advances in medicine and allied sciences and their application as an opportunity to 'conquer' and control epidemic diseases. By doing so, contagious diseases could be stopped from spreading by breaking 'chains of transmission, interrupting the circulation of carriers by means of cordons, quarantine and sequestration'.[29]

The history of quarantining and isolating patients is more than a history of preventing the global spread of a disease. It involves several, often covert, strategies which have political, social and ethical implications. Imposed initially at European ports in the fourteenth century, quarantine measures created pressure on the medical community and scientists in India to curb epidemic diseases while at the same time, they saw medical advances in medicine and their application as an opportunity to conquer and control disease and health situations.

Quarantine, as a tool through which various institutions could be operated within the imperial prerogatives, not only served colonial purpose of confinement and control but also invested authority and power in dealing with public health matters. Besides, quarantine, and the manner in which it was instituted was, thus, intricately embedded within power structures or transformed into a site of power enabling negotiations between economic and political interests. Several institutional confinements in the form of segregation camps, jails, asylums and hospitals were, thus, established to meet the requirements of colonial authority; as instruments of expansion of colonial frontiers, they also became a site of contestation for the local communities. In reality, hospitals offered better opportunities for isolation, observation and control.[30] In Calicut (state of Kerala, India), epidemic hospitals were founded exclusively for 'epidemic patients' kept in complete isolation, much 'like a jail in the name of public health'.[31] Hospital, in this sense, acted both as a place for treatment and an institution where state control and the power it got through these institutions could be exercised on the Indian peoples. In this context, within a hospital setting, as Foucault would explain it: '"biopolitics" or "biopower" and the birth rate and mortality rate etc. were the first objects of knowledge and the target it seeks to control'.[32] Similarly, the leprosaria or the houses for the poor and the asylums, became a first model of power that segregated the healthy from the sick and infirm and the deviants from the rest of the society.[33] Thus, can we then say that both medicine and medical knowledge as expressions of power are inherently 'disciplinary as well as regulatory' in their manifestations in society? Public health measures, in this context, thus, are also power-designate through which state exercises control.[34]

Inherent in quarantine was the potential to allay fears of epidemic disease. However, with a limited and uncertain understanding of the aetiology of diseases, 'state arrogance stemmed not from a (lack of) effectiveness of quarantine but from colonial conviction of racial, class and/or cultural superiority'.[35]

While trade played a very important role in colonial efforts to implement quarantine measures, it also became a reinforcing factor for conflicting views between the British colonial and the populations they ruled. India was not the only British colony where quarantine was implemented. It spread to other places including Malta and Corfu, where the plague epidemic became a serious issue of imperial concern. Elsewhere, in Congo, as Lyons argues, the threat of sleeping sickness 'forced colonial authorities to take seriously the health of their entire African populations'.[36] Between 1896 and 1906, the epidemic in the Congo basin claimed almost half-million lives which 'prompted the development of the Belgian medical service';[37] the Belgians used 'constructive imperialism through which they hoped to establish European influence'.[38] In Egypt, too, the Ottoman quarantine of 1838 to combat the cholera and plague epidemics met with vehement criticism from the European authorities, for whom the Ottoman public health authorities

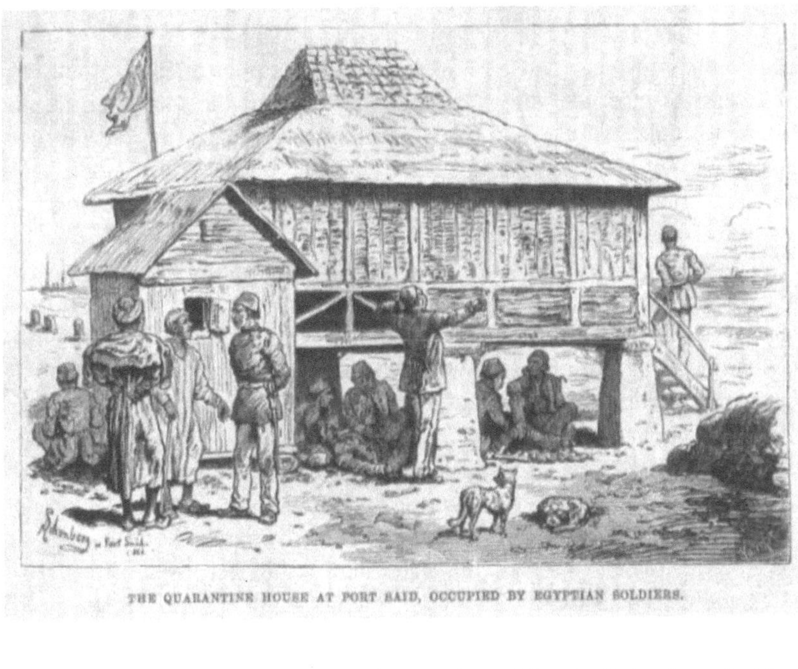
THE QUARANTINE HOUSE AT PORT SAID, OCCUPIED BY EGYPTIAN SOLDIERS.

Figure 1.1 Egypt: A Quarantine House for Egyptian Soldiers Suffering from the Plague at Port Said in 1882. Wood engraving by Kemp after J. N. Schönberg, 1882. *Source*: Wellcome Collection.

'needlessly inhibited trade and free flow of overseas traffic by imposing a ten- to fifteen-day quarantine on all traffic passing through the Straits'.[39] On the other hand, quarantine for Ottomans became a 'tool' to resist British and French commercial intrusions, and they 'remained committed to a contagionist programme of preventing plague'.[40] Quarantine, thus, became so deeply interwoven with commercial British expansion and competition that by 1865, it was perceived as 'a mere irrational derangement of commerce'.[41] In 1869, British control of the Suez Canal in 1869 and of public health institutions aggravated anti-colonial sentiments in Egypt fearing which, the British and other European powers stipulated stringent conditions that would indirectly discriminate Europeans and the Muslim pilgrims on their way to Mecca.[42] The image here depicts the suffering of Egyptian soldiers who were quarantined at Port Said (Figure 1.1).

Quarantine rules and isolation and segregation were followed in Zanzibar with equal magnitude and intensity, often with alarming consequences and popular response (Issa in this volume).

POPULAR RESPONSE, QUARANTINE AND NATIONALISTIC FERVOUR

Panic and fear gripped the British colonial authorities as threats to their colonial enterprise mounted with the perceived threat of the spread of sleeping sickness to India, 'the "jewel" of their empire'.[43] The catastrophic plague of Bombay caused much uproar and disarray in the minds of the people; quarantine tents built in public parks to isolate suspected patients faced vehement opposition from the public at large for their segregational motives (Figure 1.2).

Isolation and segregation continued as patients went through various tests and examinations even after they were discharged from the hospital.

The onset of plague epidemics, and the coercive colonial measures, making quarantine mandatory, also widened the gulf between biomedicine and indigenous medicine, Ayurveda. Practitioners of the latter became more concerned about 'professional exclusion and marginality'[44] than ever before. The Act, as noted earlier, was a historical juncture that defined the dynamic between power, authority and legitimacy in India. Similar to other policies and reforms, this too was imposed by the British authorities, and as a consequence, the dynamic of this interrelationship became a precursor to understanding the history of colonial medicine and of epidemic diseases with which it was closely entwined.[45] At the same time, the Act highlighted the 'hegemonic as well coercive processes' that lay embedded in and defined colonial power and knowledge.[46] Yet, the urgency in implementing the Act was more of a result of international pressure to contain the plague epidemic

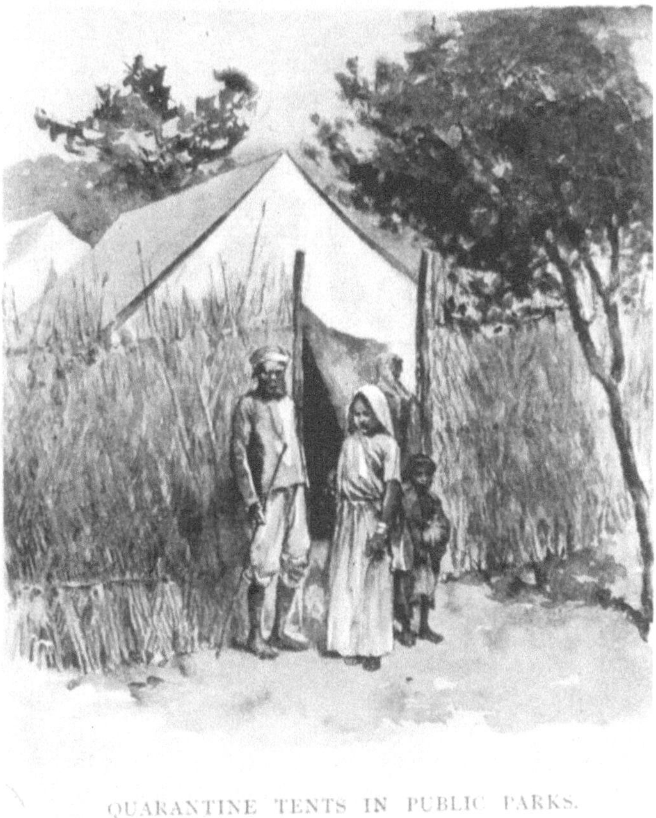

Figure 1.2 Quarantine Tents for Plague Victims in Public Parks of Bombay, 3 June 1899.
Source: National Library of Medicine.

than the actual health concerns of the civilian population, or even the British population. Accordingly, if the government

> thinks that the ordinary provisions of the law for the time being in force are insufficient for the purpose, may take, or require or empower any person to take, such measures and, by public notice, prescribe such temporary regulations to be observed by the public or by any person or class of persons as he shall deem necessary to prevent the outbreak of such disease or the spread thereof.[47]

Public health and religion in India have come face to face on several occasions but one terrain where these tumultuous engagements have resurfaced

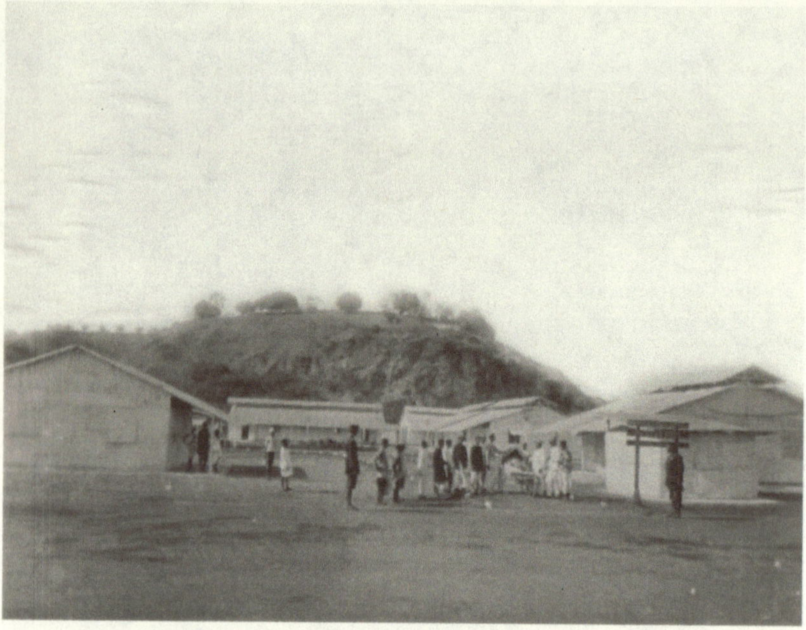

Figure 1.3 Plague Patient Who Has Just Been Discharged from Hospital Being Examined Outdoors in Bombay. Photograph, 1896/1897. *Source*: Wellcome Collection, 1896/1897.

time and again and with greater visibility is the epidemics that ravaged the country several times Figure 1.3 (above). Elsewhere, in the Cape Colony, one notices a 'religious spin' being attributed to justify and explain the smallpox epidemic among the Khoikhoi (Viljoen in this volume). The nineteenth-century epidemics of cholera and plague and their religious associations find an important place in most official and colonial administrative discussions. The spread of cholera into the West, for instance, was seen by British medical authorities as being caused by large and religious gatherings in places such as Haridwar and Puri; yet the Gangetic plains of Bengal (Presidency in colonial India) were almost wholly accepted as the areas where cholera actually originated. The public health administrators made a strong connection between the epidemic and Hindu festivals and pilgrimages. To this effect, 'the India-wide distribution of Hinduism's sacred places and the periodicity of its major festivals constituted two most important determinants of cholera epidemicity in India'.[48]

Amidst these assumptions and amidst British efforts to control the plague epidemic, public health measures became unpopular and continued to face fierce resistance from the people. Popular discontent mounted which further fuelled anti-British sentiments, especially at a time when nationalists had already formed an agenda to fight for independence from British rule. Popular unrest also collided with British authorities and their attempts to control plague which further disrupted the social and cultural environment. Quiet often,

> western medicine far outstripped popular disease comprehension, and often conflicted with social mores, a major feature of the plague ordeal.[49]

The rising political consciousness, the anti-British sentiments and respect for India's heritage and culture in need of preservation were some of the unintended consequences of colonial policies to contain the epidemic. Besides, the power and vigour with which the act was executed included coercive measures to handle the health situation. Forceful segregation of the afflicted people, personal examination or inspection by the medical officials, disinfecting them and even forceful evacuation from their homes proved inimical to public sentiments and attitude or any concern for good health (Figure 1.4 and Figure 1.5).

As plague spread to neighbouring cities, dwellings were destroyed and condemned for fear of further spread.

Any religious congregation, too, was curtailed as a preventive measure against plague. This happened at a time when research on plague was still nascent and knowledge of the aetiology of the disease was relatively fluid.[50]

Public resentment towards colonial public health measures intensified as did nationalists' goals for freedom. Generally, 'nationalism functioned as a paradigm within which nationalistic sentiments and claims for Hindu science

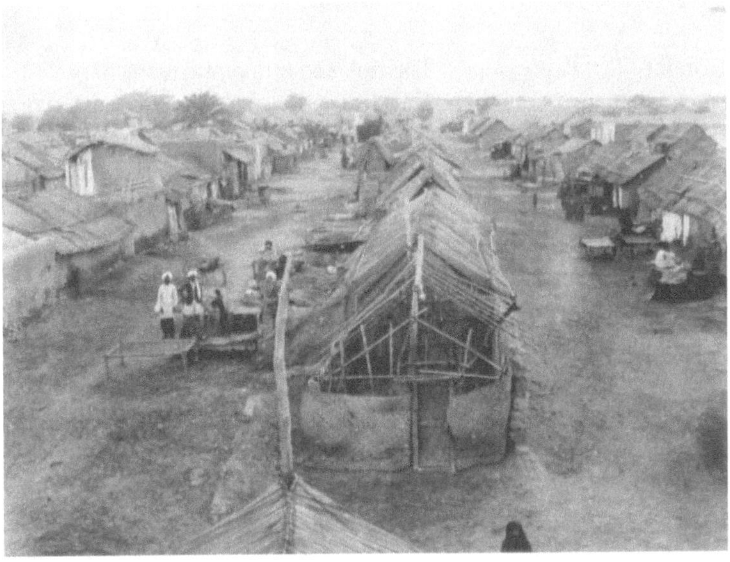

Figure 1.4 A Segregation Camp during Bubonic Plague Outbreak, Karachi, India. Photograph, 1897. (Karachi, in India until 1947, now in Pakistan). *Source*: Wellcome Collection.

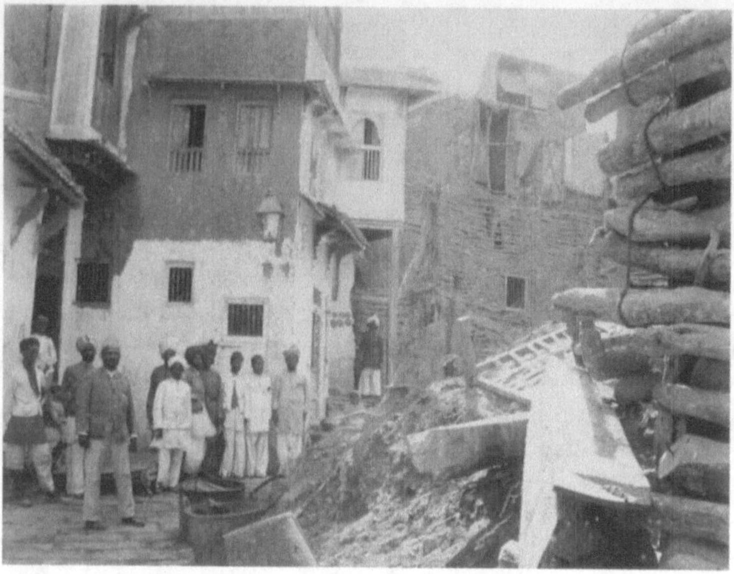

Figure 1.5 At the Height of the Epidemic in Karachi (Karachi, in India until 1947, now in Pakistan) in one week, 102 dwellings were condemned, 130 recommended for alteration and 4,000 altered. Karachi is a port in the province of Sind (subsequently in Pakistan). It was placed in quarantine in 1882, during the outbreak of bubonic plague which spread from Bombay. The Plague Committee consisted mostly of volunteers, who were organised into parties and were responsible for the segregation and inoculation of various districts. *Source*: Wellcome Collection.

and medicine were expressed'.[51] The rich and influential medical practitioners supported all claims to indigenous traditions and knowledge, incorporating them within the overarching nationalist paradigm. In this process, the encounters of Indian people with colonial authorities also meant 'limitations to medical power imposed by the "appropriation and opposition" to western medicine'.[52] Nevertheless,

> as colonial conditions turned the staging of science into a wondrous spectacle, a space opened for the subjectivity and agency of the Western-educated indigenous elite. Trained in Western schools and colleges, and employed in colonial bureaucracy and modern professions, this elite acquired a visible presence in main Indian cities and towns by the late nineteenth century. In a sense, their emergence was attributable to the colonial project of re-forming Indian subjects.[53]

'Nationalist thought in nineteenth-century India was itself a domain of contestation',[54] the very articulation of which meant 'colonization of the mind'[55] on which were premised all nationalistic assertions. The numerous nationalistic attempts at searching Indian traditions and culture were, thus, considered indispensable in the emerging thoughts about claims for a rational tradition of Indian science; P. C. Ray's masterpiece, *A History of Hindu Chemistry* (first published in 1902), adds a new dimension to the growing desire, as a result, of claims to a 'nationalist' science, cultural authority and strength in indigenous Indian knowledge. Yet, as Prakash, argues,

> The enduringly powerful identification of Hindu traditions with India's cultural texture was rooted in the colonial predicament of Hindu intellectuals. While the West was enabled by its global expansion to assert the universality of its reason in spite of its particularity, the colonized were denied this privilege; their historical fate was to assert the autonomy and universality of their culture in the domain of the nation.[56]

Through an elaborate construction of the history of classical Indian Chemistry and the science of mercury (*Rasayana*), Ray not only sought to assert the eminence of Indian culture but also added to the growing nationalist search for India's scientific culture in protest against colonial power. The science of chemistry, he argued, was 'the dominant science of a modern industrial world'[57] which 'was the real proof of the critical aptitude of a civilisation'.[58] Thus, 'in nineteenth-century contest for cultural authority, scientists had to show how and their knowledge was more reliable and powerful than other alternative traditions'.[59] Yet, another noted scientist, P. N. Bose and his illuminating work on the history of science in India, represented the changing mentality of the new and emerging Western-educated Indian intelligentsia who saw adoption of India's traditional sciences as a move to validate them in colonial India. Within the growing national movement for freedom against British rule, other prominent scientists in the nineteenth and early twentieth centuries sought to legitimate science by redefining it with new cultural and ideological paradigms. The foundation of a new journal, *The Dawn*, in 1897 by Satish Chandra Mukherjee (1868–1945) served as a voice as well as a 'forum for cultural redefinition in the light of the burgeoning struggle for independence from imperialist rule'.[60] It also was a medium through which the Western-educated Bhadralok community,[61] the 'intellectual proletariat',[62] could voice their ideas, setting a new framework 'for a constructive interpretation of the sciences of traditional India'.[63]

Other institutional confinements in hospitals as a means to prevent the spread of plague were seen as

> sudden intrusion of government authorities, the rush to Arthur Road, or other facilities, the agonised screams heard from without and the rapid announcement of collapse and death.[64]

Amidst this disorder and chaos, it was also rumoured that 'plague officers took to hospitals to make a speedy end to them there'.[65] To make matters worse, it was reported that the local inhabitants were not even aware of 'when they were going to be raided' and reported plague cases to avoid prosecution.[66] In all of this, public resistance was more akin to an antithesis to colonial coercion for hospitalization. Nevertheless, where plague interventions of 'segregation, hospitalisation and inoculation were carried out with tact and sensitivity to local feelings, they met with considerable success'.[67]

Yet, the most aggressive protest took place in 1898 in Byculla, Bombay, when some Julaha Muslim weavers set buildings on fire in a move to resist the hospitalization of a young girl suspected of plague.[68]

Besides, the extreme unpopularity and disdain for hospitals by the afflicted and their families can be gauged from a brief note that appeared in one of the leading dailies in 1897:

> The relatives of the sick man find it extremely difficult even to send word to him, not to speak of approaching him and assuaging his distress by loving attendance and affectionate words. As for attendance and nursing, how effective they might be can well be imagined from the fact that the hospital servants are at best mere strangers, invariably callous and patent mercenaries, and that the sick man, once within the hospital compound, is almost cut off from his private resources.[69]

Similar response to hospitalization was observed in the 1819 epidemic of cholera. This was particularly seen in Madras where temporary hospitals set up by the Medical Board witnessed 'a great reluctance to reside in them even for a day'.[70] As such, there was a popular feeling of 'likely violation of caste taboos and religious observance' and 'revulsion against the social isolation of a European hospital', for 'the Indian view of disease and its treatment called for family involvement and religious ministration, not secular segregation'.[71]

Besides, segregation and isolation in hospitals, post-mortem examination of afflicted or suspected plague victims by the colonial authorities met with popular opposition. This often led to 'evasion and concealment' of the sick in rooms or lofts where the chances of 'finding them' were often remote. In order to overcome this, the Government of India, in deliberating the Indian Plague Commission Report on the prophylaxis of plague, 'announced grant rewards for information regarding plague cases'.[72] Interference with funeral rites was frowned upon and as a result, corpses were often buried furtively in house compounds.

Western medicine and its negotiations within a sociocultural framework of caste, religion and gender led to new ideas of the body as subject to categories of hygiene, sanitation and purity. Best seen in the segregation and

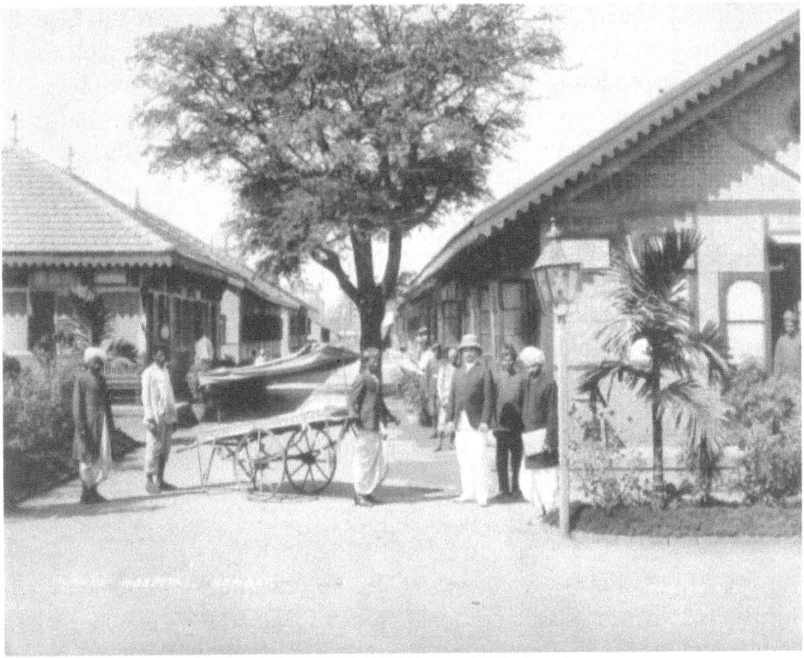

Figure 1.6 Bombay Plague Epidemic, 1896–1897: Plague Hospital, with Stretcher Carriers and Staff Standing Outside the Buildings. *Source*: Photograph by Clifton & Co. Wellcome Collection.

quarantine camps, colonial efforts also lay open pre-existing India's social hierarchies and ideas of touch, 'purity', 'pollution' and 'untouchability' (Figure 1.6). Caste, with these social connotations, provided several echelons of understanding of epidemic diseases, their varied experiences and perceptions; this also meant that in epidemic outbreaks in India, perhaps, caste, along with other social parameters of gender and religion, played a crucial role in the way plague and other epidemic health policies were implemented. Caste biases were particularly evident in the segregation camps in Punjab, for instance, which were set up according to caste and religious lines; and during the bubonic plague, it was noted that even body temperatures were checked by their own caste people.[73] While some patients were allowed to bring their own medicine and food to minimize contact with other castes. To disengage even further, there was a move to establish private and caste-specific hospitals in certain areas.

As popular expressions of resentment against colonial governmentality and public health escalated in the coming years, they were publicized through the emerging public sphere of 'native press' – newspapers and periodicals – of the late nineteenth and early twentieth centuries, thus also shaping public opinion in due course. The influenza pandemic of 1918, in particular, gained much prominence through the press as it publicized government inefficiency in handling the pandemic, punctuated by tensions between Western biomedicine and indigenous medical knowledge.[74]

Throughout the late nineteenth century and early twentieth centuries, while India became a nationalist space where collective retaliation and responses to imperial medical policies remained prominent, popular nationalism in the form of protests continued to seek to address Indian concerns for health. Amidst these happenings, as can be argued, the plague epidemic reinforced social and public health inequalities in a complex dialectic between disease and political, social and cultural modifications. Driven by Western disease paradigms and Western political, social and cultural perspectives, people's response to these transformations and to colonial policies, as Echenberg[75] remarks, remained very powerful throughout the plague.

CONCLUDING REMARKS

While both domestic and international pressure reigned supreme on the British State and her far-reaching policies to contain plague in India, the plague epidemic in India was unique for it unravelled those issues which cholera and smallpox epidemics could not. As Arnold argues, it posed important questions about the place of medical science and the authority of medical practitioners in the colonial order and about the political constraints on medical and sanitary intervention.[76]

Although quarantine started as a preventive measure against the spread of plague, it also was a marker of the challenges in devising a viable sanitary regime which would meet international and global standards of acceptance by the medical community. It also was a site within which colonial power could be exerted for economic and political advantages in international relations. In India, colonial health policies and public responses to these dominated the social and political culture of the country. Influenced largely by the prevailing nationalist agenda, some were accepted while others were dismissed as 'annihilating' the cultural boundaries. British intervention in instituting compulsory measures to exterminate plague, thus, often conflicted with Indian social mores which in itself was 'a major feature of the plague ordeal'.[77]

The role of the international pressures, the international sanitary conferences with earlier focus on cholera and its rapid spread to Europe saw plague as equally detrimental to their trade and commercial prerogatives. At the international level, there was more than the perceived threats or hurting of trade – that of undermining colonial image or damaging the economic viability in British colonies, or perhaps, undermining its visions of a successful rule.

The end of eighteenth and nineteenth centuries can also be seen as depicting a transition of both the scientific attributes and practices to contain the health conditions during epidemics. Can we say that quarantine became part of the imperial agenda which invested power, authority and hegemony in times of health crises as witnessed during the various epidemics? Can we then also say that quarantine acquired the status of disciplinary power under colonial exigencies?

Besides, the plague epidemic and the quarantine measures and other public health measures exhibited a complex interplay of colonial visions of Indian society, medical and scientific rivalries and plague administrative authorities and the people of India on whom these measures were focused.[78] In this respect, epidemic and quarantine also alluded to the start of a new chapter in political epidemiology, making obvious the differences between colonial perceptions and popular response; otherwise, how else could the epidemic continue to ravage India claiming millions of lives over decades; this was a complex situation of 'alienation and resistance' that characterized public health initiatives in colonial India. Yet, most epidemics in India lent themselves to new meanings for both the colonial administrators and the people of India, with a complex and deeper divide between the two about its gravity. These new meanings were articulated through negotiations of colonial policies with sociocultural perspectives of caste, gender and religion, among others. Western medical and sanitary policies and their engagements with India's social and cultural practices, thus, reinforced new relations and new visions of 'purity' and 'pollution' within the caste-gender-religion paradigm.

NOTES

1. Radhika Ramasubban, *Public Health and Medical Research in India: Their Origins under the Impact of British Colonial Policy* (Stockholm: Swedish Agency for Research Cooperation with Developing Countries, 1982), 4.

2. David Arnold, "Medical Priorities and Practice in Nineteenth-Century British India." *South Asia Research* 5, no. 2 (November 1985): 167–83. doi: 10.1177/02272808500208

3. The 'reserved' category included revenue, police and finance, while health matters were transferred to Indian ministers.

4. R. Nair, "The Construction of a 'Population Problem' in Colonial India, 1919–1947," *Journal of Imperial Commonwealth History* 39, no. 2 (2010): 227–47.

5. Poonam Bala, "Ayurveda (re) Invented: Engagements with Science and Religion in Colonial India," in *The Routledge Handbook of Religion, Health and Medicine*, ed. Dorothea Luddeckens, Philipp Hetmanczyk, Pamela E. Klassen and Justin B. Stein (London/New York, Routledge, 2021), 421–34.

6. Poonam Bala, "Reconstructing Indian Medicine: The Role of Caste in late Nineteenth- and Twentieth-Century India," in *Medicine and Colonialism: Historical Perspectives in India and South Africa*, ed. Poonam Bala (Routledge: London, 2016), 11–24.

7. *Proceedings of the Conference of Provincial Representative* (Simla. 24–30 June 1930).

8. W.J. Simpson. "The Evidence and Conclusions relating to the Mulkowal Tetanus Case," *Practitioner* 78 (1907): 796–812. Cited from Barbara J. Hawgood, "Waldemar Mordecai Haffkine, CIE (1860–1930): Prophylactic Vaccination against Cholera and Bubonic Plague in British India" (from jameslindlibrary.org).

9. *Proceedings of the Government of India*, Home Department, Medical Branch (July–Dec.1866).

10. J.C.Hume, "Rival Traditions: Western Medicine and Yunani-Tibb in the Punjab, 1849–1899," *Bulletin of the History of Medicine* 51 (1977): 214–31. See also J.C. Hume, *Medicine in the Punjab, 1849–1911: Ethnicity and Professionalisation in the Control of an Occupation* (PhD Thesis), Duke University (1977), 72.

11. Ira Klein, "Plague, Policy and Popular Unrest in British India," *Modern Asian Studies* 22, no. 4 (1998): 723–55, 724.

12. Detailed Statistics on this appeared in the *Indian Sanitary Proceedings*, India Office Library (IOL), v.7602 (1907): 1816–17.

13. Pratik Chakrabarti, "Covid-19 and the Spectres of Colonialism," *India Forum* (August 7, 2020).

14. Klein, "Plague, Policy and Popular Unrest," 725.

15. Warwick Anderson, *Health and History* 6, no. 2 (2004): 111–14. doi: 10.2307/40111488.

16. pp. 130–31. Rohan Deb Roy, *Malarial Subjects: Empire, Medicine and Non-humans in British India, 1820–1909* (Cambridge: Cambridge University Press, 2017), 57.

17. pp. 130–31. Rohan Deb Roy, *Malarial Subjects: Empire, Medicine and Non-humans in British India, 1820–1909* (Cambridge: Cambridge University Press, 2017), 57.

18. Klein, "Plague, Policy and Popular Unrest."

19. See Jon Arrizabalaga and Juan Carlos García-Reyes (2018). "Contagion Controversies on Cholera and Yellow Fever in mid-nineteenth century Spain: The case of Nicasio Landa," in *Mediterranean Quarantines, 1750–1914: Space, Identity and Power,* ed. David Cantor (Manchester: Manchester University Press, 2018), 170–96.

20. Klein, "Plague, Policy and Popular Unrest," 737.

21. Klein, "Plague, Policy and Popular Unrest." Cited from Vempalli Raj Mahammadh, "Plague Mortality and Control Policies in Colonial South India, 1900–47," *South Asia Research* 40, no. 3 (1 September 2020): 323–43.

22. B.W. Brown, "Plague: A Note on the History of the Disease in Hongkong." *Public Health Reports (1896–1970)* 28, no. 12 (1913): 551–57. doi: 10.2307/4569336.

23. Dr Mead's work, *A Short Discourse Concerning Pestilential Contagion, and the Methods to Be Used to Prevent It*, was a major medical contribution well ahead of its time when ideas of contagion had not become part of the medical thoughts. See n.33, p.48.

24. Arnold Zuckerman, "Plague and Contagionism in Eighteenth-Century England: The Role of Richard Mead," *Bulletin of the History of Medicine* 78 (2004): 273–308. See also Jon Arrizabalaga and Juan Carlos García-Reyes, "Contagion Controversies on Cholera and Yellow Fever in mid nineteenth-century Spain: the case of Nicasio Landa," in *Mediterranean Quarantines, 1750–1914: Space, Identity and Power*, ed. John Chircop and Francisco Javier Martinez (Manchester: Manchester University Press, 2018), 170–96.

25. For instance, Couchman ME. *Account of plague administration in the Bombay Presidency from September 1896 till May 1897* (Mumbai: Government Central Press, 1897); and Gatacre WF. *Report on the bubonic plague in Bombay: 1896–97* (Mumbai: Times of India, 1898). See also Mushtaq.

26. Restriction in mobility is imposed, for mobility will lead to contagion or punishment. Michel Foucault, *Discipline & Punish: the Birth of the Prison*, trans. A. Sheridan (New York: Vintage, 1975/1995), 195. See also, Michael A. Peters, "*Philosophy and Pandemic in the Post digital Era: Foucault,* Agamben Žižek," *Postdigital Science and Education* (29 April 2020): 1–6.

27. Zenanas constituted reserved part of a home for women of the household in the Indian subcontinent.

28. Roy Macleod, "Introduction," in *Disease, Medicine and empire: perspectives om Western Medicine and the Experience of European Expansion*, ed. Roy Macleod and Milton Lewis (London: Routledge, 1988), 7; For details and further citation, see Poonam Bala, "Ayurveda and the Raj: Agenda for a 'Nationalist Project,'" in *Medicine and Colonial Engagements in India and Sub-Saharan Africa,* ed. Poonam Bala (Newcastle upon Tyne: Cambridge Scholars, 2018), 11–26.

29. Peter Baldwin, *Contagion and the State in Europe, 1830–1930* (Cambridge: Cambridge University Press, 1999), 4. See details in Mukesh Kumar, "Question of Quarantining or Politicising the 'Plague'? Indians in the Nineteenth-Century Natal," *Proceedings of the Indian History Congress* 75 (2014; Platinum Jubilee): 996–1005.

30. David Arnold, p.61, "Touching the Body: Perspectives on Indian Plague, 1860–1900," in *Subaltern Studies* V, ed. Ranajit Guha, Subaltern Studies V, 61.

31. Yoosof U.V.Jasriya, "Epidemics and the City," *Proceedings of the Indian History Congress* 78 (2017): 549–57.

32. Michel Foucault, *Society Must Be Defended: Lectures at the College of France, 1975–76,* trans. David Macey (London: Penguin Books, 2003); see details in Jasriya, "Epidemics and the City."

33. Michel Foucault, *History of Madness* (London: Routledge, 1961).

34. Michel Foucault, *Society Must Be Defended*, trans. David Macey.

35. Jo N. Hays, "Quarantine: Local and Global Histories," *Australian Historical Studies* 48, no. 3 (2017): 459–61. doi: 10.1080/1031461X.2017.1337488

36. Maryinez Lyons, "African Sleeping Sickness: A Historical Review," *International Journal of STD and AIDS* 2, suppl 1 (1991): 20–25.

37. Maryinez Lyons, *The Colonial Disease: A Social History of Sleeping Sickness in Northern Zaire, 1900–1940* (Cambridge, Cambridge University Press, 2010), ch.5.

38. Lyons, *The Colonial Disease.*

39. Birsen Bulmus, *Plague, Quarantines and Geopolitics in the Ottoman Empire* (Edinburgh: Edinburgh University Press, 2005), 130.

40. Bulmus, 136.

41. Bulmus, 136.

42. Bulmus, 149.

43. Lyons, *The Colonial Disease.*

44. Bala, "Ayurveda and the Raj," 17.

45. Arnold, *Colonising the Body.*

46. David Arnold, "Cholera and Colonialism in British India," *Past and Present*, no. 113 (November 1986): 139.

47. Khwaja Arif Hasan provides an illustrative account of the established mores on health after the Second World War. See K.A. Hasan, *The Cultural Frontiers of Health in Village India: Case Study of a North Indian Village* (Mumbai: Manaktalas, 1967).

48. pp. 48–49, 66, 119–20 and 146–50.

49. pp. 48–49, 66, 119–20 and 146–50.

50. For details on the account of history of disease prevention in colonial India, see Muhammad Umair Mushtaq, "Public Health in British India: A Brief Account of the History of Medical Services and Disease Prevention in Colonial India," *Indian Journal of Community Medicine*, 34, no. 1 (January 2009): 6–14.

51. Bala, "Re-constructing Indian Medicine," 21.

52. Bala, "Re-constructing Indian Medicine," 23.

53. Gyan Prakash, *Another Reason: Science and the Imagination of Modern India* (Princeton: Princeton University Press, 1999): 34.

54. Pratik Chakraborty, "Science, Nationalism and Colonial Contestations: P.C. Ray and his *Hindu Chemistry,*" *Indian Economic and Social History Review* 37, no. 2 (2000): 185–213.

55. Ashis Nandy, *The Intimate Enemy: Loss and Recovery of Self under Colonialism* (New Delhi: Oxford University Press, 1983), cited from Chakraborty, Science, Nationalism and Colonial Contestation, 186.

56. Prakash, *Another Reason*, 89.

57. Chakraborty, "Science, Nationalism and Colonial Contestations," 187.

58. Chakraborty, "Science, Nationalism and Colonial Contestations," 187.

59. Jerome K. Ravetz, *Scientific Knowledge and its Social Problems* (New York: Routledge, 1996), 50 (originally published 1971 by OUP). Also cited by Pratik Chakraborty, "Science, Nationalism and Colonial Contestations."

60. Dhruv Raina and S. Irfan Habib, "The Moral Legitimation of Modern Science: Bhadralok Reflections on Theories of Evolution," *Social Studies of Science* 26, no. 1 (February 1996): 9–42.

61. Poonam Bala, *Biomedicine as a Contested Site: Some Revelations in Colonial Contexts* (Lanham: Lexington, 2009).

62. Sumit Sarkar, *The Swadeshi Movement in Bengal* (New Delhi: People's Publishing House, 1975), 150. See also Raina and Habib, "The Moral Legitimation of Modern Science." note. 10, 34.

63. Irfan S.Habib and Dhruv Raina, "Copernicus, Columbus, Colonialism and the Role of Science in Nineteenth-Century India," *Social Scientist* 17, no. 3–4 (March 1989): 51–66; note 19, 60–62.

64. Klein, Plague, "Plague, Policy and Popular Unrest," 742.

65. P.C. Snow, *Report on Bubonic Plague in Bombay, 1896–97*, IOL, 6.; cited from Ira Klein, "Plague, Policy and Popular Unrest," 742.

66. Report on Bubonic Plague in Bombay, IOL, 105.

67. Arnold, "Cholera and Colonialism," 113.

68. For details, see Natasha Sarkar, "Plague in Bombay: Response of Britain's Indian Subjects to Colonial Intervention," *Proceedings of the Indian History Congress* 62 (2001): 442–49.

69. Arnold, *Colonising the Body*, 213.

70. India Office Records, Madras, Public Proceedings (11 June 1819), Madras Medical Board to Madras Government (31 May 1819); cited in Arnold, *Cholera and Colonialism*, 137.

71. Arnold, "Cholera and Colonialism," 137.

72. Notes from India: The Government of India and the Plague Commission Report – Cholera and Plague in Bombay, *The Lancet* (18 August 1900), 545.

73. Mridula Ramanna, *Health Care in Bombay Presidency, 1896–1930* (New Delhi: Primus Books, 2012).

74. Madhu Singh, "Bombay Fever/Spanish Flu: Public Health and Native Press in Colonial Bombay, 1918–19," *South Asia Research* 41, no. 1 (2021): 35–52.

75. Myron Echenberg, *Plague Ports: The Global Urban Impact of Bubonic Plague, 1894–1901* (New York: New York University Press, 2007). See also Myron Echenberg, "Pestis Redux: The Initial years of the Third Bubonic plagues, 1894–1901," *Journal of World History* 13, no, 2 (Fall 2002): 429–49.

76. Arnold, *Colonising the Body*, 202.

77. Hasan, *The Cultural Frontiers of Health in Village India*, 48–49, 66, 119–20 and 146–50.

78. For details, see Rajnarain Chandavarkar, "Plague Panic and Epidemic Politics in India, 1896–1914," in *Epidemic and Ideas: Essays on the Historical Perception of Pestilence* , ed. Terence Ranger and Paul Slack (review of book by Mohan Rao, *Population Studies* 48, no. 3 (November 1994): 549–52.

BIBLIOGRAPHY

Anderson, Warwick. *Health and History* 6, no. 2 (2004): 111–14. doi: 10.2307/40111488.

Arnold, David. "Medical Priorities and Practice in Nineteenth-Century British India." *South Asia Research* 5, no. 2 (November 1985): 167–83. doi: 10.1177/02272808500208.

Arnold, David. *Colonising the Body: State Medicine and Epidemic Disease in Nineteenth-Century India*. Berkeley/London: University of California Press, 1993.

Arrizabalaga, Jon, and Juan Carlos García-Reyes. "Contagion Controversies on Cholera and Yellow Fever in mid-nineteenth century Spain: The Case of Nicasio Landa." In *Mediterranean Quarantines, 1750–1914: Space, Identity and Power,* edited by John Chircop and Francisco Javier Martinez, 170–96. Manchester: Manchester University Press, 2018.

Bala, Poonam, ed. *Biomedicine as a Contested Site: Some Revelations in Colonial Contexts.* Lanham: Lexington, 2009.

Bala, Poonam, ed. *Medicine and Colonialism: Historical Perspectives in India and South Africa.* London: Routledge, 2016.

Bala, Poonam. "Reconstructing Indian Medicine: The Role of Caste in late Nineteenth- and Twentieth-Century India." In *Medicine and Colonialism: Historical Perspectives in India and South Africa*, edited by Poonam Bala, 11–24. London: Routledge, 2016.

Bala, Poonam. "Ayurveda and the Raj: Agenda for a 'Nationalist Project.'" In *Medicine and Colonial Engagements in India and Sub-Saharan Africa,* edited by Poonam Bala, 11–26. Newcastle upon Tyne: Cambridge Scholars, 2018.

Bala, Poonam, ed. *Medicine and Colonial Engagements in India and Sub-Saharan Africa.* Newcastle upon Tyne: Cambridge Scholars, 2018.

Bala, Poonam. "Ayurveda (re) Invented: Engagements with Science and Religion in Colonial India." In *The Routledge Handbook of Religion, Health and Medicine,* edited by Dorothea Luddeckens, Philipp Hetmanczyk, Pamela E. Klassen and Justin B. Stein, 421–34. London/New York: Routledge, 2021.

Baldwin, Peter. *Contagion and the State in Europe, 1830–1930.* Cambridge: Cambridge University Press, 1999.

Brown, B.W. "Plague: A Note on the History of the Disease in Hongkong." *Public Health Reports (1896–1970)* 28, no. 12 (1913): 551–57. doi: 10.2307/4569336.

Bulmus, Birsen. *Plague, Quarantines and Geopolitics in the Ottoman Empire.* Edinburgh: Edinburgh University Press, 2005.

Chakrabarti, Pratik. "Covid-19 and the Spectres of Colonialism," *India Forum* (August 7, 2020).

Chakraborty, Pratik. "Science, Nationalism and Colonial Contestations: P. C. Ray and his *Hindu Chemistry,*" *Indian Economic and Social History Review* 37 no. 2 (2000): 185–213.

Couchman, M.E. *Account of Plague Administration in the Bombay Presidency from September 1896 till May 1897.* Mumbai: Government Central Press, 1897.

Echenberg, Myron. *Plague Ports: The Global Urban Impact of Bubonic Plague, 1894–1901.* New York: New York University Press, 2007.

Echenberg, Myron. "Pestis Redux: The Initial years of the Third Bubonic plagues, 1894–1901," *Journal of World History* 13, no. 2 (Fall 2002): 429–49.

Foucault, Michel. *History of Madness.* London: Routledge, 1961.

Foucault, Michel. *Discipline & Punish: The Birth of the Prison.* Translated by A. Sheridan. New York: Vintage, 1975/1995.

Foucault, Michel. *Society Must Be Defended: Lectures at the College of France, 1975–76.* Translated by David Macey. London: Penguin Books, 2003.

Gatacre, W.F. *Report on the Bubonic Plague in Bombay: 1896–97*. Mumbai: Times of India, 1898.

Guha, Ranajit, ed. *Subaltern Studies V: Writings on South Asian History and Society*. New Delhi: Oxford University Press, 1987.

Habib, Irfan S., and Dhruv Raina. "Copernicus, Columbus, Colonialism and the Role of Science in Nineteenth-Century India." *Social Scientist* 17, nos. 3–4 (March 1989): 51–66.

Hasan, K.A. *The Cultural Frontiers of Health in Village India: Case Study of a North Indian Village*. Mumbai: Manaktalas, 1967.

Hawgood, Barbara, J. "Waldemar Mordecai Haffkine, CIE (1860–1930): Prophylactic Vaccination against Cholera and Bubonic plague in British India" (www.jameslindlibrary.org).

Hays, Jo N. "Quarantine: Local and Global Histories," *Australian Historical Studies* 48, no. 3 (2017): 459–61. doi: 10.1080/1031461X.2017.1337488.

Hume, J.C. *Medicine in the Punjab, 1849–1911: Ethnicity and Professionalisation in the Control of an Occupation* (PhD Thesis), Duke University, 1977.

Hume, J.C. "Rival Traditions: Western Medicine and Yunani-Tibb in the Punjab, 1849–1899," *Bulletin of the History of Medicine* 51 (1977): 214–31.

India Office Records. Madras, Public Proceedings (11 June 1819), Madras Medical Board to Madras Government (31 May 1819).

Indian Sanitary Proceedings, India Office Library (IOL), v.7602 (1907).

Jasriya, Yoosof U.V. "Epidemics and the City," *Proceedings of the Indian History Congress* 78 (2017): 549–57.

Klein, Ira. "Plague, Policy and Popular Unrest in British India," *Modern Asian Studies* 22, no.4 (1998): 723–55.

Kumar, Mukesh. "Question of Quarantining or Politicising the 'Plague'? Indians in the Nineteenth-Century Natal," *Proceedings of the Indian History Congress* 75 (2014): 996–1005.

Luddeckens, Dorothy, Philipp Hetmanczyk, Pamela E. Klassen and Justin B. Stein, eds. *The Routledge Handbook of Religion, Health and Medicine*. London/New York: Routledge, 2021.

Lyons, Maryinez. "African Sleeping Sickness: A Historical Review," *International Journal of STD and AIDS* 2, suppl 1 (1991): 20–25.

Lyons, Maryinez. *The Colonial Disease: A Social History of Sleeping Sickness in Northern Zaire, 1900–1940*. Cambridge: Cambridge University Press, 2010.

Mahammadh, Vempalli Raj. "Plague Mortality and Control Policies in Colonial South India, 1900–47," *South Asia Research* 40, no. 3 (1 September 2020): 323–43.

Macleod, Roy, and Milton Lewis. *Disease, Medicine and Empire: Perspectives on Western Medicine and the Experience of European Expansion*. London: Routledge, 1988.

Mushtaq, Muhammad Umair. "Public Health in British India: A Brief Account of the History of Medical Services and Disease Prevention in Colonial India." *Indian Journal of Community Medicine* 34, no. 1 (January 2009): 6–14.

Nair, R. "The Construction of a 'Population Problem' in Colonial India, 1919–1947." *Journal of Imperial Commonwealth History* 39, no. 2 (2010): 227–47.

Nandy, Ashis. *The Intimate Enemy: Loss and Recovery of Self under Colonialism.* New Delhi: Oxford University Press, 1983.

Notes from India: The Government of India and the Plague Commission Report—Cholera and Plague in Bombay. *The Lancet* (18 August 1900): 545.

Peters, Michael A. "*Philosophy and Pandemic in the Post digital Era: Foucault, Agamben Žižek.*" *Postdigital Science and Education* (29 April 2020): 1–6.

Prakash, Gyan. *Another Reason: Science and the Imagination of Modern India.* Princeton: Princeton University Press, 1999.

Proceedings of the Government of India, Home Department, Medical Branch. July-Dec. 1866.

Proceedings of the Conference of Provincial Representative. Simla. 24–30 June 1930.

Raina, Dhruv, and S. Irfan Habib. "The Moral Legitimation of Modern Science: Bhadralok Reflections on Theories of Evolution." *Social Studies of Science* 26, no. 1 (February 1996): 9–42.

Ramanna, Mridula. *Health Care in Bombay Presidency, 1896–1930.* New Delhi: Primus Books, 2012.

Ramasubban, Radhika. *Public Health and Medical Research in India: Their Origins under the Impact of British Colonial Policy.* Stockholm: Swedish Agency for Research Cooperation with Developing Countries, 1982.

Ranger, Terrence, and Paul Slack, eds. *Epidemic and Ideas: Essays on the Historical Perception of Pestilence.* Cambridge: Cambridge University Press, 1992.

Ravetz, Jerome K. *Scientific Knowledge and its Social Problems.* New York: Routledge, 1996.

Roy, Rohan Deb. *Malarial Subjects: Empire, Medicine and Non-humans in British India, 1820–1909.* Cambridge: Cambridge University Press, 2017.

Sarkar, Natasha. "Plague in Bombay: Response of Britain's Indian Subjects to Colonial Intervention." *Proceedings of the Indian History Congress* 62 (2001): 442–49.

Sarkar, Sumit. *The Swadeshi Movement in Bengal.* New Delhi: People's Publishing House, 1975.

Snow, P. C. H. *Report on Bubonic Plague in Bombay, 1896–97*, IOL, 6.

Singh, Madhu. "Bombay Fever/Spanish Flu: Public Health and Native Press in Colonial Bombay, 1918–19," *South Asia Research* 41, no. 1 (2021): 35–52.

Zuckerman, Arnold. "Plague and Contagionism in Eighteenth-Century England: The Role of Richard Mead." *Bulletin of the History of Medicine* 78 (2004): 273–308.

Chapter 2

The Uncouth Woes

The Prevalence of Venereal Diseases in the British or European Troops in India (ca. 1864–1918)

Apalak Das

The present condition of the Army in India, with the enormous prevalence of venereal disease . . . yearly sending home thousands of men infected with constitutional taint, is therefore a great and growing source of danger to the whole community.[1]

Report of Departmental Committee appeared in the statement of Earl of Dunraven in the House of Lords on the Departmental Committee of the India Office (1897) on 14 May, 1897

It was not the *'Gemeinschaft'* or idea of 'community', but preserving the supposed racial potency of the 'whites', who were snivelling the menace of degeneration from venereal diseases (VD), developed into one of the prime concerns to the colonial state. Why had the preservation of 'race' become so essential to the colonial administration in India? as VD posed direct threat to health, racial supremacy and martial spirit of 'white' than the *natives*, the Raj had decided to go for 'disciplining' the European soldiers in the name of military hygiene. The recent historiography on the politico-cultural liaison between race and diseases, such as the works of Ishita Pande, Philippa Levine, Erica Wald and David Arnold, has focused on the way in which colonial discourses framed the question of racial susceptibility to the tropical maladies, vices and wickedness that crippled the British vis-à-vis European soldiers. To the Raj, the issue was whether the 'moral policing', instead of mere withdrawing Contagious Diseases (CD) Acts, would prevent the VD; amidst of the sway of liberal wind and abolitionism or anti-regulationist vibes, there was a growing apprehension in the House of Commons in 1888 regarding the practices, rules and regulations on prostitution and the treatment of VD in the cantonments and other places of British India. On 5 June 1888, a resolution was passed in the House wherein it had been settled that any sort of measly suspension of measures for compulsory examination of women and for regulating prostitution in India or the legislations that instructed and permitted the government to carry out such measures in India would be both 'insufficient' and 'ought to be repealed'.[2] However, the British Parliament was sceptical on its application in the colonies which ultimately led to the formation of a departmental committee, named after its chairman, the Under-Secretary of State for India, Mr. George W. E. Russell, appointed by John Wodehouse, the Secretary of State for India on 7 April 1893. The aim was to investigate whether the Government of India (GoI) accorded with the resolution adopted in the House of Commons or it had refashioned and restructured the legal imperatives to deal with the *native* 'consorts' (the probable source of contagion) through the enactment of new Cantonment Laws. It seems unusual that the Committee had not collected any evidence from Indian cantonments except Umballa, Meerut, Lucknow, Mean Meer (Lahore), Rawalpindi, Peshawar, Amritsar, Bareilly, Sitapur and Banaras as the inquiries must be presented in a form of a report before the end of parliamentary session. The Russell Committee found the testimonies of Mrs. Elizabeth Andrew, Dr. Kate Bushnell and several general officers as principal observations of the seven other cantonments. In relation to this, another Special Commission in India, that is Ibbetson Commission under Mr. Denzil Ibbetson, was employed by the Military Department of the GoI on 2 June 1893 which surprisingly selected only three cantonments, such as Umballa, Meerut and Lucknow, for the investigation. Both these groups had altogether accentuated the conditions of *chaklas* or brothels, the functions of lock hospitals and the periodical examination of the native women. Finally, the Russell Committee succeeded to put forth the report on 31 August 1893 in which the members in majority had concluded that all the ten cantonments largely violated the directives of the adopted resolution of the Lower House of British Parliament. Moreover, the numerous official orders and regulations were unable to abolish the old system of regulated and licensed prostitution. The Act of 1890, under the Cantonment Act of 1889, was in operation connected to the continuous system of periodical examination since 1888.[3] Therefore, the Committee was of opinion that 'this system and the incidental practices . . . did not, and the Statutory Rules, so far as they authorize or permit the same, do not accord with the accepted meaning and intention of the Resolution of the House of Commons'.[4]

The Cantonment Act of 1895 intended to resolve the matter by outlawing the periodical examinations of prostitutes and disavowing any official approval of prostitution in the Indian cantonments, although it surfaced the fissure within the imperial governance over VD, which was gradually widened in the 1890s. The Colonial Office was worried about the health of the British troops in India from the beginning; a military despatch was sent from the GoI to the Secretary of State on 4 November, 1896 where it was stated that the increasing VD cases among the European soldiers induced the empire to ruminate about the imminent pitfall. From 1876 to 1885, annually there were 258 VD patients in 1,000 in an average which escalated to 522.3 in 1895, whereas the prevalence of VD was much less in the native troops. The inference was not all 'loose' native women having VD, but a class of women were definitely responsible 'with whom the British soldier associates, there has been an increase out of all proportion to their numbers'. In that despatch, a strong and 'fresh powers' had been requested without which no restrictions could do substantial effect in reducing the VD.[5] The report of the Departmental Committee on '*the Prevalence of Venereal Disease among the British Troops in India*', which appeared in 1897, stirred up the debate between the Extentionists and Repealers once again. The controversy engendered immense tremble in the Parliament. Meanwhile, the figures had revealed unprecedented increase of VD, chiefly syphilis, in the British troops. This had impaired not only the military efficiency of the army stationed in the Raj but the health of England's civil population. Especially, when the homecoming British soldiers started to socialize with their community, the risk of infection among 'healthy' population grew manifold.[6] To the Colonial Office, the racial potency and 'discipline' of the British Army were at more risk than the health of the native consorts. Even, how far the resolution of House of Commons brought in the issues of 'choice' and 'compulsion' in case of prostitution was hitherto unaddressed in the colonial regulations later on. The native women were frequently seen as the means of contamination in the colonial legislations; however, they might not be the prime disquiet to the Raj;[7] instead, the objectification of '*germed* bodies' along with the prevention against VD was the rationale of empire, which required proper institutionalization through various health surveillances such as sanitary, departmental committee and lock hospital reports. Till the eighteenth century, the Western medical discourse identified the women's body as 'degenerated', 'depraved' and 'deformed' in contrast to the male counterpart. Subsequently, during the Victorian era, the notion was substituted with more robust surmise. The promiscuous bodies, which were by virtue supposed to be infected, were now distinguished from the 'purified' and 'moral' bodies.[8] Thence, the CD Acts had been put into practice only to control such 'promiscuity'. The mounting cases of VD in the army from 1880s proved the frailty of the preventive system. Mark Harrison has pointed out that VD control was a 'moral' problem to the similar extent of a medical crisis in the British Army. Nevertheless, the traditional perceptions of 'restraint' and 'honour' in militarism were the foundations of British Empire, materializing the moral considerations in such a way that many officers from old school perceived the VD control as undermining agency to military virtue. For them, the efficiency of a 'race' largely relied upon 'morality'; however, the pro-reformist medical officers had reversed the idea with an unyielding belief in scientific VD control for military competence rather than focusing on the nebulous concept of 'moral policing'.[9] Therefore, military hygiene was introduced in combination with successive sanitary reforms in India from the mid-nineteenth century, but these had achieved a little than expected. Transposing Philip Curtin's thesis,[10] Harrison illustrated the rate of hospital admission of the British soldiers for the treatment of malaria, typhoid and VD which remained high from 1859 to 1900; this did indicate that British troops faced higher mortality from diseases more than have they had fatalities in the battles.[11] This chapter focuses on the way in which ideas of health, hygiene and race were entangled with colonial investigations about VD in the British troops in India till the end of the First World War, and to what extent the imperial directives had succeeded to stall the prevalence of VD within the British Indian Army. It also looks at whether morality prevailed over promiscuity as the anti-regulationist movement, which was one of the frenzied debates within the medical academia vis-à-vis the Colonial Office in the nineteenth-century Britain, hovering around the politics of 'disease' (or diseased?) prevention.

PROMISCUITY, RACE AND SEX: THE VD IN THE BRITISH TROOPS IN INDIA (C. 1860s–1880s)

For the British officials, the tropical world such as India was so 'alluring' that it hardly resisted the European soldiers from becoming 'sloppy characters'. During the eighteenth century, the life of a common soldier was whirled by humid climate, tiresome early morning drill and occasional engagement with the enemies. Erica Wald has posited that drink, violence and sex turned into the 'grim trinity', associated with the young European soldiers. The Company and the Crown were equally dithered about the rising expense for maintaining the huge number of native wives, mistresses and children of European soldiers – the greatest impediments in maximizing the colonial profit. This was the reason behind the encouragement of the British East India Company towards owning native companions for sexual need by the late eighteenth century. As the European soldier was believed to be an asset, the colonial officials tried to protect them from obvious 'uncouth' hazard like VD. Unfortunately, syphilis and gonorrhea had been persistent health problems stymieing the colonial state to control the diseases even in the early twentieth century when cure of VD was possible. Medical surgeons were concerned about growing disease prevalence in the barracks. The scaling military costs had persuaded the European soldiers for more temporary sexual relations with 'lal bazaar' prostitutes. The medical faculties found an impregnable solution to restrain the venereal 'plague' by guaranteeing a band of healthy women for the soldiers in the cantonments.[12] The CD Act of 1864 had ensured the medical examination of 'diseased' women who were sent to the lock hospitals later for the treatment. In 1861, the British Army possessed 227,005 officers and men of which 82,156 belonged to Indian regiments and 144,849 to home or to the other colonial regiments.[13] The *Report of the Commissioners Appointed to Inquire into the Sanitary State of the Army in India*, in 1863, had presented the fact that the married officers were much healthier than the unmarried; moreover, the officers had not been easily driven by vices because of their improved lifestyle in comparison with the common soldiers:

> While the soldiers live together in common bedrooms in barracks, the officers generally reside in separate bungalows, where they have the due arrangements for cleanliness; their food and drink are of superior quality; their contact with the sick in hospitals is limited to periodical inspections; when ill themselves they have the advantage of separate apartments and obtain leave to resort to healthy places.[14]

As there was no reliable record on how much soldiers were affected by syphilis, the Commissioners collected the returns of the lock and other hospitals to get an inclusive image. Almost 20–25% of the total sick were the VD cases which sometimes surged to 50% at some places such as Bangalore and Roorkee and 53% at Dinapore. A considerable number of cases were so serious that they had been pronounced unfit for service and eventually sent home as invalids. For the Commissioners, the reorganization of the measures, previously taken in the three presidencies, that is, Bengal, Bombay and Madras, and cleanliness in barrack lavatories would be effective to diminish the VD significantly.[15] In the United Kingdom, the CD Act of 1866 was passed to check the ravages of VD in the army and navy and to restrict the inveterate expenses for the treatment of sailors and diseased soldiers.[16] The Indian CD Act was implemented too in 1868 with similar objective; needless to say that it was not much different from the other CD Acts, protecting the 'white race' from the tropical vice.[17] Initially, it proved effective as far as the statistics of mortality and sickness in the European troops in India was concerned. The VD admission rate in 1860–1869 was higher than 1870–1879, although the figure was still frightening. During 1870–1879, the total VD admissions in the European Army of India were 117,485 which was equivalent to admission rate of 203.5 per 1,000. In case of Bengal troop, the admission rate was 208.6 per 1,000, appearing less than that of the preceding ten years. For European Army of Madras, there was fewer, that is, 198.1 per 1,000, admittance in the hospitals in contrast to Bengal

Army but higher than the admission rate of European Army of Bombay, that is, 191.1 per 1,000.[18] On 25 July 1874, J. M. Cunningham, Sanitary Commissioner of the GoI, had submitted his report on the rules for the prevention of VD among the European troops in the Bengal Presidency in 1873. To him, the greatest difficulty for the officials was to detect the large number of 'clandestine prostitution' which had been responsible for the increase of VD cases in the European troops both in India and England. This problem was much more alarming in case of British India where the population resided adjacent to the military cantonments.[19]

The lock hospital reports have provided the admission rates of European soldiers and prostitutes evenly. There were nine military (Bangalore, Bellary, Kamptee, Cannanore, St. Thomas Mount, Secunderabad, Seetabuldee, Trichinopoly and Wellington) and four civil lock hospitals (Madras, Rangoon, Thayetmyo, and Tonghoo) in Madras Presidency. The cases of primary syphilis in the military lock hospitals had been steadily increasing since 1873. It appeared that the admission for the treatment of primary syphilis, except 1875, was more numerous among the women than the European troops. Along with this, there was a significant swell of VD cases in the European force as well. In 1873, the ratio was 149.81 per 1,000 which ascended to 231.27 in 1877. To the colonial officials, the increase of primary syphilis, which was the most dangerous of all forms of VD within the British contingents, was a serious concern. The disease was so vicious that it made the young soldiers ineffective permanently at an early phase of their career. In spite of everything, the British colonists had considered the primary syphilis as 'mild and manageable disease' if treated earlier. The most affected areas in the Madras Presidency were Bellary, Trichinopoly and Bangalore where the large number of famine-stricken women from rural areas thronged for living. They were mostly 'unregistered' prostitutes and might have carried the germ of VD.[20] Undoubtedly, there was undiminished connection between famine and prostitution reflecting in the report. The colonial officials were saying that:

> We must not be surprised if we find among the evil results of the famine an increased proportion for some years to come of cases of constitutional syphilis . . . there was, as already stated, a great influx of famine-stricken women and the increase of venereal diseases generally and of primary syphilis more particularly was due to their presence.[21]

From 1878 to 1880, the report shows trifling development as the number of primary and secondary syphilis cases and gonorrhea in the European troops furthered.[22] On 11 February 1880, the Military Lock Hospital of Trichinopoly was closed due to the withdrawal of all European troops from the station; though the total admissions in both classes of European soldiers and diseased women had marginally reduced, the surging figures of VD among the Europeans were distressing when the ratio of admission had reached 324.09 per 1,000 in 1880 in Madras Presidency.[23] The figures for 1881 displayed a sizeable decline which was momentary. It again intensified in 1882 after which the colonial officers finally had to concede that whatever the objectives might have induced the Raj to found lock hospitals for providing the gratuitous medical aid to an unfortunate class of people, these institutions to protect the British soldiers from VD were no less than catastrophe.[24] Thus, in 1888, there were 356.41 per 1,000 as ratio of admission for all forms of VD in the British troops in Madras, illustrating shrink in general VD but considerable rise in primary syphilis.[25] In Punjab province, there were sixteen lock hospitals at Delhi, Umballa, Dagshai, Kasauli, Subathu, Jullundur, Ferozepore, Mean Meer, Multan, Dalhousie, Sialkot, Rawalpindi, Attock, Murree, Peshawar and Naushahra of which ten hospital reports had been showing a reduction in VD cases among the British troops in 1887 in comparison with the figures of the previous years; however, rest of the hospitals, especially those at Delhi, Dagshai, Dalhousie, Attock and Murree, presented somewhat unsatisfactory result (see table 2.1).[26] As the report of each hospital was erroneous, A. M. Dallas, the Inspector-General of Civil Hospitals of Punjab, appealed to the Secretary to Government of Punjab for transferring this responsibility of data collection entirely to the military department which had greater control over lock

Table 2.1 Venereal Diseases among the European Troops in Punjab Province, 1886–1887

	Ratio of Admission per Mille		*Average Strength of Troops*	
Hospitals	*1886*	*1887*	*1886*	*1887*
Delhi	345.60	351.46	489	478
Umballa	287.30	222.86	1,977	1,925
Dagshai	232.09	284.83	810	804
Kasauli	No details	No details	No details	No details
Subathu	950.38	452.48	262	484
Jullundur	376.99	202.08	626	866
Ferozepore	385.75	365.69	814	1,020
Mean Meer	364.85	317.66	751	872
Multan	426.53	339.89	701	915
Dalhousie	100.70	248.27	854	866
Sialkot	255.81	212.80	1,118	1,156
Rawalpindi	448.17	212.67	2,325	2,605
Attock	244.35	330.36	106.40	112
Murree	148.55	232.26	276	310
Peshawar	390.60	237.09	1,659	1,607
Naushahra	305.03	91.62	577	698.50

Source: *Report on the Lock Hospitals in the Punjab for the Year 1887* (Lahore: Punjab Government Press, 1888), 1.

hospitals than the civil department. The proposal did not get a nod from the GoI at the end; instead, it preferred to build up cooperation between the civil and military departments in this regard. Table 2.1 shows the ratio of admission of VD cases in the aforementioned lock hospitals in Punjab province along with the average strength of the European troops in 1886–1887.[27]

The VD cases in the European troops of the North-Western Provinces (NWP) and Oudh were fairly high in the 1870s. There had been eighteen lock hospitals at Cawnpore, Agra, Bareilly, Allahabad, Meerut, Banaras, Moradabad, Ranikhet, Roorkee, Shahjahanpur, Chakrata, Naini Tal, Jhansi, Lucknow, Muttra, Fyzabad, Fatehgarh and Sitapur, providing mixed reports of success and failure. From 1874 to 1878, the mean ratio of VD cases per 1,000 was 273.1. The NWP and Oudh Government, although, seemed to be much satisfied with the way in which the local authorities intended to keep the European troops away from the native consorts. C. Robertson, the Secretary to NWP and Oudh Government, wrote a letter to the Secretary of Home Department to the GoI on 5 August 1878, while ensuring that VD was comparatively less contracted by the troops from registered prostitutes. This happened only because of the prohibition of illicit prostitution within or outside the protected areas. For example, the importance of regimental procedures of surveillance and detection was seen in most of the hospitals. At Cawnpore, where the troops stayed outside the town, the result was favourable.

Along with this, the coolie and low-caste women were staved off the cantonments.[28] Later in 1884, J. R. Reid, the Secretary to the NWP and Oudh, put forth similar view concerning the reduction of VD in the European garrison. The figure, that is, mean ratio of VD, had lessened from 273.1 in 1878 to 269.9 in 1883. Improvement was mostly observed at Banaras, Chakrata, Ranikhet and Lucknow, whereas Agra and Fyzabad could not furnish favourable result as the troops had intercourse frequently with the unregistered women while they were moving (see table 2.2).[29] To Reid, 'the various local reports explain . . . the different causes of success or failure. But, in the main, success will be found to depend on the efficiency of regimental control over the men and on the measures adopted to secure and retain a proper supply of protected women'.[30] The number of VD cases and disease prevalence among the European soldiers in 1883 are evident in table 2.2.

The departmental and lock hospital reports might have reflected the exclusive frights of the colonial officers about 'moral mayhem', caused by specific native consorts and unregistered prostitutes. This fragment of population was literally blamed for spreading Sexually Transmitted Diseases, especially syphilis, even though the problem was to constrain the 'adulterated desire' of the British vis-à-vis European common soldiers that made their 'race' impure. Karen Jochelson has articulated that individuals or groups, situating at the margins of the social hierarchy and supposedly threatening so-called societal norms, had

Table 2.2 Statement Showing the Prevalence of VD amongst the Soldiers of the European Garrisons during 1883

Lock Hospitals	Daily Average Strength of European Garrison for the Year 1883	Admission to Hospitals for VD in 1883			Ratio of Admissions to 1,000 of Strength in 1883	Mean Ratio of Preceding Five Years	Mean Ratio of Five Years Previous to the Opening of Lock Hospitals
		Gonorrhea and Allied Forms of Diseases	Syphilis	Total			
Allahabad	846	64	45	110	130.4	241.6	307.0
Cawnpore	770	73	21	94	122.1	235.9	324.0
Agra	1,134	214	156	370	325.4	322.4	212.0
Meerut	1,517	273	213	486	320.3	221.8	324.0
Lucknow	2,104	259	135	394	187.2	252.6	272.0
Bareilly	706	88	83	171	242.2	259.6	228.0
Fyzabad	712	106	142	248	348.3	164.8	287.0
Banaras	374	30	38	68	181.3	384.4	373.0
Moradabad	179	29	27	56	312.8	404.8	300.0
Shahjahanpur	206	46	39	85	412.6	286.2	364.0
Ranikhet	732	75	65	140	191.2	338.8	—
Sitapur	462	80	17	97	209.9	272.2	342.0
Roorkee	237	24	20	44	185.6	211.2	210.0
Naini Tal	254	46	30	76	299.2	280.6	244.0
Jhansi	307	27	06	33	107.5	142.8	310.0
Muttra	341	41	36	77	225.8	282.0	216.0
Chakrata	455	47	52	99	217.5	217.0	142.0
Fatehgarh	135	28	28	56	414.8	320.0	—
Total	**11,471**	**1,550**	**1,154**	**2,704**	**235.7**	**269.9**	**278.2**
Total of 1882	**13,291**	**1,738**	**1,768**	**3,506**	**263.7**	**254.7**	**278.2**

Source: Tenth Annual Report on the Working of the Lock Hospitals in the North-Western Provinces and Oudh for the Year 1883 (Allahabad: Government Press, 1884), 32.

been designated as the 'essence of disease and social corruption'. In the late nineteenth- and early twentieth-century England, VD had materialized, rather idealized, the eugenic and political fear regarding the putrefaction of morality and corrosion of family, empire and race.[31] The rise of VD cases in the European troops, even after the enactment of CD Acts, posed a fundamental question over the approach of the colonial authorities towards health of lower ranked soldiers. The British Indian Army was not a homogenous group; rather, it comprised of several officers, recruited from the upper classes or ranks and drawn from the lower echelons of the working classes. Most of the British or European common soldiers were affected by VD which, in turn, made the military profession unpopular among the civilians of Victorian England. The soldiers were differentiated as a 'stigmatized group' from the healthy civil population.[32] From Foucauldian point of view, the Cantonment Acts embodied the 'disciplining of public space' through supervision while enclosing the 'public consorts' from 'normal Indian women'.[33] The movement for repealing the CD Acts, bolstered by Josephine Butler and Florence Nightingale, got momentum in 1880s that forced the GoI to defunct the CD Acts completely. Nevertheless, the surveillance over the 'bodies' continued to function in the name of new Cantonment Acts. Besides, quarantine and isolation policies were often seen as interfering strategies of private spaces during the plague epidemic and hence, did not win popular favour in colonial India and Zanzibar (Bala and Issa, respectively, in this volume).

LIBERALISM, EMPIRE AND HEALTH: THE CONTENTIONS ON THE EFFECT OF VD ON THE EUROPEAN TROOPS IN INDIA (C. 1890s–1910s)

The criticism of the liberal groups over the CD Acts in the British Empire was gradually dominating the political debates in England. The liberals were demanding explanation to the colonial administration about the prevalence of VD in the British Indian Army. On 14 November 1871, the Ladies National Association (LNA) had published the *Report for the Repeal of the Contagious Diseases Acts* in which the members clearly condemned the functioning of CD Acts and addressed the personal rights of women. The organization was also incredulous to the investigation of Royal Commission in December, 1870 while saying:

> We hold that it is a dangerous precedent to allow any Government . . . to assume that the good name and personal rights of women are subordinate to the necessity of protecting soldiers from the physical disease which is the consequence of licentious indulgence. The issuing of a Royal Commission proceeds on this fatal assumption, and we therefore urge our friends everywhere, emphatically to protest against it, as they would against the shameful Acts themselves.[34]

After the submission of the Royal Commission's report in July 1871, the LNA had accused the first Gladstone Ministry (which is known for its various economic and political reforms) for retaining these 'cruel', 'unjust' and 'immoral' laws.[35] Despite a split within the repeal movement, Josephine Butler and her LNA had succeeded to garner popular support against the CD Acts to a large extent. Paul McHugh has viewed the movement of LNA as one of the decisive junctures in the history of feminism. From 1870 to 1890, there was a considerable shift from militant form of protest to 'social purity wave' in the repeal movement which raised the fundamental issue of 'morality'. This premeditated changing stance had influenced the opinions in the British Parliament during 1890s.[36] What is more intriguing is the advancement and progression in medical knowledge related to VD in this time. The English venereology had witnessed significant transformation between the repeal of the CD Acts in 1886 and the inference of the Royal Commission on VD (RCVD) in 1916. Although the government intervention was minimal, the venereological knowledge of doctors, midwives and nurses came to be materialized through the adoption of new diagnostics, the growing emphasis on the centrality of laboratory-based medicine and therapeutic expertise. Therefore, the English medical academia had already found the answers of quite a lot of inquiries related to pathology of gonorrhea and syphilis. Both these diseases were acknowledged as the serious intimidations to health, fertility and national efficiency.[37] On 4 July 1890, the Military Department of GoI issued a notification in continuation with the earlier notice, which was published on 20 December 1889. In this new order, the Governor-General in Council had decided to include some rules under section 26 (clause 21) and section 27 (subsections 2 and 4), mostly connected to treatments of soldiers, in the Cantonment Act, 1889. The hospitals, within or outside the limits of the cantonment, should be maintained partly or wholly at the expense of the cantonment fund to provide treatments to the infected cases. A medical officer had been assigned to every hospital. If an infected person had refused to go to the hospital or left the hospital before being pronounced as cured by the medical officer, the Cantonment Magistrate might not only remove that person from the cantonment within 24 hours, he could punish him by fining maximum Rs. 50 or imprisoning him as long as eight days for re-entering or residing in the cantonment without written permission.[38] Later, the Raj sought to incorporate all CD altogether. The particular stress was laid on the facts that the VD was not to be treated by regimental authorities in any way differently from other CD, and prostitutes were not permitted to dwell in regimental bazaars or to accompany the army contingents on the march. These directives, issued on 11 July 1892 by Colonel W. L. Dalrymple, the Quarter-Master-General to India, were for the regimental and station authorities whose observance had been earnestly requested by the commander-in-chief.[39] In this regard, Major General E. H. H. Collen, Secretary to the GoI, Military Department, had extended his willingness to implement these rules in a letter to the Secretary to the Government of Madras and Bombay, Military Department. For Collen, this concept of founding new cantonment general hospitals to remove the exclusivity of VD was desirable as it rendered service also to others, suffering from infectious diseases like smallpox; nevertheless, this did not refrain him from making a difference between VD and other CD as far as the treatment was concerned. He had proposed a separate building for the VD cases. The new regulation aimed at widening the civil dispensary system to military cantonment than establishing new military hospitals having inflexible discipline for which, as Collen said – 'it being understood that the popularity and consequent stability of the system will depend to a very great extent on the successful personal effects of those officers to win the confidence and respect of the native population'.[40]

The GoI was under pressure due to the political stand of liberal government in home.

Thus, once again, on 18 July 1893, a confidential memorandum was released by E. Stedman, the Quarter-Master-General for India, where the GoI had expressed its reservation on the growing misapprehension and misinterpretation of the cantonment regulations related to infectious diseases. It was stated that disregard of the rules and regulations, appeared in the earlier circulars of 11 July 1892 and 8 July 1893, would be observed 'apart from discipline' and 'short-sighted and harmful', putting the entire system of prevention of the disease among the troops in jeopardy. The deviations, such as paying *mahaldarnis* from public funds, ensuring compulsory examination of women, providing residence to prostitutes in regimental bazaars, blackmailing the prostitutes by subordinate medical staff and taking penalties for non-attendance at examinations, were strictly prohibited.[41] H. Daly, the Assistant Secretary to the GoI, on 2 August 1893, desired to know whether any or all circulars and orders, issued frequently by the Military Department of GoI, had been in force in the cantonments of Hyderabad, Central India, Rajputana, Baluchistan, Ajmer-Merwara and Baroda. Except Baroda, which was under the jurisdiction of Bombay Presidency, the reports of other cantonments seemed to be satisfactory for the GoI as most of them were abide by the given directives (no such orders were in force in the cantonments of Erinpura and Kherwara or in the Sanitarium at Mount Abu, Rajputana).[42] There was no periodical examination in Oudh, Bundelkhand and Bengal in 1893, although some of the cantonments, that is, Cawnpore and Meerut, voluntarily organized such inspection. Thus, E. Stedman had notified that these voluntary examinations too must be brought to an end without delay.[43] Did the new cantonment regulation at all significantly reduce the VD cases in the

European troops in the British Raj? After a sudden plummet in 1891, the VD cases mounted steadily till 1895 (see table 2.3).

H. R. Whitehead, the Army Medical Staff and Surgeon-Major of Royal Victoria Hospital, Netley,[44] had submitted a medical report on the cases of syphilis from India on 21 August 1896. For him, the disease appeared more virulent than before and it was the sole reason for continual increase of invalid in-service soldiers from India and the other colonies. From 1 October 1891 to 30 September 1894, almost 1,151 men had been invalided of which 242 were syphilis cases or 20% of the total number of invalidation were due to syphilis. The cases reduced in 1895, but the percentage of syphilis amplified nearly 40%. Whitehead was of opinion that the health and efficiency of the soldier were mostly destroyed by this malignant form of VD and it might occur again if they joined the service after the recovery.[45] He said:

> No one can imagine a sadder sight than the reception here of a batch of poor fellows suffering from this disease, from one of the troopships, utterly broken down in health, hardly able to crawl, covered with scabs and sores, with the foul odour of the disease about them, objects of disgust and loathing to themselves and all around them, their condition is indeed pitiable and shocking.[46]

Table 2.3 is comprehensively presenting the admission rate of VD among the British troops in India from 1860 to 1895 accompanied with some acts and observations.

In 1896–1897, the Principal Medical Officer of Netley registered 363 cases out of which 196 or almost 74% had a history of syphilis from India and 100 were declared unfit for service.[47] On 20 March 1899, Major Rasch, one of the members of British Parliament, asked the Secretary of State for India, George Francis Hamilton, whether the increasing virulence of secondary syphilis in the British Army in India had revealed that the patients did not go through early treatment, and they were only removed from the cantonments to spread the disease elsewhere. In his reply, Hamilton was quite sceptic about the Rasch's conclusion. He countered that as there was a considerable reduction in the admission rate due to the treatment of European soldiers in the barracks, it would be wrong to arrive at any definite inference in this regard.

Further, on 23 October 1899, Hamilton had set forth the statistics of admission rate for VD among British troops in India. In 1898, there had been 363 VD cases out of 1,000 against 486 cases in 1897 and 522 in 1895. To Hamilton, this was a significant fall since 1887. On the other hand, the total number of VD admissions in 1898 was 24,286 in comparison with 32,768 in 1897 and 36,058 in 1896.[48] Some cantonments in India had confirmed a trivial growth of VD cases in the British troops during 1899, such as Dum Dum, Barrackpore, Meerut and Delhi of Bengal Command; Mean Meer, Sialkot and Attock of Punjab

Table 2.3 Venereal Disease among British Troops in India, 1860–1895

Year	Admission Rate per 1,000 Strength					
	Primary Syphilis and Simple Venereal Ulcer Combined	Secondary Syphilis	Gonorrhea and Other Venereal Diseases	Total	Increase or Decrease Compared with Previous Year	Remarks
			Bengal			
1860	118.7	25.8	174.3	318.8	+33.4	1860. weekly inspection of men for venereal diseases discontinued
1861	140.4	28.7	183.1	352.2	–45.3	
1862	116.4	26.9	163.6	306.9	–26.5	
1863	98.1	30.2	152.1	280.4	–24.9	1864. Bengal Act XXII, authorized Lock Hospital system
1864	87.4	33.1	135	255.5	–40.6	
1865	64.8	28.7	121.4	214.9	–8.5	
1866	64.6	25.5	116.3	206.4	–46.2	1865. lock hospitals began to be opened
1867	51.4	23.7	85.1	160.2	+33.8	
1868	56.2	25.4	112.4	194	+13.1	1870. Army Enlistment Act introducing short service system
1869	69.8	23	114.3	207.1	–12.3	
1870	40.7	25	129.1	194.8	+27.6	
1871	73.3	24.2	124.9	222.4	–25.2	
1872	62.3	22.8	112.1	197.2		
			All India			
1872	61.4	22.4	107.2	191		1873. Proportion of unmarried soldiers began to increase.
1873	53.4	20.4	107.9	181.7	–9.3	
1874	67.5	25.2	104.8	207.5	+25.8	
1875	67.1	25.1	121.3	213.5	+6	1877. Annual arrivals of new troops began to increase
1876	59.8	23.9	119.8	203.5	–10	
1877	65.2	22.1	137.1	224.4	+20.9	
1878	95.4	22.1	174.1	291.6	+67.2	1879–80. large numbers of troops were on active service in Afghanistan
1879	81.6	24.1	147.6	253.3	–38.3	
1880	87.4	23	138.6	249	–4.3	

1881			92	23.1	144.5	259.6	+10.6	1882. Married
1882			87.6	23.2	154.7	265.5	+5.9	establishment, India,
1883			87.2	23.5	160.6	271.3	+5.8	reduced.
1884			90.2	24.4	178.9	293.5	+22.2	1885. Fifteen lock
1885			122.1	28.7	191.8	342.6	+49.1	hospitals experimentally
1886			157.9	33.3	194.6	385.7	+43.1	closed, 1st January 1885.
	Primary Syphilis	*Simple Venereal Ulcer*	*Total*					
1887	75.5	66.6	142.1	29.4	189.9	361.3	–24.4	1887. Closed lock
1888	72.1	70	142.1	32.4	197.7	372.2	+10.9	hospitals reopened early
1889	134.3	90.9	225.2	51.2	205.1	481.5	+109.3	in the year.
1890	135.6	85.1	220.7	66.3	216.6	503.6	+22.1	1888. Lock hospital
1891	104	55.2	159.2	60	181.5	400.7	–102.9	system abolished in
1892	102.6	58.5	161.1	57.8	191	409.9	+9.2	latter half of the year.
1893	129.3	84.3	213.6	61.6	190.8	466	+56.1	
1894	173	75.1	248.1	74.6	188.7	511.4	+45.4	
1895	174.1	64.9	239	84.9	198.4	522.3*	+10.9	
	178.6	66.8	245.4	86.8	204.6	536.8**		

(*) including troops on field service, (**) excluding troops on field service

Source: *East India (Contagious Disease), no. 1, Report of a Departmental Committee on the Prevalence of Venereal Disease Among the British Troops in India* (London, 1897), 15.

Command; Colaba, Mount Abu, Quetta and Khandalla of Bombay Command; Port Blair, Mandalay, Mallapuram and Wellington of Madras Command.[49] Still, the memorandum, by the Army Sanitary Commission on the report of the Sanitary Commissioner to the GoI, had illustrated a general diminution in VD figures in 1899. The recorded admission rate was 313.4 per 1,000 in 1899 in contrast to 362.9 per 1,000 in 1898. For the British authority, this gradual reduction of VD cases had only been achieved due to the efficacy of cantonment hospitals, regular examinations and thorough inspections of soldiers.[50] However, not everyone was convinced by the continual decrease of VD. A. G. Wyman, colonel of Late Dorset Regiment, reacted on Hamilton's claim that the figures were prepared on the basis of active service, that is, the regiments in frontier campaigns who were less exposed to VD than the troops in cantonments.[51]

This attenuation continued in 1900 when the admission rate of European soldiers was 298.1 against 313.4 in 1899. Bombay Command had witnessed large increase of VD, whereas Bengal and Madras Commands shared less than that of Bombay.[52] The situation reversed in 1902 while the total admission rate of VD cases increased 281.4 per 1,000 as compared with 276.0 in 1901. It happened largely because of new arrival of regiments from field service in South Africa – some regiments carried the diseases with them. Secondly, the soldiers contracted VD while marching through the stations to Delhi and to the hills. There were some stations having sizeable amount of cases, such as Cannanore, Fort Fulta, Muttra, Taragarh, Calcutta and Fyzabad. This time the Bengal Command had the highest rate of admission for gonorrhea, and Madras Command for primary syphilis.[53] The increase of VD cases in Burma division had drawn attention of the Raj in 1904, that is, 344.5 per 1,000. In general, there were 200.3 cases per 1,000 in the British troops in India in 1904 much lower than 1903, but it was rather surprising that, despite the development in the VD diagnosis in the early twentieth century, yet substantial number of VD patients was found in the British or European troops in India.[54] Often, sanitation classes for soldiers, especially for Non-Commissioned Officers and men in sanitary duties, were arranged by the Royal Army Medical Corps (RAMC) and Divisional Sanitary Officer in which the instructions on the effects of VD on military efficiency and its prevention had been incorporated.[55] The improvement of army health did not underscore the 'moral' upgrading of the British soldiers in India. Since 1907, the Wesleyan Methodist Church was concerned about the 'moral' degeneration of the British soldiers. Reverend Joseph Reed, General Superintendent of Wesleyan Church, Bombay, Punjab and Lucknow Districts, had submitted a memorandum to the Social Purity Committee of the Wesleyan Methodist Church on 23 September 1910 in which he criticized the Indian Army authorities, becoming hostile to his works on moral interests.

Particularly while the Army had been trying to provide sanitary conditions for preventing the VD, there was neither any consultation with the

Ecclesiastical Department nor Reed and his associates were allowed in the places as chaplains. It was concluded, by Reed, that the army authorities in India preferred the 'immoral' measures for the disease prevention more than the moral influence.[56] He even continued to add: 'The army authorities seem to utterly ignore the moral aspect of the sexual problem and only direct their attention to the physical questions involved'.[57]

Nonetheless, Reed repeatedly called attentions to the War Office concerning the irregularities in the Indian cantonments. To the missionaries, the sanitary sexual intercourse or personal prophylaxes to prevent the VD, which often appeared in the lectures given by the RAMC in the European barracks, were detrimental to the 'moral' health of the European soldiers.[58] This grievance was accorded and forwarded by H. Bisseker, the Secretary of the Social Purity Committee to India Office. John Morley, the Secretary of State for India, took this accusation very seriously. On 28 October 1910, he wrote to the Earl of Minto, Governor General of India in Council, to investigate whether such alleged irregularities were in reality made by the military authorities in India.[59] On 2 March 1911, Lord Hardinge, G. Fleetwood Wilson, J. L. Jenkins, R. W. Carlyle, H. Butler, Syed Ali Imam and W. H. Clark had sent a letter to Earl of Crewe, the Secretary of State for India by denying each indictment of Reed.

Voluntarily women were treated as outpatient in the cantonment general hospitals, but no special privileges were extended to European prostitutes who had been under same restrictions like the native women. Hardinge and his fellows had assumed that a reduction of admission rate from 371.4 per 1,000 in 1898 to 67.8 per 1,000 in 1909 indicated a general improvement of 'morality' among the British troops in India. However, they seemed to be aware of the sexual impurity existing among the unmarried men, both soldiers and civilians; the commander-in-chief and his predecessors had always attempted to boost the moral tone of the Indian Army.[60] Harrison has shown that during the First World War the British Army sought to control VD in a peculiar way which was a blend of 'moralism' and 'pragmatism'. As the senior British officers and a few medical men were disinclined to accept the preventive measures that ignored the sense of 'immorality', the medical management against VD was invoked in the British Army at a snail's pace in contrast to the other armies of allies or enemies.[61] The treatment of VD was not uninhibited from penal stigma; moreover, during the war, the authority had imposed penalties over the British and Indian soldiers irrespectively to discourage the illicit sex.[62] In 1917, there were 4,201 VD admissions with three deaths in European troops in India. The ratio of admission varied from 1913 to 1917, reflecting in table 2.4. In this table, ten stations, that is, Peshawar, Rawalpindi, Lahore, Quetta, Mhow, Poona, Meerut, Lucknow, Secunderabad and Burma, were put under consideration.

Table 2.4 Ratio per 1,000 of Strength for All VD by Divisions for the Years 1913–1917

Divisions	*1913*	*1914*	*1915*	*1916*	*1917*
Peshawar	30.1	21.4	30.8	24.5	17.8
Rawalpindi	30.4	37.9	32.3	35.7	26.7
Lahore	47.7	43.3	10.1	16.9	27.4
Quetta	37.2	43.1	33.0	35.0	36.4
Mhow	48.7	58.6	33.1	47.1	44.2
Poona	65.6	74.7	32.9	58.7	85.2
Meerut	43.4	51.3	36.7	32.6	44.7
Lucknow	73.5	65.7	22.3	56.8	71.4
Secunderabad	62.7	59.1	34.9	26.1	81.1
Burma	105.1	103.7	44.5	57.7	58.0

Source: Annual Report of the Sanitary Commissioner with the Government of India for 1917 (Calcutta, 1919), 15

Apart from that, a few larger stations had shown the highest admissions rates of VD, for example, Calcutta, Colaba, Poona, Meerut and Kirkee. The officials even believed that most of the cases had been contracted outside the station. To counter the habitual vices of the European soldiers, numerous lectures were organized, and sports as well as pastimes had been provided. With recurring inspection of new arrivals and surprise scrutiny, the cases were detected at the earliest for the treatment.[63]

CONCLUSION

How far the moral fabric of the health propaganda was effective to stall the prevalence of VD among the British or European soldiers in India is a contentious ground to be probed, but the approach of the colonial state in relation to VD was subject to contradiction. Probably, preserving the 'racial potency' of the whites while satisfying the sensual needs of the British soldiers at the same moment was not the only arduous duty of the Raj; it put the empire in perpetual conundrum. As VD had a little impact over the native soldiers, the British Indian Army was entirely fretted about the moral degeneration of the white race. Both the liberal and pro-CD Act factions had taken the 'moral obligation' of the army into account in the name of either individual freedom or constraint. Philippa Levine has pointed out that prostitution vis-à-vis promiscuity was placed under the colonial retribution. The colonized, precisely the native women, had been alleged as 'immoral' that could threaten the British imperialism. On the other hand, the CD Acts of 1860s–1880s and the movement of the liberals for the repealment of the CD Acts shaped the perceptions of military medicine. To Levine, colonial medicine ultimately helped the empire to extend and reconcile its power.[64] But, the Raj had to readjust its standpoint on the disease prevention besides the changing contour of 'home' politics. Thus, the dynamism of colonialism acted in a complex relation of opposition.[65] It is true that at the onset of the twentieth century, the incidence of VD cases among the British troops declined, albeit in a punctuated speed, with the development of military medicine, newer diagnoses and treatments.

The native women were perceived as probable source of harbouring VD even after the revocation of CD Acts in the 1880s. Under the modified cantonment acts in India, the examination of the infected bodies continued. David Arnold has rightly argued that the disciplinary and medical requirements of the army facilitated inclusive medical power of the Raj to chastise Indian women at the time when there were few medical facilities accessible for general populace.[66] Besides, ideas of quarantine and discipline reigned supreme in the wake of the pandemics (Bala in this volume). The 'bodily' regulations were manifested through the 'western metaphors of disease and health' in British India.[67] Uncouthness associated with the VD was frequently 'politicized', rather, 'criminalized' in the course of moral reform.

NOTES

1. See House of Lords Debate, HL Deb 14 May 1897, vol. 49 cc 467-91: DOI: BRITISH TROOPS IN INDIA (HEALTH). (Hansard, 14 May 1897) (parliament.uk).
2. See *Report of the Committee appointed by the Secretary of State for India to Inquire into the Rules, Regulations, and Practice in the Indian Cantonments and Elsewhere in India with regard to Prostitution and to the Treatment of Venereal Disease* (London: Eyre and Spottiswoode,1893), v.
3. Ibid., v–xxv.
4. Ibid., xxv.
5. See *Report of A Departmental Committee on the Prevalence of Venereal Disease Among the British Troops in India* (London: Eyre and Spottiswoode, 1897), 21; Military Despatch from the Government of India to the Secretary of State for India, No. 184, dated Simla, 4 November 1896.
6. Ibid., 5–14.
7. Philippa Levine, "Rereading the 1890s: Venereal Disease as 'Constitutional Crisis' in Britain and British India," *The Journal of Asian Studies* 55, no. 3 (August 1996): 585–612.
8. Mary Spongberg, *Feminizing Venereal Disease: The Body of the Prostitute in Nineteenth-Century Medical Discourse* (New York: New York University Press, 1997), 1–14.
9. Mark Harrison, "the British Army and the Problem of Venereal Disease in France and Egypt during the First World War," *Medical History* 39, no. 2 (1995): 135.
10. Philip D. Curtin, *Death by Migration: Europe's Encounter with the Tropical World in the Nineteenth Century* (New York: Cambridge University Press, 1989), xvii.

11. Mark Harrison, *Public health in British India: Anglo-Indian Preventive Medicine 1859–1914* (New York: Cambridge University Press, 1994), 228.

12. Erica Wald, *Vice in the Barracks: Medicine, the Military and the Making of Colonial India, 1780–1868* (Basingstoke: Palgrave Macmillan, 2014), 1–5.

13. See *Report of the Commissioners Appointed to Inquire into the Sanitary State of the Army in India* (London: Eyre and Spottiswoode, 1863), 10.

14. Ibid., 38–39.

15. Ibid., 126–28.

16. J. Brendon Curgenven, *The Contagious Diseases Act of 1866 and its Extension to the Civil Population of the United Kingdom* (London: Victoria Press 1868), 3; this paper was read at a Meeting of the Health Department of the "National Association for the Promotion of Social Science", March 30, 1868.

17. Andrew Lyon, *the Law of India, vol. 2* (Bombay: Thacker, Vining & Co., 1873), 194–99.

18. James L. Bryden and Arthur Stephen, *Vital Statistics of the Bengal Presidency: Sickness and Mortality in the European Army of the Bengal Presidency from 1870 to 1879* (Simla: Government Central Branch Press, 1882), 15–16.

19. IOR/P/525, Dec 1874, Pros. Nos. 18-19, Notes on the Working of the Rules for the Prevention of Venereal Disease among European Troops in the Bengal Presidency in 1873.

20. See *Annual Report on the Lock Hospitals of the Madras Presidency for the year 1877* (Madras: Madras Government Press, 1878), 1–11.

21. Ibid., 11.

22. See *Annual Report on the Lock Hospitals of the Madras Presidency for the year 1878* (Madras: Madras Government Press, 1879), 5–6.

23. See *Annual Report on the Military Lock Hospitals of the Madras Presidency for the year 1880* (Madras: Madras Government Press, 1881), 3–4.

24. See *Annual Report on the Military Lock Hospitals of the Madras Presidency for the year 1882* (Madras: Madras Government Press, 1883), 4–7.

25. See *Annual Report on the Military Lock Hospitals of the Madras Presidency for the year 1888* (Madras: Madras Government Press, 1889), 6–7.

26. See *Report on the Lock Hospitals in the Punjab for the year 1887* (Lahore: Punjab Government Press, 1888), 1–2.

27. Ibid., proceedings of the Hon'ble the Lieutenant-Governor of the Punjab in the Home (Medical and Sanitary) Department, no. 340, dated 21st July 1888.

28. See *Fourth Annual Report on the Working of the Lock-Hospitals in the North-Western Provinces and Oudh for the year 1877* (Allahabad: North-Western Provinces and Oudh Government Press, 1878), 112.

29. See *Tenth Annual Report of the Working of the Lock Hospitals in the North-Western Provinces and Oudh for the year 1883* (Allahabad: North-Western Provinces and Oudh Government Press, 1884), 32.

30. Ibid., 32.

31. Karen Jochelson, *The Colour of Disease: Syphilis and Racism in South Africa, 1880–1950* (New York: Palgrave, 2001), 4.

32. Lesley A. Hall, "'War always brings it on': War, STDs, the military, and the civilian population in Britain, 1850–1950," in *Medicine and Modern Warfare*, eds. Roger Cooter, Mark Harrison, and Steve Sturdy (Amsterdam: Rodopi B.V, 1999), 205–208.

33. Stephen Legg, "Governing prostitution in colonial Delhi: from cantonment regulations to international hygiene (1864–1939)," *Social History* 34, no. 4 (November 2009): 451–52.

34. See *Report of the Ladies National Association for the Repeal of the Contagious Diseases Acts* (Liverpool: T. Brakell, Printer, 1871), 5–8.

35. Ibid., 10.

36. Paul McHugh, *Prostitution and Victorian Social Reform* (New York: Routledge, 1980), 16–29.

37. Anne R. Hanley, *Medicine, Knowledge and Venereal Diseases in England, 1886–1916* (New York: Palgrave Macmillan, 2017), 3–4.

38. National Archives of India (NAI), Government of India (GOI), Pros. Nos. 36-88, Foreign Department, Secret-I Branch, October, 1894, Working and treatment of venereal and other contagious diseases in Cantonment Hospital.

39. Ibid., Confidential no. 20, Office of Quarter-Master-General in India, Army Head-Quarters, Simla, the 11th July, 1892.

40. Ibid., Pros. No. 41, dated Simla, the 8th November 1892.

41. Ibid., Pros. No. 55, Confidential no. 11, Office of Quarter-Master-General in India, Army Head-Quarters, Simla, 18th July 1893.

42. Ibid., Pros. No. 58, Simla, the 2nd August, 1893.

43. Ibid., Pros. No. 83, Confidential no. 24, Office of Quarter-Master-General in India, Army Head-Quarters, Simla, 26th October, 1893.

44. See *East India (Contagious Diseases), no. 1, Report of a Departmental Committee on the Prevalence of Venereal Disease among the British Troops in India* (London: Eyre and Spottiswoode, 1897), 30.

45. Ibid., 31.

46. Ibid., 30.

47. Ibid., 31.

48. NAI, GOI, File. No. Defence A 1900 Mar 309-311, Defence Department, Sanitary A Branch, March, 1900, Simla Records, Prevalence of Venereal Disease in the British army in India. comparison of statistics for the years 1897 and 1898.

49. NAI, GOI, File. No. Defence A 1901 May 366, Defence Department, Sanitary A Branch, May, 1901, Simla Records, Reports regarding increase of Venereal Disease among British troops during the Year 1899.

50. NAI, GOI, File. No. Defence A 1901 Aug 3088-89, Defence Department, Sanitary A Branch, August, 1901, Simla Records, Memorandum by the Army Sanitary Commission on the Report of the Sanitary Commissioner to the GoI for 1899.

51. A. G. Wyman, "the Decrease of Venereal Disease in the Indian Army," *the British Medical Journal (BMJ*), dated 6th January, 1900, 48.

52. NAI, GOI, File. No. Defence A 1902 Jan 2486-2492, Defence Department, Sanitary A Branch, January, 1902, Simla Records, Statistics of Venereal Disease among British and Native Troops in India during 1900.

53. NAI, GOI, File. No. Defence A 1904 Jul 838-840, Defence Department, Sanitary A Branch, July, 1904, Simla Records, Statistics of Venereal Disease among British and Native Troops in India during 1902.

54. NAI, GOI, File. No. Defence A 1905 Dec 697-698, Defence Department, Sanitary A Branch, December, 1905, Simla Records, Statistics of Venereal Disease among British and Native Troops in India during 1904.

55. Major Robert J. Blackham, "Sanitation Classes for Soldiers," *Journal of the Royal Army Medical Corps* 14, no. 1 (January, 1910): 77–83.

56. NAI, GOI, File no. Defence A 1911 Mar 1705-1706, Defence Department, Sanitary A Branch, March, 1911, Calcutta Records, Alleged Irregularities in the Action taken by the Military Authorities in India for the Prevention of Venereal Disease among British Troops.

57. Ibid.

58. Ibid.

59. Ibid.

60. Ibid., Pros. No. 1706, Confidential, No. 44, March, 1911.

61. Harrison, "the British Army and the Problem of Venereal Disease," 156.

62. Kaushik Roy, *Indian Army and the First World War 1914–1918* (New Delhi: Oxford University Press, 2018), 85.

63. See *Annual Report of the Sanitary Commissioner with the Government of India for 1917* (Kolkata: Superintendent Government Printing India, 1919), 15–16.

64. Philippa Levine, *Prostitution, Race, and Politics: Policing Venereal Disease in the British Empire* (New York: Routledge, 2003), 9.

65. Ibid., 13.

66. David Arnold, *The New Cambridge History of India, vol. 3, part 5: Science, Technology and Medicine in Colonial India* (New York: Cambridge University Press, 2000), 90.

67. Judy Whitehead, "Bodies Clean and Unclean: Prostitution, Sanitary Legislation, and Respectable Femininity in Colonial North India," *Gender & History* 7, no. 1 (April 1995): 41.

BIBLIOGRAPHY

Annual Report on the Lock Hospitals of the Madras Presidency for the year 1877. Madras: Madras Government Press, 1878.

Annual Report on the Lock Hospitals of the Madras Presidency for the year 1878. Madras: Madras Government Press, 1879.

Annual Report on the Military Lock Hospitals of the Madras Presidency for the year 1880. Madras: Madras Government Press, 1881.

Annual Report on the Military Lock Hospitals of the Madras Presidency for the year 1882. Madras: Madras Government Press, 1883.

Annual Report on the Military Lock Hospitals of the Madras Presidency for the year 1888. Madras: Madras Government Press, 1889.

Annual Report of the Sanitary Commissioner with the Government of India for 1917. Kolkata: Superintendent Government Printing India, 1919.

Arnold, David. *The New Cambridge History of India, vol. 3, part 5: Science, Technology and Medicine in Colonial India.* New York: Cambridge University Press, 2000.

Blackham, Major Robert J. "Sanitation Classes for Soldiers." *Journal of the Royal Army Medical Corps* 14, no. 1 (January 1910): 77–83.

Bryden, James L., and Arthur Stephen. *Vital Statistics of the Bengal Presidency, Sickness and Mortality in the European Army of the Bengal Presidency from 1870 to 1879*. Simla: Government Central Branch Press, 1882.

Curgenven, J. Brendon. *The Contagious Diseases Act of 1866 and its Extension to the Civil Population of the United Kingdom*. London: Victoria Press 1868.

Curtin, Philip D. *Death by Migration: Europe's Encounter with the Tropical World in the Nineteenth Century*. New York: Cambridge University Press, 1989.

East India (Contagious Disease), no. 1, Report of a Departmental Committee on the Prevalence of Venereal Disease among the British Troops in India. London: Eyre and Spottiswoode, 1897.

Fourth Annual Report on the Working of the Lock-Hospitals in the North-Western Provinces and Oudh for the year 1877. Allahabad: North-Western Provinces and Oudh Government Press,1878.

Hall, Lesley A. "'War always brings it on': War, STDs, the Military, and the Civilian Population in Britain, 1850-1950." In *Medicine and Modern Warfare*, eds. Roger Cooter, Mark Harrison, and Steve Sturdy, 205–208. Amsterdam: Rodopi B.V, 1999.

Hanley, Anne R. *Medicine, Knowledge and Venereal Diseases in England, 1886-1916*. New York: Palgrave Macmillan, 2017.

Harrison, Mark. *Public Health in British India: Anglo-Indian Preventive Medicine 1859-1914*. New York: Cambridge University Press, 1994.

Harrison, Mark. "The British Army and the Problem of Venereal Disease in France and Egypt during the First World War." *Medical History* 39, no. 2 (1995): 135.

Jochelson, Karen. *The Colour of Disease: Syphilis and Racism in South Africa, 1880-1950*. New York: Palgrave, 2001.

Legg, Stephen. "Governing Prostitution in Colonial Delhi: from Cantonment Regulations to International hygiene (1864-1939)." *Social History* 34, no. 4 (November 2009): 451–52.

Levine, Philippa. "Rereading the 1890s: Venereal Disease as 'Constitutional Crisis' in Britain and British India." *The Journal of Asian Studies* 55, no. 3 (August 1996): 585–612.

Levine, Philippa. *Prostitution, Race, and Politics: Policing Venereal Disease in the British Empire*. New York: Routledge, 2003.

Lyon, Andrew. *The Law of India, vol. 2*. Bombay: Thacker, Vining & Co., 1873.

McHugh, Paul. *Prostitution and Victorian Social Reform*. New York: Routledge, 1980.

Oldenburg, Veena Talwar. *The Making of Colonial Lucknow, 1856-1877*. Princeton: Princeton University Press, 1984.

Report of a Departmental Committee on the Prevalence of Venereal Disease Among the British Troops in India. London: Eyre and Spottiswoode, 1897. *Report of the Commissioners Appointed to Inquire into the Sanitary State of the Army in India*. London: Eyre and Spottiswoode, 1863.

Report of the Committee appointed by the Secretary of State for India to Inquire into the Rules, Regulations, and Practice in the Indian Cantonments and Elsewhere in India with regard to Prostitution and to the Treatment of Venereal Disease. London: Eyre and Spottiswoode, 1893.

Report of the Ladies National Association for the Repeal of the Contagious Diseases Acts. Liverpool: T. Brakell, Printer, 1871.

Report on the Lock Hospitals in the Punjab for the year 1887. Lahore: Punjab Government Press, 1888.

Roy, Kaushik. *Indian Army and the First World War 1914-1918*. New Delhi: Oxford University Press, 2018.

Spongberg, Mary. *Feminizing Venereal Disease: the Body of the Prostitute in Nineteenth-Century Medical Discourse*. New York: New York University Press, 1997.

Tenth Annual Report on the Working of the Lock Hospitals in the North-Western Provinces and Oudh for the year 1883. Allahabad: North-Western Provinces and Oudh Government Press, 1884.

Wald, Erica. *Vice in the Barracks: Medicine, the Military and the Making of Colonial India, 1780-1868*. Basingstoke: Palgrave Macmillan, 2014.

Whitehead, Judy. "Bodies Clean and Unclean: Prostitution, Sanitary Legislation, and Respectable Femininity in Colonial North India." *Gender & History* 7, no. 1 (April 1995): 41.

Wyman, A. G. "The Decrease of Venereal Disease in the Indian Army." *The British Medical Journal (BMJ)*. Dated 6 January 1900, 48.

Chapter 3

Bubonic Plague and State Control in Zanzibar (ca. 1897–1905)

Amina Ameir Issa

By September 1896, bubonic plague had occurred in Bombay, the major port city in India. The plague entered India from either China or the Gulf areas, where the disease had devastated the regions since the eighteenth century. From Bombay, the plague then spread to Pune, Karachi and Calcutta.[1] Between 1896 and 1914, the bubonic plague had killed more than 8 million Indians.[2] By the end of 1897, the plague was transmitted to other Indian Ocean port cities of Africa to Mauritius and it reached Madagascar in 1898. In the same year, the bubonic plague reached Mombasa port in Kenya. Through the same Indian Ocean trade routes, the plague had reached Natal, South Africa, in 1902 carried by Indian indentured labourers. The bubonic plague was conveyed through merchandise from India to Zanzibar and it arrived in 1905. Generally, the plague was mainly extended through commercial expansion and movement of goods and people. The first case of bubonic plague in East Africa occurred in 1897 with the arrival of Indian indentured labourers to Mombasa port for the construction of the Uganda Railway. In 1890, Sir William Mackinnon, Chairman of Imperial British East African Company (IBEA Co.), wrote a letter to Lord Salisbury, Secretary of the Foreign Department in London, requesting a subsidy to construct the Uganda Railway which completed in 1902 costing £5.3 million. It became an important instrument for the transportation of raw materials and labourers in the British colonies of Kenya and Uganda and it aimed to fulfil the Brussels Agreement between European powers. The Brussels Act of 1890 had proposed measures to be taken in order to stop slave trade in the interior of Africa and to improve the living conditions of the people in Africa. However, the act became hazardous as about 2,493 out of 32,000 Indian labourers died of cholera and 6,454 became disabled during the construction works.[3] The mass migration of indentured labourers led to the spread of bubonic plague from India to East Africa, whereby Indians and local people of East Africa died of these epidemics.

From the early 1897, with the eruption of bubonic plague in India, the colonial authorities in East Africa took caution on incoming vessels from India. The British and German colonial governments met to discuss the issue of the plague and it was decided to send Medical Officer (MO) to Lamu to inspect all vessels coming from India. On 16 January 1897, Lloyd Mathews, the first minister of Zanzibar between 1891 and 1901, required Captain Agnew, port officer, to check all crafts from India, Arabia and the Persian Gulf. Mathews also instructed police officers at Mkokotoni, Mangapwani and Chuini, the local ports in north part of Zanzibar Island, not to allow any passengers or crew to land in these ports from dhows coming from the northern ports of Mombasa, Lamu, Kismayu and Mogadishu.[4]

Further measures were taken by the state in Zanzibar, which immediately increased its staff in the Sanitary Department, fearing that the plague might spread to Zanzibar. A staff of 120 sweepers under 19 supervisors and 2 inspectors cleaned the town daily. That the number of staff in the department was huge compared with other departments within the administration goes to show how important health and medical matters were considered by the government in a time of perceived emergency.

Lime and other disinfectants were distributed by the government in all quarters of the town. Mr Sorabji Manekji, the head of the Sanitary Department, reported to Lloyd Mathews that twenty-two pushcarts were daily employed in carrying away all dirt and rubbish of the town. Passengers who arrived at the Zanzibar port from Madagascar were isolated at Prison Island, whereby a small building was kept for isolating people during epidemics. The precautions were taken as Madagascar was another subsequent port for the Indian indentured labourers beside Natal and Mombasa. This was reported in the *Zanzibar Gazette* of 16 March 1898 and 4 January 1899, respectively. In 1894, Alexandre Yersin, a Franco-Swiss microbiologist and a student of Pasteur, suggested that rat was the major factor in the transmission of the disease. Aware that in 1897, Paul-Louis Simond, a French biologist, and Waldemar Haffkine, a Calcutta bacteriologist, had proved that the plague-carrying fleas were distributed through rats every precaution was taken to eliminate rats in Zanzibar Town. In 1896, when bubonic plague started to ravage in India, it was not yet established that black rats were the main carriers of the disease. It was thought that 'the human body and the conditions of human habitation and sanitation were . . . primary factors in the spread of the disease'.[5] Simond published a paper in 1898 identifying it 'as a rat disease and postulating that its transmission to man occurred through rat fleas. The case was not experimentally proven to the satisfaction of his fellow bacteriologists and least of all the Indian Plague Commission'.[6]

Despite the control measures taken to stop the spread of the bubonic plague from India and East Africa, the plague reached Mombasa port in December 1898. The British authorities in East Africa reacted to the occurrence of the epidemic by introducing several public health measures to halt the spread of the plague. One of the major efforts was the establishment of the Quarantine Station in Zanzibar in 1899. These measures were given greater urgency by the incident of the SS *Bhundara*, which carried Indian indenture labourers for the construction of the Uganda Railway. At the end of 1898, a telegram from the colonial government in Mombasa was sent to the Colonial Office in London informing them that the steamer SS *Bhundara* from the port of Bombay with 1,000 Indian indentured labourers had arrived at Mombasa with a cargo of 700 tons of rice to be transported to Zanzibar. Moreover, it was reported that six people had died of the plague on board.[7] The colonial authorities in both Mombasa and Zanzibar required the *Bhundara* to return to India. In response, captain of the *Bhundara* requested 120 tons of water necessary for the journey back to India but neither Mombasa nor Zanzibar authorities reacted to that requirement.[8] Within a few days, it was decided to retain the *Bhundara* in East Africa fearing more deaths would occur if the ship returned to India.

Further tension evolved over plague affairs in Mombasa on 30 December 1898, when a telegram from Mr George Mackenzie of Smith Mackenzie & Co., a British trade agency, informed the Foreign Office that the Captain of *Bhundara* feared a mutiny would occur on his steamer if prompt steps could not be taken to satisfy his passengers.[9] The *Bhundara* problem was resolved in the early weeks of January 1899 when a plague camp, to act as a temporary Quarantine Station, was established at Manda – an Island in the Lamu Archipelago off the Northern Kenyan coast. It became the first public health measure to involve the whole British East African colonies since each country introduced its own measures. In 1898, the Plague Regulations for Zanzibar and East Africa, prompted by the *Bhundara* case, were sanctioned by the authorities in London.[10]

The detention of *Bhundara* caused a distress to the individual traders and to the commercial agents in India and in Zanzibar. A case in point was that of the Bengal Chamber of Commerce which addressed a strong protest to the Indian government when *Bhundara* was detained. The chamber condemned the restrictive measures which were taken by the Zanzibar and Kenyan governments against the plague-stricken steamer *Bhundara*. The chamber officials stated that 'every possible precaution was taken at Karachi in connection with the embarkation of "coolies" proceeding to Africa by the SS *Bhundara*'. This was reported in the *Zanzibar Gazette* of 15 March 1899.

At the same time, the British colonial administrators in East Africa feared that the situation might worsen as the plague was also ravaging Tamatave, one of the Madagascan ports.[11] The plague in Madagascar was also linked with the Indian labourers and merchandises which were sent there. The German officials in Tanganyika (Tanzania Mainland) made it clear that 'they would not allow the German mail ship to enter Dar es Salaam, even with the clean Bill of Health because she [the mail ship] had touched Madagascar where plague was introduced by Indians'.[12]

Between January and June, the British Protectorate authorities in Zanzibar and Mombasa organized several meetings to discuss on how Zanzibar and East Africa in general could fight the threatening bubonic plague. In early June 1899, a meeting was held at the Foreign Office at Whitehall, London, attended by Mr Bertie, Sir Thorne Thorne, the former MO of Health in London in the 1860s, who became a health adviser at the Colonial Office, London, in the 1890s. Others present were Sir C. Hill from the British government in London; Sir John Kirk, a former British Consul in Zanzibar in the 1870s; and Sir Arthur Hardinge who in 1894 was appointed as a Consul General to Zanzibar being promoted to Colonial Head, 1895–1900, at the British East Africa Protectorate, overseeing there the construction of the Uganda Railway. Besides, the meeting considered Dr Charlesworth's views, an Edinburgh graduate who was among the senior MOs of the Medical Department of Zanzibar at that time.[13] The meeting decided that a joint Quarantine Station for East Africa had to be established on Prison Island opposite Zanzibar Town.[14] The island had been used before as a prison for those convicted of smuggling slaves after the abolition of the slave trade in 1873 and for the European convalescent. The meeting ascertained that if plague cases occurred in more than one ship, Bawe, another small island near Prison Island, could be used.

It was resolved in that meeting that the cost for maintaining the Quarantine Station had to be divided into four. One-fourth was to be paid for by the East African Protectorate, one-fourth by the Zanzibar Government and one-half was to be paid by the 'Uganda Railway Authority',[15] since it frequently used Mombasa port for the transportation of labourers, who might introduce more epidemics in East Africa. It was agreed that

> Zanzibar Government should be prepared to accept [the] entire responsibility for the control of the joint Quarantine Station on Prison Island. The Zanzibar Government should undertake the whole of the initial outlay, amounting to £2,800 in addition to what had already been expended on the purchase of the Island from the Omanis Sultanate, and the erection of buildings, and should provide for the proper supervision of the station and for maintaining it in an efficient state of repair, whilst on the other hand the East African Protectorate and Uganda Railway administrations should be jointly responsible for the expenditure arising out of salaries, medicines etc. The cost should be divided equally between the East African colonies.[16]

Zanzibar was chosen to station the Quarantine Station for the East African British colonies for various reasons. First, the Zanzibar port was a busy port at that time receiving ships to and from Asia and Europe. It became important to have a station to act as surveillance of any incoming epidemics. Second, it was established at the meeting in London that 'there was [is] no island in the neighborhood of Mombasa which could be utilized as a quarantine station'.[17] Likewise, in other western Indian Ocean area, the quarantine stations were established at the northern and southern ends of the Red Sea during the mid-nineteenth-century cholera epidemics.

These measures were introduced at a time when quarantine measures were still controversial. Resistance against quarantine rules occurred in many countries as they interfered private spaces. Fierce opposition in colonial India was further aggravated by the rising national consciousness against British rule (Bala in this volume). People were required to open their houses and belongings to the public health officers. Moreover, since the mid-nineteenth century, in Britain, social movements had pressurized the government to stop the quarantine practices which were thought to interfere with free trade and imperial commerce. According to Anne Hardy, the opposition to quarantine as well as the development of sanitary reforms led to a shift in practices: public health measures in the ports were to be administered, not by the custom officials, but by MOs.[18] From 1872, Port Sanitary Authorities had been introduced in Britain to prevent the entry of dangerous communicable diseases into the country. Port health officers became responsible for checking for any suspected cases.

In the later 1870s, this port authority system was also adopted in India. As in Britain, in India, it was feared that the quarantine would interfere with trade. The Port Health scheme under a port health officer was first instituted in Calcutta and was extended to other ports in India. Mark Harrison stated that in India:

> Based on the British scheme, established on the recommendation of John Simon, the port health officer was charged with responsibility for the sanitary condition of the port and its environs, and with the medical inspection of ships. Instead of quarantining all persons arriving from infected ports, he was to isolate and detain only those suspected of carrying diseases.[19]

This new practice was adopted in Zanzibar in 1898, in the fear that Indian indentured labourers might introduce plague. In Natal, MOs adopted the 'English Quarantine' system whereby they recorded the details and future whereabouts of passengers disembarking from the vessels for the purposes of monitoring them for signs of illness.[20]

The Quarantine Rule in Zanzibar was proclaimed by Sultan Humoud b. Mohammed (r. 1896–1902) in the *Zanzibar Gazette* of 20 November 1899.

The rule was framed in accordance with the provisions of the Venice Sanitary Convention of 1897 for the Port of Zanzibar.[21] The rule was according to Article 45(1) of the East Africa Order-in-Council, 1897, whereby Her Majesty's Commissioner and Consul General had the power to make regulations relating to public health. This also led to the introduction of the East African Infectious Diseases Regulation. The regulations ordained that

> (n)o person or goods coming from an infected or suspected port shall be permitted to land at any port or place in the East African Protectorate, hereinafter called the Protectorate, except Mombasa, Lamu, or Kismayu, until they have obtained, at one of the three ports aforesaid, a clean bill signed by the Medical Officer of the Province, or by a qualified Medical Officer empowered to act on his behalf.[22]

The Venice Sanitary Convention of 1897 was attended by European countries and Egypt, which faced several smallpox, cholera and bubonic plague outbreaks during the nineteenth century. The objective of the conference was on controlling the bubonic plague which had started in China in 1894. The Venice Convention settled the incubation period for plague and the period for quarantine to be adopted for administrative purposes. After much discussion ten days was accepted by a large majority. The principle of disease notification was unanimously adopted. Each government had to notify other governments on outbreaks of plague and at the same time, they had to state measures of prevention being carried out to prevent its spread. These conventions were important in bringing about international cooperation and they reached agreements on prophylactic measures against diseases such as cholera, plague and yellow fever.

Thorne, who commented on the earliest draft of the Quarantine Rules of Zanzibar in 1899, objected to the way the colonial authorities in Zanzibar had introduced new clauses which had not been mentioned in the Venice Sanitary Convention of 1897. He observed that some of the proposed clauses of the Quarantine Rules of Zanzibar 'find no place either in the Venice Convention of 1897, or any modern Conventions dealing with the prevention of diseases'. He disputed the use of the term Sanitary Camp and preferred the use of the term Sanitary Station.[23] Responding to this, Sir Lloyd Mathews, in a letter to Lord Salisbury, the secretary of state in London, stated that 'it is inadvisable to insist in a country such as this (Zanzibar) on the strict and literal application of every provision of the Venice Convention'.[24] Hardinge also had commented that:

> My humble opinion has always been that we ought not in these Protectorates [Kenya and Zanzibar] to be tied down too closely to the Venice Rules. These rules, as I have before had the honor to point out, were not only drawn up

> without any consideration for the peculiar local conditions of East Africa which at the time when they were drafted was threatened by plague, but admit of differential application in Europe, the Red Sea and the Persian Gulf.[25]

Other ideas and views which influenced the adoption of quarantine rules in Zanzibar came from the British officers who worked in India during the plague period. Sir Lloyd Mathews wrote to R. W. Hornabrook, a former British officer who worked in India in 1896 and who in 1899 became a plague officer for the Transvaal Chamber of Mines in South Africa, in order to seek opinion on how Zanzibar could apply quarantine measures. Hornabrook informed that the dangers of importation of plague by ships coming from the plague-infected ports were threefold: the occurrence of the plague among passengers, the landing of rats from the plague-infected ships and the importation of infected cloth.[26] The medical and health authorities in Zanzibar had therefore concentrated on checking merchandises and passengers who arrived at the port from the infected areas in order to control the epidemics.

In the early period of the establishment of the Quarantine Station, Dr Johnson, an assistant MO from Mombasa, was dispatched to Zanzibar to take charge of the station.[27] At the same time, Lloyd Mathews applied to India for plague or hospital assistants, who could carry medical supervision of plague victims. These were hospital assistants, a category of medical helpers first introduced in India in 1835 at the Calcutta Medical College. The posts of plague assistants were inaugurated to help plague victims from the mid-1880s. Mathews did not succeed in his bid, however, as many Indian hospital assistants were employed in South Africa during the South African War of 1899 which ended in 1902.

Mathews appointed Dr Henry Alfred Spurrier, a Director of Health Services of the Zanzibar Government, to be a chief MO for the station. He was required to take responsibilities for everything connected with boarding ships from infected or suspected ports, or from wherever plague was rumoured to exist. Among his duties was to see that the 'Venice Convention' was strictly carried out, despite Mathew's belief that this was not necessary. He had to cooperate with the medical doctors of the Government Hospital, Drs Nariman and MacDonald, and to report monthly on the sanitary condition of the town. Spurrier took charge of all duties of port health officer, inspecting vessels, including dhows of every kind and superintending the completion of the necessary buildings at Prison Island.[28] The Quarantine Station, which in addition had fumigation facilities, was established to monitor and quarantine people and incoming vessels and goods from any port in the world, which passed through East Africa. Generally, steamship transport accelerated the transmission of bubonic plague infection in the Indian Ocean ports, despite all these measures. This could be seen with the eruption of bubonic plague in 1905.

THE OUTBREAK OF BUBONIC PLAGUE IN ZANZIBAR TOWN IN 1905

Regardless of the establishment of the Quarantine Station and the introduction of Port Health Services, bubonic plague broke out in Zanzibar Town in 1905, details of which are covered in the Zanzibar colonial records. These reports indicated that the epidemic led to an expansion of the colonial government's intervention on the life of the population under the name of public health. It increased the role of the state but was finally beneficial to both the people and the state who needed secure and healthy labourers to work on the economic field such as in clove and coconut plantations which were the backbone of the economy.

The first suspected case of plague to be noticed by the MOs occurred in the Stone Town area on 3 August 1905 from a German trader, Herr Ratje, who dealt with the transportation of hides from East Africa to Germany. Stone Town evolved from the early nineteenth century due to its role in the international trade and it played a major role in receiving and transmission of plague and other diseases. Ratje died a few days from excessive body temperature and heart failure. Dr Friedrichsen, a private German doctor who treated him, sent the material from Ratje's 'post mortem' to the German bacteriologist, Professor Robert Koch, who was in Tanganyika (Tanzania Mainland) at that time, investigating anthrax. Medical doctors in Zanzibar thought that the case might be anthrax as the deceased dealt with hides. Professor Koch did not believe the case was anthrax.[29] He suspected it was bubonic plague.

Within a month, on 31 August, Dr Howard of the Universities' Mission to Central Africa (UMCA) Hospital, a British Protestants mission centre, found plague bacilli in an African patient who was an employee of one of the Indian traders near the port. Afterwards, many of the plague cases occurred in apartments and shops around Malindi, near the port and at bazaar centres owned mainly by Indian traders. The total number of people who were affected with the disease was 154, out of an estimated number of the town population which reached 100,000. About 123 people died and 31 recovered. The epidemic became more severe in Stone Town, where 133 cases were reported. Very few cases had occurred in Ng'ambo (the 'Other Side') of the town where only fourteen cases were reported. Only seven cases were noted in rural areas, far away from the busy and commercially active Stone Town. It took one month for the Health Department to announce the presence of the plague in the town because of the uncertainty as to whether the disease was bubonic plague or anthrax, which was reported in the south of Pemba Island, a sister island, at that time. Finally, the colonial authorities announced the presence of plague in the town on 1 September 1905.[30]

The attitudes of the British and the linkage of local culture with disease continued unchallenged due to lack of medical data. The British colonial administrators and medical doctors in Zanzibar, however, blamed the urban population for ignoring sanitation measures.

They pointed out that the plague occurred since the town was dirty. They did not consider the imperial expansion and the development of the capitalist economy, which led to the free movement of goods and people, as reasons.

Soon after the confirmation that bubonic plague had broken out in the town and not anthrax as expressed by a few number of medical officers, several sanitation measures focusing on removal of rubbish which according to the reports of Health Officers attracted rats became apparent. The officials were of opinion that enormous amount of rice and cereals in the bulky godowns (warehouses) throughout the town provided rats with abundant food. The wood and iron rooftops and match-boarding partition work of the houses gave them nesting facilities. Stables and cow houses too, scattered thickly through the town, were for the most part floored with loose boards gave the rats sustenance under the same roof.[31]

The medical authorities in Zanzibar were not clearly able to explain when and where the bubonic plague originated. But it was 'traceable in the opinion of Dr. Friedrichsen to a cargo of rice brought by the Deustch Ost Afrika Line, (D.O.A.L) *S. S. Sultan* on her voyage from Bombay to Durban in June 1905. The ship arrived in Zanzibar port on June 16 and left for South on June 20'.[32] It was also maintained by the MOs that 'the greater part of the cargo of rice brought to Zanzibar on the voyage from Bombay was stored in a catacomb-like godown of an Indian and thence distributed to other godowns and shops. Some of the first cases occurred amongst Indian's clerks and godowns'.[33] This was a time when colonial scientific knowledge was not advanced enough which made control measures to become vague.

GOVERNMENT'S REACTIONS TO BUBONIC PLAGUE

The colonial authorities in Zanzibar took immediate actions of declaring Zanzibar Town and the port as plague-infected areas on 2 September 1905. This was followed by the publication of a 'Plague Decree' in the Official Gazette (*Zanzibar Gazette*) on 3 November; a decree gave powers to the medical authorities to detain suspected plague victims, to segregate, to hospitalize them and to destroy the property of plague victims. In addition, 'the town was divided into 14 districts and each placed in charge by an European Inspecting Officer and a Medical Officer who were supplied with gangs of men and carts to assist the Sanitary Department in a thorough simultaneous cleaning up of the town, visiting all houses and seeing them emptied of all hoarded rubbish, and carrying out general whitewashing'.[34] Lime was supplied freely and houses were limewashed at government expenses. A shop-to-shop inspection of foodstuffs was done by the sanitary inspector aided by the district officers. At the port, all passengers and crews of every ship were detained at the Quarantine Station for ten days before being allowed to leave steamers or dhows.[35]

Also, 'considerable use was made of the Press in imparting information and in attempting to stir up the householders, merchants and shopkeepers generally to cleanse their premises and surroundings. Leaflets in Gujarati, Arabic, English and Swahili using the Arabic script were left at every house, their matter and form being varied from time to time to invite fresh attention'.[36] Dr MacDonald was assigned a task of delivering special lectures in English through Indian and Swahili interpreters to the town dwellers and to the representatives of the different communities on practical measures to be taken in combating plague.[37]

The colonial violated religious instructions by announcing that 'all deaths should be reported at the Health Office and no burial was to take place until the body had been inspected by medical officers and all sick persons were to be reported and to be permitted to be seen by a medical man'.[38] Of course this was done to ensure no further deaths occurred but the notice itself required the town people to open their privacy to officials. This decree was enforced by heavy penalties for non-compliance.[39]

Sick people, mostly Indians, were identified and removed swiftly to the Government Hospital and their relatives were segregated in an 'Observation Camp' at Ziwani in the south-east of the town under the charge of Dr F. Paul, an MO at the Government Hospital. A hospital was opened outside the town at Maruhubi, on the north road, being an extension of the regular hospital for smallpox cases. We do not know to what extent the 'Observation Camp' or 'Isolation Camps' (lazarettos) were used to detain people infected with the plague virus in other East African colonies. We assume that the camps existed there.

The 'Plague Hospital' at Maruhubi in 1905 was under the authority of Dr MacDonald, another MO of the Government Hospital. He was assisted by Miss Brewerton, a matron at the UMCA Hospital, and other UMCA Hospital staff. Other staff included Durgadas Soni, an Indian hospital assistant, and eight African 'Ward boys'.[40] Similarly, in India, health camps were introduced immediately in order to respond to the massive death rate of plague victims.[41] Moreover, supplies of Haffkine's Plague Prophylactic were telegraphed for to India and the stock of disinfectants reinforced by orders to Bombay and London. W. M. Haffkine, a Bombay and Calcutta bacteriologist, developed a plague prophylactic in 1896 during the plague period. He started to produce large quantities of this prophylactic in 1902. The vaccine produced by Haffkine was met with resistance in India due to the idea that it had been prepared using pig and cattle flesh, a combination which was met with disgust by the Muslim and Hindu communities in Bombay and in the Bengal area.

As the disease was associated with fleas from rats, the catching and killing of rats was insisted on. A reward of two annas for sending a live or dead rat to the Department of Health Office was announced at the onset of the outbreak of the plague in 1905. Rat dissection works and the laboratory for chemical works were carried on at the Health Department building to simplify the fights against the plague.[42]

The killing of rats however caused substantial ill feeling among Hindus, both in India and in Zanzibar, whereby a plague notice, which ordered the killing of rats, was seen as interference with Hindu belief which prohibited killing anything, from insects to animals. The 'rat killing' had little success among high-caste Hindus in the Punjab area.[43] An example of this was the resistance by devout Hindus who sabotaged the traps.[44] In most cases in Zanzibar Town they responded negatively, leaving rats to increase. An anonymous writer, presumably a European, wrote in the *Central Africa*, a UMCA Journal of October 1905, pointing out that:

> In the first place, we trusted to the extermination of rats to do away with the most common germ-carrier. This work has been carried on for several years by the government, which has paid hard cash for every rat delivered at the Police Barracks. But there are Indians whose religious conscience forbids the killing of a rat. Therefore, in very many houses rats run free and in some cases pious Asiatics have been known to redeem rats from the Africans who wished to slay them.

Other methods used included the application of carbolic powder and Jeyes Fluid in houses to kill the fleas from rats. Sometimes the town fire engine was used to spray the fluid. Houses were disinfected and sprayed with perchchloride of mercury solution. 'Clayton Gas' was used to drain the town. During the plague time rat poisoning was carried out. The chief poison brands were 'Common Sense', 'Rough on Rats', 'Grosboisine Paste and Powder' and 'Danzy Rat Virus'. All were supplied by the MOs. The disinfecting staffs were led by a European officer, T. S. Shaw and a Goan officer, F. de Souza, and twenty-two Africans.

Meanwhile, the combined efforts to halt the plague in Zanzibar involved the cooperation of British medical authorities from Kenya and the Colonial Office in London. Six nurses from the Colonial Nursing Institution were applied for from London and arrived on 28 October 1905. A British female doctor and inoculators were obtained from Nairobi. Nursing staff was borrowed from the UCMA Hospital and from the Roman Catholic Sisters of St Joseph, both of Zanzibar.[45] Miss Margaret Catherine Roseburg, an experienced nurse who had worked in Bombay and Sitara in 1899 during the plague period and was employed thereafter to work at the British South African Company Hospital in Rhodesia, was recruited to Zanzibar in 1905 to nurse plague victims. The letter of her appointment indicated that she was required to take care of both European and 'native' victims.[46]

RESPONSES OF THE URBAN POPULATION

The responses of the Zanzibar Town population to the plague measures were often violent. Cases of violence were reported among Indians who were severely affected by the epidemics. There is substantial evidence drawn from the other writings on the social history of bubonic plague elsewhere in the world which shows that many of the states used coercive measures to fight plague. These provoked the people to react fiercely.[47] In India, in Bombay, Calcutta and in the Punjab Presidencies, fierce fighting with police and other colonial officers occurred as Indians resisted anti-plague measures. Violent protests and resistance were characteristic of popular response to colonial health measures (Bala in this volume). Arnold demonstrated that 'because of the manner in which it was perceived by the colonial authorities and the nature of the sanitary and medical measures deployed against it, bubonic plague provoked an unparalleled crisis in the history of state medicine in India'.[48]

In urban Zanzibar, people fled to the rural areas after the declaration of an outbreak of plague and the publication of the decree. The bazaars were closed in protest and rioting by the different Indian communities.[49] Commercial activities had stopped due to the enforcement of the public health measures. Imported goods from outside Zanzibar, especially from India where the plague had broken out, were stopped from entering the port.

Bishop Dr Hine of the UMCA mission station in Zanzibar, who was in the town during the plague period, wrote to William Traves, a UMCA secretary in London, on 5 September 1905 informing him of the plague in Zanzibar. Hine reported that he met an excited crowd at Malindi, and in one of the Indian houses where a plague victim was identified. His family refused to let him be moved to the Plague Hospital. Hine noted that the urban dwellers roamed in the streets with knives with intentions of stabbing anyone who might remove plague victims, while the UMCA Hospital was almost empty as the town people feared to come to the hospital, thinking that Dr Howard might send them to the Plague Camp.[50] The character of the urban population responses to plague epidemic measures suggested how alien the Western public health measures in Zanzibar were at that time.

This reluctance to allow the removal of plague victims hindered the government's efforts to stop the spread of plague. Indeed 'different castes objected to go to the one general Government Hospital for all and wished for their own community hospitals, a proposal welcomed by the Government when the right to inspect to secure efficiency was conceded'.[51] However, some of these community hospitals did not meet the required standard as reported by Dr Spurrier that 'those belonging to the Ismaili Khoja community were transferred to the Hospital got ready by that community, formerly Livingstone's house. The Banyans' and Ithnasheri Khojas' Hospitals were not convenient for the reception of convalescents'.[52] So, the health authorities had to use force to hospitalize the victims at the Government Hospital. Objection was made too to the covered cots used for conveying cases to the hospital as being in shape like the Mohammedan [Muslim] burial biers. This was overcome by permission to take the sick on 'native' beds, which remained in the hospital.[53] The grievance was issued by the Hindu community.

The whitewashing of houses caused problems as many properties were damaged in the process. The townspeople were not happy with these anti-plague measures and resisted them. One anonymous author wrote in *Central Africa* of October 1905 that Indians in the town resisted sanitary measures as most of them refused to obey orders that were issued by the medical and health authorities. The author further commented about the sanitation by showing that 'whitewash was provided for the poorer classes;every effort was made to keep the town sanitary. But the Indian population prefers dirt, so what can a government do?' It is unlikely that the people preferred dirt but they resisted government interference.

During the plague, the Indian and Arab Association leaders criticized the medical and health authorities who prevented the families of the plague victims from visiting their ill relatives. It was reported that 'exclusion from visiting the sick was strongly objected to and permission to enquire at the hospital entrance where a daily bulletin announcing the condition of each patient was posted with a provision that when very ill the cases could be visited in the wards under supervision went some way to silence this objection'. Any examination of the dead for diagnostic purposes remained to the end strongly objected to by Arab leaders, who perceived this as interference with their religion.[54] In India, corpse inspection had been instituted in order to register the plague cases and as a check to further spread of the disease. However, the inspection of Muslim corpses fuelled riot and protest in Bombay Presidency in 1898.[55]

The treatment of plague victims caused deep concern not only by the local people but by medical doctors too. This could be seen when Bishop Hine of UMCA, who was trained as a medical doctor at the University College, London, in the 1870s, commented on the way the bodies of plague cases were examined by showing that:

> To me it seems that the modern scientific medical training is much more brutalizing that it was in my time. The sick person is nothing. He is only an anatomical specimen – his tissues forming material for myopic examination – himself of no

> account. The great thing is to see some kind of micrococcus – a something with or without a flagellum that perhaps has not been seen before. Pathogen is the only thing considered and ruled the medical mind. The sick individual is merely case X or case XII. This doctor is simply scientific – he has no human feelings.[56]

At the same time the quarantine restriction interrupted the movement of people from one area to another as reported by Bishop Hine who feared would considerably hamper their movements to the mainland, where they had another two stations.[57]

Likewise, in Zanzibar Town, many communities preferred privacy for their female members and they objected to the visiting and inspection of houses, which in most cases was done by the male MOs, who alone were available at that time.[58] Similarly, several violent episodes happened in India when women were physically examined by European male doctors. It was feared that 'most doctors were male as well as white; their touch was considered polluting or worse, as tantamount to sexual molestation. This was especially so when, in searching for the bodily signs of plague, doctors tried to examine women's necks, thighs, and armpits'.[59]

Compulsory vaccination was introduced during the plague period in Zanzibar. Initially, the urban population was not ready to be vaccinated. The composition of Haffkine's serum remained a debatable subject to the end among very strict Indian caste members.[60] Sources are not clear on the reasons behind such resistance. Possibly, as in India, resistance to vaccination was associated with the belief that the lymph had been prepared using pig and cattle flesh. Additionally, in many parts of the world where Haffkine's Plague Prophylactic was introduced, it led to fever, painful swellings of the lymph nodes and soreness at the point of inoculation.[61] In Zanzibar, community leaders were approached by the MOs, which was a successful move. Instructions to be followed after inoculations were posted in many places in the town. The inoculation with Haffkine's Plague Prophylactic was begun on 26 September 1905 and up to 30 September 1905, 23,422 people in the town were inoculated. Since the population census had not begun at that time, it is unknown to what percentage of the population this represented. The population of the town as estimated by Oscar Baumman, an Austrian Consul in 1895, was 100,000.[62]

Sometimes, however, community leaders assisted in mitigating tension. Indeed, there were reports that occasionally, urban people collaborated with the colonial government in the evacuation of plague victims. In 1905, during the bubonic plague, Aga Khan, the Ismail spiritual leader, supported the government efforts to control the epidemic. He visited Zanzibar and urged his followers to be inoculated. The same case happened in India when Aga Khan advised his followers to obey the government's plague regulations and to accept inoculation against the disease.[63]

Much of the damage resulting from destruction of property was compensated. Moreover, the Indian communities suffered loss in their business when the port was declared infected. A Compensation Board, led by J. H. Sinclair, the British consul and assisted by H. Lascari, a British Barrister, one MO and one disinfecting officer, was set up to investigate the claims. The government decided to pay for goods which were destroyed during the events.[64]

By the end of epidemic which lasted for three months, the Ismaili Community of Zanzibar delivered an address to show their gratitude towards Dr Alfred Spurrier and Dr Archibald Donald Mackinnon, a Scottish medical doctor, who was employed in IBEA Co. in Kenya as a staff surgeon during the British expansionism period in East Africa from the early 1880s in preventing the spread of plague. He served in medical works in Kenya, Uganda, Zanzibar and India. He was a senior MO in Zanzibar during the plague period.[65] The Khoja organized the meeting and invited friends from different nationalities to honour them.[66] It was generally agreed that the bubonic plague in early colonial Zanzibar, which was an outcome of the development of colonial economy, spearheaded the enforcement of many public health decrees and laws. The colonial state in Zanzibar had opportunities to interfere in the life of the town people through these public health laws and decrees. It did, however, carry out its obligations and duties in protecting the population who were important and suitable for the development of colonial economy.

CONCLUSION

This chapter has discussed that the integration of East Africa with international economy led to the spread of bubonic plague. From the late 1890s, as more people and goods were imported in East Africa, the spread of bubonic plague and other diseases was very common. This could be proved with the importation of Indian indentured labourers in the construction of Uganda Railway who brought the plague in East Africa. The British colonial authority in East Africa introduced surveillance measures in order to stop the expansion of the disease. Public health measures, including the construction of the Quarantine Station, were launched in order to respond to the spread of the bubonic plague. These measures were introduced since it was feared that commercial and administrative life in East Africa would be paralysed. The main concern of the colonial authorities in East Africa was that the plague would cause a substantial loss of population necessary for the economic expansionism. Plague arrived in Zanzibar in 1905 in which there were a number of deaths that took place. The population of Zanzibar Town objected against the plague measures as deliberate move to extend colonial control over them.

NOTES

1. David Arnold, *Colonizing the Body: State Medicine and Epidemic Disease in Nineteenth-Century India* (California: California University Press, 1993), 201.

2. For the history of Bubonic Plague in India, see Catanach, I. J, 'Plague and the Tensions of Empire: India 1896–1918', in David Arnold (ed.), *Imperial Medicine and Indigenous Society* (Manchester: Manchester University Press, 1988), 149–71; Rajnarayan Chandavarkar, 'Plague Panic and Epidemic Politics in India, 1896–1914', in Terence Ranger and Paul Slack (eds.), *Epidemics and Ideas: Essays on the Historical Perception of Pestilence* (Cambridge: Cambridge University Press, 1992), 203–40; Arnold, *Colonizing*, 200–39; Nafisa Essop Sheik, 'This Most Perilous and Epidemical Disease' Plague Precautions and Public Politics in Natal, 1896–1903 (B.A. Honours Thesis, Department of Historical Studies, University of KwaZulu-Natal, 2004).

3. Jan Jelmert Jørgensen, *Uganda A Modern History* (London: Croom Helm, 1981), 42–43.

4. Zanzibar National Archives, ZNA AC 1/ 33, Foreign Office Correspondence, 1897, January–April.

5. Arnold, *Colonizing*, 210.

6. Chandavarkar, 'Plague', 215–216. See Myron Echenberg, *Black Death, White Medicine, Bubonic Plague and the Politics of Public Health in Colonial Senegal, 1914–1945* (Oxford: James Currey Ltd, 2002), 20.

7. Public Record Office (PRO), London, FO 2/433 Africa, 'Telegram from Mombasa to London, 26 December, 1898', Case of the "Bhundara," Claim for Detention of, at Zanzibar and Mombasa-Plague and Quarantine Regulation 1898–1900, 22.

8. 'From Marquess of Salisbury to Hardinge, 27 December 1898', Case of the "Bhundara", PRO FO 2/433, 81.

9. FO 2/433 Africa, 82.

10. FO 2/433 Africa, 259.

11. PRO FO 2/912, Africa (East) 'Quarantine Station on Prison Island Zanzibar 1894–1904', 1.

12. PRO FO 2/433, 'Case of the "Bhundara"', 81.

13. PRO FO 2/912, 'East Africa Plague Precautions – A Meeting at the Foreign Office, 9 June 1899', Quarantine Station on Prison Island Zanzibar 1894–1904, 147.

14. PRO FO 2/912, 'East Africa', 147.

15. PRO FO 2/912, 'East Africa', 147.

16. Zanzibar National Archives (ZNA) AJ16/11, 'Quarantine Station, 1899', 'Quarantine Station Equipments, Repairs.'

17. PRO FO 2/912, 'From Hardinge to Marquess, 15 December, 1898', Quarantine Station on Prison Island Zanzibar 1894–1904, 3.

18. Anne Hardy, 'Cholera, Quarantine and the English Preventive System', *Medical History*, 37 (1993), 250–269.

19. Mark Harrison, *Public Health in British India: Anglo-Indian Preventive Medicine, 1859–1914* (Cambridge: Cambridge University Press, 1994), 120.

20. Sheik, 'This Most Perilous', 2004, 11, 54

21. PRO FO 2/912, 'East Africa', 46.

22. PRO FO 2/912, 'East Africa', I47.
23. PRO FO 2/912, 'East Africa', 28–29.
24. PRO FO 2/912, 'East Africa', 46.
25. PRO FO 2/912, 'East Africa', 47.
26. PRO FO 2/912, 'East Africa', 71.
27. PRO FO 2/912, 'East Africa', 71.
28. ZNA AB 2/286, 'Quarantine Station at Zanzibar'; ZNA AB 86/53, Personal File 'Dr. A. H. Spurrier Medical Officer, Letter from Lloyd Mathews 28-8-1899 to Dr. Spurrier'; R. H Crofton, *Zanzibar Affairs, 1914–33* (London: Francis Edwards Limited, 1953), 137–38.
29. ZNA BA 8/1, Alfred Spurrier, 'Report for the Outbreak of Bubonic Plague, Zanzibar' (Zanzibar: Government Press, 1905), 2.
30. Spurrier, 'Report for the Outbreak of Bubonic Plague', 1–2.
31. Spurrier, 'Report for the Outbreak of Bubonic Plague', 2.
32. Spurrier, 'Report for the Outbreak of Bubonic Plague', 5.
33. Spurrier, 'Report for the Outbreak of Bubonic Plague', 6.
34. Spurrier, 'Report for the Outbreak of Bubonic Plague', 3.
35. Spurrier, 'Report for the Outbreak of Bubonic Plague', 11–14.
36. Spurrier, 'Report for the Outbreak of Bubonic Plague', p 11; The same measures were applied in Uganda during 1920 bubonic plague. See Megan Vaughan, *Curing their Ills, Colonial Power and African Illness* (Cambridge: Polity Press, 1991), 40–41.
37. Spurrier, 'Report for the Outbreak of Bubonic Plague', 11.
38. Spurrier, 'Report for the Outbreak of Bubonic Plague', 3.
39. Spurrier, 'Report for the Outbreak of Bubonic Plague', 3.
40. Spurrier, 'Report for the Outbreak of Bubonic Plague', 3.
41. Chandavarkar, 'Plague', 207. See also Catanach, 'Plague', 154, 159 and John Hays, *The Burdens of Disease, Epidemics and Human Response in Western History* (Rutgers: Rutgers University Press, 1998), 199.
42. Spurrier, 'Report for the Outbreak of Bubonic Plague', 3. Catanach, 'Plague', 154, 159 and Hays, *The Burdens of Disease,* 199.
43. Catanach, 'Plague', 162.
44. Hays, *The Burdens of Disease,* 197.
45. Spurrier, 'Report for the Outbreak of Bubonic Plague', 3.
46. ZNA AE 16/3, Agreement with Nurse (Miss Margaret Catherine Roseburg) to serve on Plague Duty in Zanzibar for six months.
47. For this discussion, see the work of Catanach, 'Plague', 149–71; Chandavarkar, 'Plague Panic', 203–40; Nancy Elizabeth Gallagher, *Medicine and Power in Tunisia, 1780–1900* (Cambridge: Cambridge University Press, 1983); Carol Benedict, *Bubonic Plague in Nineteenth-Century China* (California: Stanford University Press, 1996); Echenberg, *Black Death;* John T. Alexander, *Bubonic Plague in Early Modern Russia, Public Health and Urban Disaster* (Oxford: Oxford University Press, 2003).
48. Arnold, *Colonizing*, 202.
49. Spurrier, 'Report for the Outbreak of Bubonic Plague', 3–4.
50. Rhodes House Library (RHL) Mss., 'From Hine to Travers, Mkunazini, 9 September, 1905', Bishop Hine 1905–1906, Box A1 XIII, 299.

51. Spurrier, 'Report for the Outbreak of Bubonic Plague', 4.
52. Spurrier, 'Report for the Outbreak of Bubonic Plague', 13.
53. Spurrier, 'Report for the Outbreak of Bubonic Plague', 4.
54. Spurrier, 'Report for the Outbreak of Bubonic Plague', 4.
55. Arnold, *Colonizing*, 216–17.
56. RHL Mss. 'From Hine to Travers, Mkunazini, 5 September, 1905', Bishop Hine 1905–1906, Box A1 XIII, 299.
57. RHL Mss. 'From Hine to Travers, Mkunazini, 9 September, 1905', Bishop Hine 1905–1906, Box A1 XIII, 329.
58. Spurrier, 'Report for the Outbreak of Bubonic Plague', 4.
59. 59 Arnold, *Colonizing*, 214.
60. Spurrier, 'Report for the Outbreak of Bubonic Plague', 44.
61. Echenberg, *Black Death*, 103–104.
62. In 1895, Oscar Baumman, the Austrian consul in Zanzibar, did survey of the town. He estimated the number of the inhabitants to be 100,000. See Oscar Baumman, *Die Insel Zanzibar* (Leipzig: Duncker and Humblot, 1897).
63. Arnold, *Colonizing*, 272.
64. Spurrier, 'Report for the Outbreak of Bubonic Plague', 13.
65. For the history of the British Colonial MOs, see the work of Anna Crozier, 'The Colonial Medical Officer and Colonial Identity: Kenya, Uganda and Tanzania Before World War Two' (PhD Thesis, University College London, 2005).
66. ZNA CA 1/10, 'Misc. Spurrier.'

BIBLIOGRAPHY

Alexander, John. *Bubonic Plague in Early Modern Russia, Public Health and Urban Disaster*. Oxford: Oxford University Press, 2003.

Arnold, David, ed. *Colonizing the Body: State Medicine and Epidemic Disease in Nineteenth Century in India*. California: California University Press, 1993.

Baumman, Oscar. *Die Insel Zanzibar*. Leipzig: Duncker and Humblot, 1897.

Benedict, Carol. *Bubonic Plague in Nineteenth-Century China*. Stanford, CA: Stanford University Press, 1996.

Catanach, I. J. "Plague and the Tensions of Empire: India 1896–1918," In *Imperial Medicine and Indigenous Society*, edited by David Arnold. Manchester: Manchester University Press, 1988.

Chandavarkar, Rajnarayan. "Plague Panic and Epidemic Politics in India, 1896–1914," In *Epidemics and Ideas: Essays on the Historical Perception of Pestilence*, edited by Terence Ranger and Paul Slack. Cambridge: Cambridge University Press, 1992.

Crofton, Richard. *Zanzibar Affairs, 1914–1933*. London: Francis Edwards Ltd, 1953.

Crozier, Anna. 'The Colonial Medical Officer and Colonial Identity: Kenya, Uganda and Tanzania before World War Two.' PhD dissertation, University College London, 2005.

Echenberg, Marion. *Black Death, White Medicine: Bubonic Plague and the Politics of Public Health in Colonial Senegal, 1914–1915.* London: Heinemann, 2002.

Gallagher, Nancy. *Medicine and Power in Tunisia, 1780–1900.* Cambridge: Cambridge University Press, 1983.

Gilbert, Erick. *Dhows and the Colonial Economy of Zanzibar, 1860–1970.* Ohio: Ohio University Press, 2004.

Hardy, Anne. "Cholera, Quarantine and the English Preventive System." *Medical History*, 37 (1993): 250–69.

Harrison, Mark. *Public Health in British India: Anglo-Indian Preventive Medicine, 1859–1914.* Cambridge: Cambridge University Press, 1994.

Hays, John. *The Burdens of Disease, Epidemics and Human Response in Western History.* Rutgers: Rutgers University Press, 1998.

Jørgensen, Jan. *Uganda A Modern History.* London: Croom Helm, 1981.

Spurrier, Alfred. Report for the Outbreak of Bubonic Plague, Zanzibar, September–November, 1905. Zanzibar: Government Press, 1905.

Chapter 4

Cape of Contagion

Cape Town, Contagion and the Curse of Smallpox (ca. 1713, 1755 and 1767)

Russel Viljoen

'As to the Hottentots, they died as if by hundreds, so that they lay everywhere along the roads as if massacred as they fled inland with kraals, huts and cattle, all cursing the Dutch who they said had bewitched them, hoping to be free from this evil sickness'.[1] These observations translated from Dutch into English were authored by François Valentyn, an ordained Dutch minister and colonial sojourner. Published in 1726[2] subsequent to him visiting the Cape of Good Hope, South Africa, in early 1714, Valentyn had alluded to the very first outbreak of smallpox that struck in the Cape Colony in 1713. Direct reference to the indigenous Khoikhoi people of South Africa suggests that smallpox had affected them most and had blamed the Dutch for its introduction to the Cape Colony. As such, the Dutch had intentionally cast an evil spell over them akin to bewitchment. If these remarks are to believed, it not only reflects the state of panic that reigned among the Cape Khoikhoi as the 'curse' of smallpox took effect on the Cape Colony, but it articulated views of mistrust and antagonism towards the Dutch at a particular juncture of their history. In no uncertain terms, it represented an extreme form of resentment towards Dutch colonialism and viewed it as a ploy to subjugate them. From a Khoikhoi perspective, smallpox was a human-manufactured disease fortuitously used by the Dutch to eliminate and alienate them from the Cape and its resources. As a disease, smallpox was deemed a 'curse', and as recently argued by medical scholars, disease is often interpreted as 'an external invader' of an otherwise reasonably healthy person and 'an unwarranted intrusion, accompanied by anxiety and a sense of helplessness'.[3] As far as the Khoikhoi were concerned, the Dutch not only settled their country and occupied their land, but also sought, based on the 'bewitchment' claim, to poison their bodies with foreign and unknown diseases. Threats to their health and overall well-being naturally posed a serious threat to their overall existence as well.

Regarded as key historical moments in documenting the epidemiological narrative of disease in colonial Cape Town, this chapter revisits how three smallpox epidemics disrupted Cape colonial society during course of the eighteenth century with particular reference to the indigenous Khoikhoi. As such, it contributes to the existing historiography of smallpox and the social history of disease at large in early Cape colonial society.[4] As a point of departure it investigates the initial impact of smallpox on Khoikhoi and the emerging Cape-Dutch society at the point of infection and transmission among the Cape population. It argues when smallpox struck periodically during the course of the eighteenth century, it signified a tipping point which threatened Khoikhoi autonomy regionally, a trend that continued throughout the eighteenth century.

PRELUDE TO SMALLPOX

Mark Harrison recently argued how since the Black Death, Africa, Europe and the rest of the world 'became epidemiologically intertwined'.[5] As the world became more 'intertwined' since the sixteenth century brought about by frequent oceanic travel and the founding of new colonies, it naturally expedited the transmission of disease in human history. William McNeill called it, the 'free exchange of infections'[6] between old and new societies. Labelled by Valentyn as 'the most famous southern part of Africa',[7] the strategic and geographical location of the Cape and its incorporation into the major oceanic sea routes and commercial trading networks of the Dutch East India Company (VOC) facilitated the introduction and transmission of contagious diseases to African shores.[8]

Although the Cape shores were rounded by European navigators in 1488 and then intermittently until 1652, the introduction of disease to the Cape seemed far and in between as contact between Europeans and indigenous Khoikhoi was less than sporadic owing to the lack of person-to-person contact. The burgeoning triangle of trade between Amsterdam in Europe, the Cape in Africa and Batavia in Asia since colonial conquest undoubtedly heightened possibilities of the introduction of infectious diseases and illnesses. Cape Town was a developing VOC halfway station which treated sick sailors and travellers travelling between Europe and the Far East.[9] Inbound ships that docked in Table Bay always posed a threat and soon links would develop between sea routes, ships and sickness. In an era of 'transoceanic exchanges',[10] colonial contact also implied the introduction and spread of contagious colonial diseases. This trend was noted throughout the emerging colonial and imperial world, notably, the Indian and Pacific Oceanic indigenous communities (Van Heyningen, Briskey and Samanta in this volume).

Introduction of 'new' diseases brought here by arriving ships, sailors and sojourners, to which both the existing settler, slave and servile indigenous populations had no or little previous exposure, heightened risks of an epidemic.[11] For strategic reasons, Cape Governors monitored and recorded the modus operandi of Khoikhoi pastoralists, their movements and trek patterns. As such, they witnessed and recorded patterns of sickness prevalent among the Cape Khoikhoi population as and when it occurred. Trade negotiations and bartering implied physical contact which brought Khoikhoi herders and colonists into direct contact with each other and created new channels of transmission of new diseases to Khoikhoi communities.

Outbreak of smallpox was, however, preceded by many other illnesses unknown to the Khoikhoi. In 1658, six years following Dutch colonial settlement of the Cape, an array of contagious diseases, many to which Khoikhoi communities had low or no immunity, came to be identified. In early October 1658, Doman reported that the Cochoquas Khoikhoi 'have suddenly been seized with a great sickness'.[12] Later that month, as the disease prevailed, news reached Jan van Riebeeck, the first Cape Commander, that the Cochoquas was 'much incensed against' the Dutch and threatened to 'burn our houses' and 'kill our people'. Prevalence of the disease caused much resentment as the Cochoquas blamed the Dutch for the introduction of unknown diseases for which no traditional medicine and treatment existed. As far as the Cochoquas were concerned, 'they were now almost all sick, and at their weakest'.[13] The introduction of disease had angered the Cochoquas as the illness not only weakened them physically, but exposed them politically, making them vulnerable to cattle raids executed by rival clans owing to their inability to defend themselves as a result of their illness.

Between June and July of 1659, Oedasoa, his child and wife contracted the virus which suggests that the infection prevailed much longer among the Cochoquas in some form or another[14] as they remained susceptible and disease prone owing to continued trade relations with the Dutch.[15] Four years later in November 1663, 'an infectious or contagious disease, which had for some time back carried off many people'. The high mortality rate threatened their political stability and feared future attacks as the Sonquas 'threatened to make war on them'.[16] Exposure to disease over a period of time and related deaths significantly reduced the numbers of the Cochoquas Khoikhoi to the point that it threatened their independence. In September 1666, as the outgoing Cape Governor, Zacharias Wagenaar, reflected on the state of the colonial project and briefed his successor, Cornelis van Quaelberg, the impact of diseases on Khoikhoi communities was a central point of discussion. He, for instance, singled out how the once strong 3,000 Cochoquas from which the Dutch 'procured the greatest quantity of livestock' and nine other Khoikhoi clans had 'some time ago, very much diminished and melted away by a sickness which prevailed among them'.[17] The evidence suggests clearly how contagion affected and disrupted the social, economic and political stability of Cochoquas and other clans over a short period of time.

Eleven years later, on 12 December 1674, Captain Dorha of the Chainoqua Khoikhoi noticed the sudden appearance of 'an infectious disease among his people of whom 9 or 10 males or females had already died very suddenly'. The leadership regarded this 'as bad omen, for no particular severe sicknesses are known among them and Death usually contends himself with old worn out people'. Periods of uncertainty not only triggered unusual responses but spawned the acceptance of peculiar religious beliefs. The entanglement of religious beliefs with the epidemic crisis was paramount in colonial India (Bala in this volume). The unexplained deaths no doubt baffled the Khoikhoi and contracting the illness was seen as a bad omen, which according to tradition was associated with the work of the devil.[18] Thirteen years later in 7 April 1687, an infectious fever was rampant among VOC slaves and on 19 April 1687, the Governor Simon van der Stel 'received intelligence that one half of Hottentot kraal had died, and that other half lay sick'. Two days later, another report confirmed an outbreak of a 'very severe and deadly sickness among the Hottentots, who do not know what to do for it, and although they decamp and move from place to place, the sickness still pursues them'.[19] Towards the end of the seventeenth century, the introduction and exposure to various colonial diseases remained a constant threat to Khoikhoi society and their existence under colonial rule. As such, Khoikhoi communities remained alert and apprehensive about the constant introduction of 'severe and deadly' colonial diseases and the threat it posed to their health and autonomy. It further amplified Khoikhoi susceptibility to foreign illnesses and an admission, that they 'do not know what to do for it' except to 'decamp and move from place to place'. The latter seemed a rational strategy to avert contamination and a form of self-isolation. Moreover, to 'decamp and move from place to place' was in line with pastoralism and the practise of transhumance.[20]

SMALLPOX IN CAPE TOWN, 1713, 1755 AND 1767

Though prevalent in many parts of the ancient and early modern world,[21] the Cape Colony as a conquered territory remained smallpox free for a considerable number of years since colonial settlement began in April 1652. The characterization of smallpox as the 'Angel of Death'[22] and 'Speckled monster'[23] finally made its appearance in Cape Town during the month of

February 1713, six decades after the VOC settled and colonized the region in April 1652. Existing literature on smallpox suggests that the virus shares a long history with humanity and the African continent. Smallpox in Africa dates back 3,000 years and as trade with Africans increased throughout the centuries, smallpox was periodically reintroduced to many African societies across the vast continent.[24]

Scientifically known as either *variola major* or *variola minor*, depending on the variant, smallpox was a virus and dreaded disease, notoriously associated with suffering and death. Of the two strains, *variola major* proved more lethal. The mortality rate of this strain averaged 20%, but could be as high as 50%.[25] According to the bacteriologist, T. H. Pennington, 'smallpox had no animal reservoir and spread person to person by a respiratory route'.[26] Transmission occurs through a cough, sneeze in the form of droplets released into the air. As an airborne disease, the sprayed droplets enter the lungs and bloodstream of the host and infection is brought about. By means of its clinical composition, the virus was highly infectious and had an incubation period of between ten and fourteen days before human hosts and carriers develop symptoms such as fever, headache, backache, nausea and levels of delirium.[27] 'During the first few days of the fever', explains Pennington, in a scientific manner, 'the virus multiplied in skin epithelial cells leading to the development of focal lesions and the characteristic rash. Macules [flat red spots] progressed to papules, vesicles [blisters] and pustules [pus], leaving permanent pockmarks, particularly in the face'.[28]

Epidemiologists, microbiologists and virologists have written about the relationship between 'hosts' and 'susceptibles' in the context of contagious and communicable disease, of which smallpox formed part.[29] Jones and Moon[30] identified the 'process of infection' and quoting this process seems worthwhile. They wrote: 'at individual level (and taking the simplest case with person-to-person transmission) we can recognise susceptibles who have not yet but can be infected, (infectives) who have the disease and can transmit it to others, and immunes who have recovered from the disease and are, temporarily or permanently, immune from further infection'.[31] Cape society, be it indigenous and colonial, however, like any other societies, too was subjected to a 'process of infection' which unfolded when smallpox was introduced to the Cape Colony.

Smallpox was incurable and those that contracted the virus were at risk to die within days of contamination depending on the strain of the virus. Much of the infection 'had taken place behind the scenes and passed unnoticed by the victim' to new susceptible hosts, and as Gareth Williams has stated, it is 'often missed especially in sporadic cases with no ongoing outbreak to raise suspicions'.[32] The Khoikhoi did not understand the science, biology and epidemiology of foreign diseases and disorders prevalent among them. From the outset, they were confronted with an invisible disease, an unknown illness and a medical phenomenon which 'they have never seen' before. Under these circumstances, it completely disrupted their entire social organization and political structures including neutralizing their medical knowledge and forms of indigenous treatment.[33] In their world and understanding, smallpox experienced periodically since 1713 inflicted an inexplicable premature death on people of all ages for which no cure existed. Historically each time, smallpox struck periodically in 1713, 1755 and 1767, it transitioned into an epidemic and as such, shaped the future of the Khoikhoi and early Cape society in a profound manner. Similar pattern was observed in colonial India and Zanzibar when colonial measures to control epidemic situations provided a platform for popular resistance and indigenous means of alleviating suffering as a result (Bala and Issa in this volume).

The introduction of smallpox in Cape Town was linked to the arrival of Johannes Van Steeland,[34] a Commissioner and member of the Council of the Indies (*Raad van Indië*) in February 1713.[35] He was the commander of a return fleet comprising nine vessels that left Batavia bound for Rammekens, in The Netherlands. The Dutch vessel *Zandenburg* departed from Batavia on 26 November 1712 and arrived seventy-eight days later in Cape Town on 12 February 1713. Onboard the *Zandenburg* was the master, Adriaan Timmerman, forty-five seafarers, thirty-five soldiers and seven passengers comprising the Van Steeland family, including his children. While in the service of the VOC, Van Steeland was married twice. His first wife was Wilhelmina Frontenius and Anthonia Nilo, his second. Both wives died in India which suggests that he was a widower when he left India in 1710 and later Batavia in 1712.[36] The *Zandenburg* was a crew and cargo ship and not a slave ship per se transporting slaves from Batavia to the Cape. The virus was either originally brought from Batavia by an infected person or persons who had presumably recovered during the seventy-eight-day journey. According to ship record of the *Zandenburg*, two persons had died during the journey and it is not certain whether or not the deaths were smallpox related.[37] In any event, as those of onboard develop immunity to smallpox during the journey or through previous exposure, the virus attached itself to the clothing items worn by the infected. This was not uncommon. Bedding or clothing often infected with pus dispersed from blisters could remain infectious for several days.[38] Upon arrival, it appears that neither Adriaan Timmerman as captain, or Van Steeland, as commander of the fleet and VOC Commissioner, had fully disclosed to the Cape authorities ashore about the sick and the mortalities suffered at sea. Therefore, upon arrival, as Valentyn had written upon further probing, the infected clothes of the Van Steeland family, specifically 'the laundry-goods of the children', were brought ashore and washed at the Company Slave Lodge.[39] Slave washerwomen – who had had no previous exposure to smallpox – handled the infected clothes and contaminated other slaves in the Slave Lodge. As Gareth Williams has written: 'Viruses are not alive: they lack all the machinery of life and are totally dependent on hosts for survival'.[40] Within a slave society and the conditions slaves were subjected to suggest that 'hosts' were plentiful. 'Hosts' were found in vulnerable human beings owned as slaves at the Cape. The congested and confined living space to which Company slaves were subjected proved conducive for the virus to be transmitted and thrive. Valentyn described the shape and size of the Slave Lodge in 1714 as follows:

> Very large Slave House, this being a building of one story, about 30 feet high, flat-roofed, 77 paces long and 46 deep, where dwell a great number of slaves of the Hon. Company, about 600 when we were there, under the rule of a Mandoor and an Under-Mandoor.[41]

Because person-to-person contact among slaves in the Company Slave Lodge was frequent and inevitable, the virus secured at once multiple 'hosts' of all ages and gender, which allowed for the rapid transmission of the virus within a short space of time. Though the movement of slaves was restrictive, they initially only infected each other, but as the circle of transmission widened, smallpox spread beyond the confines of the Slave Lodge. Soon, the virus found its way into mainstream Cape Town community and infected burgher households residing in Table Valley.[42] In 1714, Valentyn personally counted 254 large and small houses.[43]

Accommodated in the Cape Castle, along with other Cape dignitaries, the Van Steeland family did not contract smallpox throughout the duration of their stay at the Cape. As Commissioner, he went about his business for the duration of his stay at the Cape[44] and remained oblivious to the fact their smallpox-infested dirty laundry had caused an outbreak of smallpox and thus responsible for the introduction of the virus to the Cape Colony. Following their departure to Amsterdam, they had left behind a lethal disease about to infect a diverse colonial community, incapable of handling an outbreak of this magnitude.

By early March 1713, acting Governor Willem Helot reported that smallpox had broken out among company-owned slaves and by 30 March infection rates had increased substantially. The *Dagh Register* (Daily Journal) became the main source of information which included updates on how the smallpox outbreak of 1713 had unfolded. The Helot administration provided day-to-day accounts as best they could, of how the first wave of smallpox struck and spread throughout the colonial city. Inhabitants and would-be sufferers soon experienced that smallpox was highly contagious and above all, incurable. Between March and April 1713, the number of cases escalated on a daily basis and soon 150 people were declared deceased. Another 200 people were infected and became sick within days. The authorities called the virus a *slim soort van kinderpokjes siektes*[45] (smart kind of smallpox illnesses) and labelled it a sickness that had never been diagnosed at the Cape before. It soon became apparent that the virus was highly transmittable and spread mainly through person-to-person contact. As such, contact with infected individuals had to be avoided at all costs.

The large VOC-owned slave community housed in the overcrowded and confined Company Slave Lodge became the epicentre of the disease and had borne the brunt of the early infections and mortality rates which had soon risen to 441. Slaves residing in the Slave Lodge found themselves at the coal-face of an emerging epidemic and proved most vulnerable affecting all slaves irrespective of gender and age, including the elderly. One slave, aged 100, contracted and succumbed to smallpox in April 1713.[46] The overcrowded environment and congested living spaces created ideal conditions in which the transmission of the virus thrived.

The gradual introduction of 'new' infectious diseases, and especially its deceptive incubation period, caught many unaware and thus difficult to respond to. By May 1713, focus shifted towards the indigenous Khoikhoi population of the Cape. The acting Governor Helot also reported that smallpox (*kinderpokjes*) penetrated the ranks referred to as '*Africaense* indigenous' (*Africaense inboorlinge*) at the Cape, which either referred to the indigenous Khoikhoi or Cape-Dutch individuals born at the Cape.[47] The Cape authorities also monitored the spread of smallpox among slave and Khoikhoi population closely and provided daily updates. In subsequent days and months, the rate of infections increased exponentially among the servile population. By 3 May 1713, the infection rate among the '*Africaenen* had increased' (*Africaenen toe te neemen*), to quote the colonial record.[48] The Cape authorities later reiterated that 'the poor Hottentots are not spared, but disastrously do not know the disease and have never seen it'.[49] And as a result, 'of this medical ignorance are thus very disastrously affected'.[50] The information confirmed three observations. In the first instance, the Khoikhoi did not know that smallpox existed, have never seen it before and did not know how to treat it. Like the slave and colonist community, the Khoikhoi too began to suffer the brunt of human losses and faced the dilemma to either fight or take flight. As the Khoikhoi discovered that their indigenous medicines proved unresponsive, they chose the latter and saw flight as the only viable option in an environment where their own traditional healing practices and medicines had no effect whatsoever to cure smallpox.

Based on the description given by Valentyn and corroborated by the colonial record, the Khoikhoi people experienced and faced a severe medical crisis. The surveillance and intelligence gathered by the Cape authorities confirmed this view. In their opinion, the outbreak of smallpox among the

Khoikhoi was deemed 'catastrophic' (*ramspoedig*) and worsened by the fact that Khoikhoi medical practitioners, like European practitioners, lacked the medical expertise to treat smallpox.[51] As shown elsewhere, Khoikhoi prioritized their health. Indigenous practitioners could treat known illnesses and injuries.[52] Unknown illnesses, however, were bound to create chaos, fear and blame. Sudden and prolonged illnesses affected their daily economic routine of hunting, gathering and herding livestock. Sudden changes in the human body brought about by infection, especially the onset of clinical features and symptoms, notably, fever, nausea, vomiting, resulted in the deaths of many Khoikhoi with compromised immune systems. As the virus manifested itself among Khoikhoi communities, it plunged them into a deep medical crisis and forced many families and individuals to face an unknown medical, health and wellness dilemma. As such, Khoikhoi and Cape colonial society was exposed to a disease, bound to disrupt every aspect of human life. As Banister et al. have written, 'disease is not a static event, or an alien presence within us. Rather, it is a conflict of opposing forces different strengths which can be expressed on different levels: physical, psychological, social or spiritual'.[53]

As a medical condition and disease, smallpox was soon rendered as an unknown medical entity among the Khoikhoi and Cape society at large. The Khoikhoi struggled to make sense of smallpox, its causes and symptoms, susceptibility and transmission. What did become apparent was that within days of contracting the virus, victims develop skin rashes, experience severe difficulty in breathing followed by death. At best, it remained a mysterious illness that brought about death and because it was incurable, it was regarded as a curse, as articulated by Valentyn. By cursing the Dutch, the Khoikhoi believed that the outbreak was deliberately orchestrated by the Dutch to bring about their demise.

Wim van Damme and Wim van Lerberghe have argued that epidemics often triggered mixed responses from those affected, ranging from shock to fear.[54] Similar studies by Curtin highlight the combination of fear, fight and flight as common responses resorted to by those affected by an epidemic disease.[55] Khoikhoi response was characterized at first by fight (by means of experimenting with indigenous medicine, which proved futile), followed by fright (panic, anxiety, fear) and finally, flight. As their fight using indigenous medicines proved ineffectual, flight seemed the only logical response. Flight not only brought distance between those infected, but also much-needed isolation. As fleeing into the vast interior seemed rational and therefore a practical strategy to escape contamination, it also took them away from Dutch proximity and influence. Many sought refuge and recovery by occupying new territories distant from colonial influence. It naturally triggered a period of migration and movement of Khoikhoi from Cape Town, leading to depopulation of certain areas. Khoikhoi who 'fled' from Cape Town across the Hottentots Holland Mountains with a view to join other unaffected Khoikhoi groups lost their lives in clashes. For fear of contracting smallpox, Khoikhoi groups, who had remained unaffected, defended their territory by not allowing those infected with smallpox to join or penetrate their ranks.[56] It seems that Khoikhoi communities beyond Hottentots Holland Mountains who remained unaffected by the 1713 outbreak did everything in the power to remain smallpox free and even turned on other Khoikhoi groups to safeguard themselves and clans.

As transmission of the virus spiralled out of control, infections and mortality among the colonist population of Cape Town and its hinterland escalated. For instance, the wheat farming region of Drakenstein, the high mortality rate among the Khoikhoi population residing and working in that region sparked fears of immediate labour shortages. The farming community which had relied on seasonal Khoikhoi labourers were subsequently deprived of a stable labour force owing to the rise of smallpox-related deaths among the Khoikhoi.[57]

Although flight seemed the preferred strategy to avoid contracting smallpox, it also contributed to its transmission. Those on the run had in fact become new carriers and spreaders of the virus to new potential 'hosts'. Such individuals or groups had effectively 'carried' the virus into the interior. Moreover, the direction in which Khoikhoi fled also determined the path of infection. The parameters and radius of infection had thus expanded in line with the movement of people. For instance, by June 1713, smallpox reached Drakenstein[58] and by the early 1714, it had reached Piketberg, situated 130 kilometres from Cape Town.[59]

The epidemic of 1713 which began in March peaked in October and then subsided towards mid-December 1713 in Cape Town, but active cases of smallpox were still recorded in February 1714 in the rural parts of Drakenstein, especially among the Cochoquas Khoikhoi. Evidence suggests that the *Caabse Hottentots* (Cape Khoikhoi) or Peninsular Khoikhoi groups were the ones adversely affected by smallpox and it appeared that inland communities were relatively unaffected by the 1713 outbreak. Other than (7 May 1713) when it was reported that nine Khoikhoi were buried by company officials,[60] accurate mortality rates of *Caabse Hottentots* were never determined, or made available, except maybe among the Piketberg Khoikhoi, which will be referred to later again.

An absence of four decades saw smallpox return to the Cape Colony in the mid-1750s. Globally, however, smallpox still thrived and continued to take its toll. Canada and its indigenous Indian population suffered an outbreak of smallpox in 1755 and lasted until 1757.[61] Its reintroduction to the Cape in May 1755 when a ship that left colonial Ceylon (Sri Lanka) bound for Amsterdam via the Cape brought the colony on the brink of yet another epidemic. Sri Lanka, a VOC-controlled island colony located within the Indian Ocean, was identified as the source of smallpox that reappeared in Cape Town in 1755. In 1754–1755, according to Zameer-Careem, smallpox struck in Maritime Provinces of Sri Lanka and the scourge took its toll claiming many lives on the island. So severe was the epidemic that the Dutch Governor, Joan Loten, reported that smallpox sufferers were often abandoned by their relatives and left to die.[62] Travel and trade links between Sri Lanka, Cape Town and the Netherlands proved instrumental in dissemination of smallpox across the vast Indian Ocean to the Cape. It appeared that cargo, clothing or persons infected with the virus boarded the ship that left the shores of Sri Lanka. In all likelihood, the infected person or persons confined for months on a congested ship aided transmission of the virus. Those infected had presumably reinfected each other for the duration of the journey, until new 'hosts' were found at the Cape when the ship docked in Table Bay in May 1755. The new generation of people born at the Cape, between 1713 and 1755, were therefore unexposed to smallpox and thus more susceptible. The reintroduction of the infectious virus suggests that the 'curse' of smallpox still reigned within the contours of the colony. At first, it only infected privately owned slaves belonging to Jan de Waal in the vicinity of Table Bay. It then gradually infected the small Khoikhoi population in Cape Town. Improved travelling routes from Cape Town into the interior accelerated the dissemination of smallpox into the interior and brought it to previously unexposed communities. The Cape winter season experienced between May and August accelerated the transmission of smallpox. Smallpox and fever coexisted as separate illnesses and both thrived in cold weather conditions accompanied by coughing and sneezing. Colds and fever compromised the immune systems of individuals and made many susceptible to contracting smallpox.[63]

Smallpox, known as *kinderpocken* (children's pox) or *pokjes* (pox), was dispersed beyond Stellenbosch and the Hottentot Holland Mountains. Contact with Cape Town was to be avoided as far as possible to reduce the infection rate. Farmers in Soetendaals Valley and Buffelsjagts River regions were cautioned not to allow visitors from Cape Town to enter their homes until the efficacy of the virus subsided. In the district of Swellendam, reports reached the Castle that 'many slaves died, but even a greater number of Khoikhoi had died'.[64] In the midst of these circumstances, 'their livestock owned by the Khoikhoi (*Hottentotten*) were left unattended, scattered far and wide in the grazing pastures'. The fact that the Khoikhoi left their herds unattended was either a sign that they fled their respective kraals and left their livestock behind, or became so ill, that they could not attend their cattle, or had died having contracted the virus.

One could also assume that many farmers in the vicinity exploited the situation and plight of the Khoikhoi. Many raided cattle left unattended by the fleeing Khoikhoi as well as land left vacant as a result.

Regular registration of mortality rates had given the Cape authorities a new angle to monitor the curve of infections and devise measures to restrict further infections. In 1755, for instance, documentation of infections and fatalities improved significantly compared to 1713 when it was recorded in a haphazard fashion. As the epidemic peaked between June and July of 1755, Governor Ryk Tulbagh and the Council of Policy announced stringent measures and interventions in an effort to curb the spread of smallpox. In June 1755, the number of deaths stood at 270 and spiked to 1,102 in July 1755. This represented an increase of 832 deaths in only one month. Tulbagh also sought divine intervention and encouraged all to pray. By calling smallpox one 'plague' (*plaag*), he too labelled it a curse. As head of the Colony, during the 1755 and 1767 epidemics, he placed considerable trust in God through prayer and urged Christian believers and clergymen to do likewise.

Administratively, the Cape authorities seemed better organized to manage the prevailing smallpox crisis by implementing a range of regulations to curb *pokkies te stuiten* (stop the spread of smallpox).[65] Enforcements through the promulgation of *placaats* (decreed public notices) gatherings were prohibited, shops closed and movement of people restricted.[66] Two houses were hired and renovated as hospitals. Slaves were paid one guilder to watch over the sick and the poor.[67] Calculation of mortality rates was good indicator to gauge the trajectory of smallpox infections and related deaths. By keeping accurate record of recorded deaths and by making it known publicly positioned them to monitor the curve of smallpox trends and patterns.

The information extrapolated from recorded deaths suggested that the Cape authorities devised a system to track and trace those infected and recorded death rates as it happened on a weekly and monthly basis. In certain cases, victims, whether slaves or colonists, were often even mentioned by name. The number of deaths recorded during the month of July 1755 suggests that the epidemic peaked during winter. In subsequent months it bottomed out completely and subsided visibly towards the advent of spring and summer months of 1755.[68] There was no resurgence or second wave and the smallpox curve found itself in decline. Figures from far-flung magisterial districts were less accurate than in Cape Town. Though the mortality rates proved startling, it provided evidence of lives lost and a shattered Cape society, socially and economically. By calculating and measuring smallpox in terms of mortality rates on a monthly basis and strict adherence to the adopted regulations suggested somehow that epidemic could be managed to an extent. Statistics and mortality rates, however, still revealed indeed a grim picture of the impact of smallpox on Cape society. In total 2,072 people died between May and October of 1755 of smallpox-related complications.

In May 1767, smallpox struck again as the 'speckled monster' returned to the shores of Cape Town. A Danish vessel *De Kroonprins* docked in Cape Town harbour. Despite the strict precautionary measures implemented by the Council of Policy following the 1755 outbreak, smallpox returned to the Cape in May 1767 and claimed lives of slaves, colonists and children. In total 878 people perished of which fifty-three were Khoikhoi. Once again the disease spread beyond the immediate contours of Cape Town and affected the interior of the Colony, especially spaces occupied by Khoikhoi communities.[69] Compared to the recorded deaths, the 1755 proved much more severe than in 1767. Total had hardly reached those that succumbed in 1755.

In 1767, smallpox infiltrated Cape interior, particularly the district of Swellendam inhabited by Khoikhoi groups. Written reports explained the severity of smallpox in the interior and revealed that several Khoikhoi individuals perished. In order to prevent further contamination, victims were buried immediately and their clothing items burned. Two years later, by 1769, the effect and impact of smallpox was evident in the region. Backleij Plaats near Swellendam, an area inhabited by the Hessequa Khoikhoi for decades, was completely deserted. Many had died, but survivors were completely impoverished having lost their resources (livestock and land). Unable to restore their livelihood following the death of many leaders, members of the kraal settled and worked on colonial farms as farm servants.[70] Statistically the outbreak of 1767 was less fatal than the one of 1755 and possibly even 1713. From a commercial and trading point of view, the 1767 outbreak which lasted until 1769, the induction of Cape Town into the world of commercial trade, provided a gateway for the introduction of disease to the Cape Colony. As McNeill has written, the 'transoceanic exchanges'[71] and ocean economy during the eighteenth century duly promoted the introduction of 'new diseases' to the Cape Colony of which smallpox was most profound at this stage.

CURSE OF SMALLPOX

S. L. Kotar and J. E. Gessler[72] identified a connection between smallpox and spirituality. In their view, it justified the emergence of smallpox gods and goddesses in India, China and Africa. At the Cape, however, disease per se soon became synonymous with superstitious behaviour, omens and curses. In December 1674, the Khoikhoi leader, Dorha, interpreted the sudden death experienced by his people as a 'bad omen' and the work of external forces. It was labelled a 'bad omen, for no particular severe sicknesses are known among them and Death usually contends himself with old worn out people'.[73]

Similar utterances re-emerged in 1713. It suggests that all of diseases introduced to the Cape by Europeans since Dutch settlement, smallpox was the worst of the worst and therefore labelled a curse, quite frankly, an 'evil sickness'. The vocabulary used by Valentyn, notably, 'cursing', 'evil sickness' and 'bewitched', resonates not only with the religious beliefs, but unearthed deep-seated resentment of unresolved Khoikhoi-Dutch political power relations and tension. The association of smallpox with spirituality suggests that the comment made by Valentyn 'all cursing the Dutch who they said had bewitched them, hoping to be free from this evil sickness' deserves deeper analysis. How then are we to interpret and understand the comment made by Valentyn with reference to 'cursing' and 'bewitchment'? Did Valentyn actually hear these comments himself? Was it perhaps related to him in a translated private conversation with a Khoikhoi leader? Or did he merely encapsulate a common view held among the Cape Khoikhoi at the time when smallpox struck in 1713? Valentyn does not say, but we can assume it was a combination of what he witnessed first-hand as an observer and an articulation of sentiments expressed and views held by survivors trying to make sense of a merciless disease and a desperate cry for help.

Valentyn arrived at the Cape in 1714, which meant that smallpox had been prevalent among the Khoikhoi people and Cape-Dutch society, for least eight months. During this time, it caused great distress and destruction among the Khoikhoi people. Of course, the Khoikhoi themselves could have formulated their own opinion of smallpox, which became common knowledge at the time. Either way, it reflected Khoikhoi dissent towards the Dutch. Outbreak of smallpox had clearly a devastating effect on the Cape Town Khoikhoi. Valentyn too carried first-hand knowledge of Khoikhoi and their history. The advent of smallpox bought about traumatic experiences to the fore and during this period of uncertainty, it reinforced mistrust between Khoikhoi and colonists. Belief existed that the Dutch brought smallpox to the Cape and deliberately released it among the Khoikhoi people. It was a deliberate act of sabotage and shrewd manner to gain access to their land and livestock. In the event of their demise, the Dutch would be given free access to their land and livestock. It was bound to undermine Khoikhoi existence and in the case of death due to contracting smallpox, colonists were given uncontested access to their land and livestock. Colonialism, meaning the presence of the Dutch, was a curse in itself and sparked the introduction of smallpox. It handed the Dutch an unfair edge. By cursing the Dutch, the Khoikhoi believed that smallpox was deliberately orchestrated by the Dutch to expedite their demise. The curse of smallpox implied more than a religious utterance, but assumed overtones of a political statement and strained power relations.

Smallpox and its introduction to the Cape Colony, as articulated by Valentyn, occurred as a direct consequence of colonial conquest. It became a strategy by the Dutch to alienate the Khoikhoi and by implication the Dutch were seen as the 'evil one' – the equivalent of *Gaunab*.[74] In Khoikhoi religious belief system, *Gaunab* was the initiator and provider of 'bad luck' and one that often pronounced of an evil spell or bad omen over Khoikhoi people. The curse and bewitchment was a deliberate attempt to disrupt, displace, dispossess and finally, alienate them from their land and livestock using smallpox to achieve their goals. The curse of smallpox was clearly more than a medical disaster and a mental menace. Disease was interpreted as a political ploy and colonial curse to destabilize Khoikhoi society. Smallpox affected Khoikhoi society in its entirety and effectively threatened their entire future as an independent group. By fleeing the Cape, some Khoikhoi survivors deflected and neutralized smallpox in an effort to develop immunity and as such hoped to triumph over the curse. For the Khoikhoi people to have reasoned in this manner was not far-fetched, but rational. The disease was brought to the Cape by the Dutch, onboard Dutch-owned ships and introduced to a country that was settled and colonized by the VOC since 1652. It was a knee-jerk reaction by the Khoikhoi to protect their identity, status and preserve their autonomy in the land of their birth.

The Dutch Governor, Ryk Tulbagh, in particular, placed trust in God for deliverance from smallpox. In 1755, Tulbagh described smallpox as a *vernielende plaagen* (destructive plague) which could only be defeated through prayer, in addition, to strict adherence to the adopted Council of Policy regulations such as prohibition of large gatherings. In his prayer, he specifically requested God, '*over ons te willen ontfermen en dit land af wenden van de droewige en al vernielende plaagen – Amen*' (to have mercy on us and turn this land away from the sad and destructive plague – Amen).[75] Tulbagh, too, labelled smallpox a 'destructive plague' and a curse. As Cape governor, he too put a religious spin on the epidemic by prioritizing prayers as panacea for smallpox. In order to defeat smallpox, Tulbagh urged the church as an institution, ministers and congregants to pray for an end to the '*vernielende plaagen*' (destructive plague). Religious sermons were used to comfort bereaved families on how to deal with their losses.[76] On Sunday, 13 July 1755, Rev. Gerhardus Coetser preached about the '*quaadaardige kinder pocken*' (evil children's pox/smallpox) which continued to cause havoc among the burgher population of Cape Town[77] and by end of July 1755, the entire Table Valley region were infected with smallpox.[78] Rising death toll in Cape Town soon reduced the church membership and kept churchgoers from attending. By August 1755, the church in Cape Town experienced a drastic decline in their attendance of Sunday services.[79]

In at least one recorded incident, the Dutch attached superstitious beliefs to the 1713 smallpox epidemic. In 1713, the discovery of two pigeons that had fallen from the roof of the Cape Castle and had mysteriously died was linked to the prevailing epidemic.[80] The inexplicable death of the two pigeons served as an omen for the prevailing smallpox epidemic and troubled times ahead. Decades later, however, under British rule in November 1798 when 'numerous shoals of fish being washed on the Beach' and the shores of Cape Town, 'the inhabitants look on this matter as ominous' and prelude to 'some disastrous event'. Andrew Barnard, a British colonial official, then recalled, 'in the memory of the oldest man do they remember a circumstance of this kind, and it was the forerunner of a most dreadful disease which swept away nearly half the inhabitants of this Colony (the Small Pox)'.[81] Though Barnard jokingly accused the inhabitants of Cape Town 'of superstition and absurdity' he, nevertheless, suggested that epidemics and natural disasters were linked to curses, superstitious beliefs and peculiar behaviour for a considerable period of time during the eighteenth century.

EPILOGUE

On 31 July 1755, when the Cape Governor, Ryk Tulbagh, prayed for spiritual intervention, the death toll of smallpox-related deaths peaked considerably. Compared to the month of June 1755, it represented a major resurgence of smallpox deaths. When he contemplated the recorded statistics, for the month of July, he noticed that 489 colonists, 418 privately owned slaves and 195 VOC slaves died of smallpox. In total, during the month of July 1755, the fatalities climbed to a staggering 1,102. This by all means represented a great loss of life. In the months that followed, however, the mortality rate subsided considerably. Tulbagh's prayers were either answered or smallpox infections and related deaths had declined naturally owing to fewer infections. Either way, the curve of new infections dropped sharply and so did the death rate.

The mortality rate of smallpox-related deaths among the Khoikhoi population remained inaccurate and recorded in a haphazard fashion. At best, the assessment of mortality rate remained speculative. Khoikhoi mortality rates were therefore with good reasons, either under-recorded or completely unrecorded. It is a fact, however, that Khoikhoi communities were infected and affected differently and all cannot be assessed in the same manner. Travelogues, at best, provided sweeping statements of Khoikhoi mortality rates often years after smallpox had struck. Without providing accurate figures of Khoikhoi deaths, Carl Thunberg wrote how smallpox 'exterminated the greater part of them'.[82] Valentyn claimed that the Khoikhoi 'died as if by hundreds, that they everywhere along the roads as if massacred',[83] while O. F. Mentzel informed his readers how 'thousands of . . . Hottentots perished' which lead to their 'annihilation'.[84] The colonial records proved equally vague, if not, inaccurate. It claimed how bad smallpox affected the Khoikhoi and how regions traditionally occupied by them in significant numbers previously were left vacant as a result. In 1755, the *Landdrost* (Magistrate) of Swellendam, Andries Horak, had penned a letter to the Cape Governor, informing him of 'a greater number of Khoikhoi had died' compared to slaves and colonists.[85] In all fairness and in his defence, it was not his responsibility to provide an accurate headcount and record of Khoikhoi deaths, especially of those still attached to their respective clans and kraals, unless of course, they came across deceased Khoikhoi, in which case, they were obliged to dispose of, for hygienic purposes and for fear of possible contamination. Given how infectious smallpox was, a fact many came to accept, many had presumably avoided as far as possible contact with Khoikhoi kraals, fearing contamination. Moreover, the Khoikhoi were not VOC subjects per se, but seen as an independent nation. The Cape authorities therefore were not obliged to track and trace Khoikhoi mortality rates as was the case with Company-owned slaves and colonists. For instance, when smallpox re-emerged at the Cape in 1767, the mortality rates of both free blacks (freed slaves) and Khoikhoi were recorded together in the monthly statistics. Again, an inaccurate total mortality rate concerning the Khoikhoi was recorded.[86]

Such commentaries clearly suggest that although Khoikhoi mortality rates remained undeterminable, its impact remained immense nonetheless and not negligible in any way. Even though the mortality rate among the Khoikhoi could not be accurately and consistently recorded, it did not imply that smallpox was less severe among the Khoikhoi either and therefore less catastrophic. However, in order to determine the impact smallpox had on a Khoikhoi community, the mortality rate as recorded among the Piketberg Khoikhoi (Cochoqua) community in February 1714 serves as a good barometer. It provides concrete evidence as to what damage smallpox caused among a particular village and kraal. A delegation of Khoikhoi survivors that arrived at the Cape Castle stating that 'one out of ten members of their society had survived' serves as ample evidence to assess the impact of smallpox on a clan.[87] In this particular case, which is probably, the exception rather than the rule, the mortality rate stood at a very high 90% based on the word of the survivors. The Khoikhoi leaders themselves calculated the mortality rate among their followers. In their assessment, the death toll was severe and concluded that 'one out of ten members' survived smallpox.[88] In other words, assuming a clan comprised of ten individuals, nine had died and only one survived. It suggests that an entire clan or clans had been decimated, leaving behind only a few survivors. Here, the recovery rate was essentially zero, assuming that the remaining 10% was not even infected, but yet still affected by smallpox on so many other levels, of which their political organization was one. In this particular case, the death of four Khoikhoi leaders, notably, Asdrubal, Jason, Hartloop and Kounga, left a leadership vacuum among the Piketberg Khoikhoi. Travelling to Cape Town was a matter of necessity rather than an act of irresponsible behaviour and risk contracting smallpox. In the end, the journey to Cape Town in the midst of an epidemic was undertaken for at least three reasons. In the first instance, they could report to the Cape authorities that although smallpox may have subsided in Cape Town and life returned to some degree of normality, within the interior, however, specifically the Piketberg region, smallpox infections were still rife and a major threat among the Khoikhoi. Second, they reported the severity of the situation and losses suffered by the Khoikhoi. Third, they requested that the acting Cape Governor, Willem Helot, appoint and approve new Khoikhoi leaders. Despite the fact that smallpox was highly infectious and fear of transmission a real possibility, the acting Governor granted their request and allowed the Khoikhoi delegation access to the Castle. At the Cape Castle, Scipio Africanus succeeded Asdrubal, Hannibal succeeded Jason, Hercules succeeded Hartloop and Kounga succeeded his father, also named Kounga.[89] Helot had merely continued a tradition started by the Van der Stel family (Simon and later Willem Adriaan) when they governed the Cape during the latter half of the seventeenth century until the early eighteenth century in 1707.[90] The ratification of Khoikhoi leadership by another political force – a Governor representing the VOC – suggests that the Piketberg Khoikhoi had fallen politically apart before the 1713 epidemic and were therefore no longer as autonomous as they had hoped to be. Moreover, the fact that four different captains were appointed suggests that more than a solitary clan was affected, but several clans or sub-clans. In this case at least four. Elphick writes that these Khoikhoi leaders that arrived at the Castle were part of a 'cluster of clans' spread across the region of Piketberg.[91] This scenario painted an even bleaker picture, which suggests that the impact of smallpox was much more severe. According to the historian Dan Sleigh, the impact of the 1713 was clearly visible among the Khoikhoi of the Drakenstein Mountains towards Vier-En- Twintig Rivieren and cited the destructive nature of epidemic as a factor for the reduction of the Khoikhoi people in the region.[92] Later in November 1714, a company trader, David Feijerabend, who directed a trade expedition into the same region, witnessed the devastation brought about by smallpox. He reported that he encountered several depleted and scattered Khoikhoi kraals and a few impoverished survivors. Despite witnessing their plight, he still exploited their dire situation and managed to trade 391 head of cattle.[93] Among the few survivors, economic recovery seems appeared to have been slow among the regional Khoikhoi. When another VOC trade expedition entered the same region two years later in 1716, the impoverished Khoikhoi communities headed by several equally impoverished Khoi leaders, notably, Scipio and six others, were not in a position to trade at all which suggests that the Khoi affected by the epidemic battled to recover economically and possibly on many other fronts.[94] As far Africanus Scipio was concerned, his wealth seems to have been depleted very quickly since 1712. Elphick writes that Kaij Jesse Slotsboo, a VOC official, noted that during an expedition he led to the region in 1712, Scipio was fairly wealthy and owned at least 2,000 sheep.[95] Six years later, in 1716, he was completely impoverished, which suggests that the combination of pressurized trade and smallpox had taken its toll on Scipio personally and other leaders of associated clans, let alone their respective followers.

We can only assume that many more such examples existed, including the very high mortality rate of 90% when the average mortality rate of smallpox was usually set between 20% and 50% as mentioned earlier. Presumably in the same vicinity Khoikhoi kraals and villages suffered a similar fate or worst, and simply went by unnoticed and unrecorded. For instance, in 1767, according to the Cape records, fifty-three Khoikhoi died of smallpox. These Khoikhoi were presumably employed by colonists in Cape Town or eeked out a living in and around Cape Town. Their deaths were easily recorded as they were known within the immediate community and labour economy of Cape Town. Clearly, based on the colonial correspondence between the local *Landdrost* (Magistrate) of Swellendam and Cape Governor, more than fifty-three Khoikhoi died countrywide where its impact was much more severe in the interior. Exactly how many Khoikhoi had died was not accurately recorded in the same manner as colonists, slaves and free blacks. Deceased colonists had left behind relatives, friends, wills and testaments and slaves had owners. One would imagine in both cases, relatives and slave owners had notified the authorities of smallpox-related deaths.

Mortality figures were recorded along racial and ethnic lines. It exposed how racially and ethnically divided Cape society had become. The recorders of the mortality rates in 1755 and 1767 had categorized the deceased along racial lines. Those that died of smallpox were separately categorized as colonists/burghers (European origin), VOC slaves (property of the VOC, mixed Asian/Oriental ancestry), free black community (freed slaves, mixed Asian/Oriental ancestry) and Khoikhoi (African and indigenous ancestry).[96] Indicative of how racially divided the Cape had become that even during an epidemic, categorization of people along class, racial and ethnic lines had to be maintained by the Dutch rulers. It appears as though 'racial immunity' as argued by Mark Harrison[97] had existed at the Cape, even though the statistics told a different story.

Smallpox transformed the geographical and political landscape of the interior and expedited the transition of the Khoikhoi into becoming a labour force during the eighteenth century. The virus struck among the Khoikhoi at the worst possible time in their history. Though the epidemic only lasted at most a few months of the year when it struck, the aftermath was often too severe to readjust and rebuild their lives and livelihood as autonomous pastoralists and hunter-gatherers. Unoccupied land left vacant by Khoikhoi who fled deeper into the interior was eventually reoccupied by a new generation of colonial stock farmers, called *trekboers*. Leonard Guelke argued that key areas settled by *trekboers* before 1720 included the Berg River region which incorporated the Piketberg region.[98] The possibility exists that these areas had become depopulated owing to colonial expansion and intrusion, but also through flight when impoverished Khoikhoi herders were left without livestock and a future livelihood, so much so that they sought alternative ways in order to survive, of which becoming farm servants was an alternative.

Equally, so, not all Khoikhoi communities or clans were as strong as the next one and often differed in size and numbers. Towards the end of November 1714, the livestock-less sub-clans of Piketberg Khoi had shown signs of economic disintegration. Recovery patterns of larger clans were much better than smaller clans. For instance, though smallpox affected the Namaqua Khoikhoi in 1755, their record of recovery appeared impressive and soon became 'again numerous'. Their size as a group ensured their survival and greater recovery rate. In 1761, the trader, explorer and traveller, Hendrik Hop 'noticed that the chickenpox ([*sic*] smallpox) which visited the Cape in 1755 has the same time raged here to a great extent among these tribes. This notwithstanding, these Namaquas are again numerous, they live scattered in small kraals and villages and for the rest lives without any captain, always in peace with one another'.[99]

In some Khoi communities, cracks caused by poverty were visible prior to the arrival of smallpox. Prior to smallpox, Khoikhoi had already entered the colonial labour market as farm servants.[100] Smallpox brought about irrevocable change and as such, it engulfed every aspect of Cape society. Each time it struck, it brought into being an abnormality which disrupted the lives, lifestyles and livelihoods of people from all walks of life and nationalities. All Cape communities suffered losses, however; the rich, the poor, *trekboers* in the interior, indigenous Khoikhoi, slaves, men, women and children succumbed to a disease that knew no age, class, colour, culture, race, gender and religion. Wealthy and middle-class Cape burghers that died of smallpox bequeathed their possessions and wealth in their wills and testaments to next of kin and named beneficiaries.[101] Others, especially slaves and Khoi, died without a trace and even anonymously. For the Khoikhoi, graves covered with small stones became the only visible epitaph and reminder of the departed and timely reminder of the unknown and uncountable victims of smallpox. In the interior, 'graves' and 'stones' represented those that died of smallpox, but also served as a grim reminder of a traumatic period of their history and how disease changed the course of their future and possibly even their existence.[102] It reinforced and revealed the unlikely and bitter bond that existed between smallpox and Khoikhoi society.

While the Dutch sought spiritual intervention to end smallpox, the Khoikhoi had held the Dutch directly responsible for its introduction to the Cape in 1713. In Khoikhoi society, a direct association existed between colonial conquest and smallpox. By holding the Dutch accountable for the introduction of smallpox, they had in fact alluded to disease as a form of colonial conquest. By implication, European conquest and contact was the real curse and the introduction of smallpox a direct consequence of colonial rule.

The post smallpox period of recovery and reintegration of survivors was either very slow or non-existent. The *Caabse* (Cape) Khoikhoi communities that fled from Cape Town in 1713 never returned. The Peninsular Khoikhoi communities thus disappeared from this landscape in the post-smallpox era. At each juncture of a particular post-smallpox period, as seen in 1713, 1755 and 1767, Khoikhoi society found itself in a state of transition as survivors – left without livestock and land – offered their services to white farmers as many found themselves on the brink of poverty. In many instances, it led to the depopulation of indigenous communities within certain areas. Although the Khoikhoi remained a factor within Cape society, their autonomy remained under pressure. At the very least, smallpox exposed fault lines within their own internal social, political and economic structures.

The Cape Khoikhoi had failed to reinvent themselves in the post-epidemic years as evidence suggests that post-smallpox period of recovery following each outbreak of smallpox appeared extremely challenging. Loss of their land and livestock invariably meant loss of their livelihood and a life of poverty. Many individuals and families fled without their livestock or their possessions in an effort to survive. If nothing else, it plunged, if not hurried, the Khoikhoi into a phase of economic destruction rather than one of reconstruction. Invariably, each post-smallpox period of recovery was characterized by poverty and dislocation. In the absence of land and livestock, it forced the Khoikhoi to sell their labour as herders and shepherds in the emerging stock farming economy and as menial labourers in the agrarian sector of the economy. Sadly, for many Khoikhoi, it became their only means of survival in a changing labour-intensive economy and society.

The backlash of smallpox far exceeded fatalities, however. Each post-smallpox period of recovery seemed worse than the one before and suggests that after each epidemic, Khoikhoi society appeared more politically destabilized, physiologically infertile, physically scarred, psychologically broken, economically poverty stricken and socially ruined. If nothing else, it accelerated the assimilation and integration of survivors and the generation thereafter into colonial society and redefined their independent status within the confines of the Cape Colony. During each outbreak, though it appeared periodically throughout the course of the eighteenth century, it initiated new challenges and on each occasion, the consequences of smallpox epidemics were far more unforgiving than the previous time. Smallpox, indeed, proved a curse in more ways than one. The Khoikhoi generation of 1713 and the ones that followed, however, despite harbouring hope, never materialized politically, economically or otherwise. The Khoikhoi were, therefore, never 'free from this evil sickness', known as smallpox. And neither would humanity be totally freed from the scourge of smallpox. The arrival of smallpox in 1713 had put the Cape Colony and its inhabitants on alert of future outbreaks and epidemics. Prior to and since the eighteenth century, it would periodically appear, disappear and reappear until deep into the twentieth century and strike when it was least expected. Allan Ingram's recently-written and chapter title: "How Small is Small?: Small pox and Large Presence" is very thought-provoking indeed. It encapsulates the "Large Presence" of smallpox in human history.[103] As smallpox *variola* is a minute virus transmitted through often invisible droplets, face-to-face contact with humans and infected clothing, its presence, within our global world and in the history of humanity, remained and loomed large.

NOTES

1. François Valentyn, *Description of the Cape of Good Hope with the Matters Concerning It,* eds. P. Serton, R. Raven-Hart, and W.J. de Kock (Cape Town: Van Riebeeck Society, Part 1, Second Series, no. 2, 1971), 217.

2. The book authored by François Valentyn is titled: *Oud en Nieuw Oost-Indien, Beskrywing van Malabaar, Japan, Kaap der Goede Hoop, en 't Eyland Mauritius,* vyfde deels, tweede druk (Joannes van Braam & Gerard Onder de Lingen, Amsterdam & Dordrecht, 1726). François Valentyn was born in 1666, Dordrecht, The Netherlands. He was a trained minister of religion and was employed by the VOC since the age of nineteen in the Moluccas. He later moved to Ambon as a field chaplain. He remained in the service of the VOC his entire life and returned to the Netherlands in 1714. He died in 1727 aged sixty-one, a year after his book, *Oud en Nieuw Oost-Indien,* was published in 1726. Valentyn stayed over at the Cape four times in 1685, 1695, 1705 and for the last time in 1714. Over a period of twenty-nine years, he stayed at the Cape for a period six months. See introduction of *Description of the Cape of Good Hope with the matters concerning it,* for an English summary of his biography by Prof P Serton, 3–30.

3. Eric W, Banister, Murray Allen, Samia, Fadl, Gordon, Bhakthan, Dawn Howard, *Contemporary Health Issues* (London, Boston: Jones and Bartlett Publishers, 1988), 10.

4. See Robert Ross, "Smallpox at the Cape of Good Hope in the eighteenth century", in *African Historical Demography,* vol.1, eds. C Fyfe and D McMasters (Centre for African Studies: University of Edinburgh, 1977), 416–428; Achmat Davids, "'The Revolt of the Malays': A Study of the reactions of the Cape Muslim

to smallpox epidemics of nineteenth-century Cape Town", in *Studies in the History of Cape Town,* vol.5, ed., Christopher Saunders (Cape Town, UCT,1983), 47–79; Elizabeth van Heyningen, "Epidemics and Disease: Historical Writing on Health in South Africa", *South African Historical Journal*, 23 (1990):122–133; Andrew Smith, "Khoikhoi susceptibility to virgins soil epidemics in the 18th century", *South African Medical Journal,* 75, 7 (January 1989):25–26; Russel Viljoen, "Disease and Society: VOC Cape Town, its people and the smallpox epidemics of 1713, 1755 and 1767". *Kleio,* XXVII (1995):22–45; Howard Phillips, "Smallpox, 1713–1893", in *Plague, Pox and Pandemics,* Howard Phillips, (Auckland Park: Jacana, 2012), 1–37; Russel Viljoen, "Debating and Debunking Some Myths surrounding the Decline of the Overberg Khoikhoi with reference to the smallpox epidemics of 1755 and 1767", Unpublished conference paper, South African Historical Society, Rhodes University, 1995). See Sumner La Croix, "The Khoikhoi Population 1651–1780: A Review of the evidence and Two New Estimates", *Studies in Economics and Econometrics*, 42, no. 1 (2018):15–34.

5. Mark Harrison, *Contagion: How Commerce Has Spread Disease* (New Haven and London: Yale University Press, 2012), 16.

6. Willam H McNeill, *Plagues and Peoples* (London: Penquin, 1976), 185ff.

7. Valentyn, *Description of the Cape of Good Hope*, 33.

8. Harrison, *Contagion*, see chapters 1 and 2.

9. Maurice Boucher, *The Cape of Good Hope and the foreign contacts 1735–1755* (Pretoria: University of South Africa Press, 1985), 12–13.

10. McNeill, *Plagues and Peoples*, 185ff.

11. Boucher, *The Cape of Good Hope*, 12–13.

12. Donald Moodie, *The Record or Series of Official Papers Relative to the Condition and Treatment of the Native Tribes of South Africa (*Amsterdam and Cape Town: AA Balkema, 1960), 143. H.B. Thom, ed., *Journal of Van Riebeeck Vol 2, 1656–1658* (Cape Town, Amsterdam: AA Balkema, 1954), 346.

13. Moodie, *The Record*, 146.

14. Moodie, *The Record*, 176–178.

15. Moodie, *The Record*, 291.

16. Moodie, *The Record*, 272.

17. Moodie, *The Record*, 291.

18. Moodie, *The Record,* 336.

19. Moodie, *The Record,* 420.

20. Richard Elphick, *Khoikhoi and the Founding of White South Africa* (Johannesburg: Ravan Press, 1985), 47 and 58; Leonard Guelke and Robert Shell, "Landscape of Conquest: Frontier water alienation and Khoikhoi strategies of survival, 1652–1780", *Journal of Southern African Studies*, 18, no. 4 (1992):803–824; Andrew Smith, "One becoming Herders: Khoikhoi and San ethnicity in Southern Africa", *African Studies*, 49, no. 2 (1990):51–73; See special issue in *Southern African Humanities*, (December 2008), titled: "Khoekhoe and the origins of herding in southern Africa", eds. Francois-Xavier Fauvelle-Aymar and Karim Sadr, 1–248.

21. Donald R Hopkins, *The Greatest Killer: Smallpox in History* (Chicago: The University of Chicago Press, 2002), 22–102.

22. Gareth Williams, *Angel of Death: The Story of Smallpox* (Basingstoke: Palgrave Macmillan 2010), 2.

23. Jenifer Lee, Carrell, *The Speckled Monster: A Historical Tale of Battling Smallpox* (New York: Dutton, 2003); John R Smith, *The Speckled Monster: Smallpox in England 1670–1970 with particular reference to Essex* (Chelmsford: Essex Record Office, 1987).

24. Frank Fenner, Donald Henderson, Arita, Isao, Jezek, Zdenek and Ivan Ladnyi, *Smallpox and its Eradication* (Geneva: World Health Organization, 1988), 233–234.

25. Williams, *Angel of Death,* 24; TH, Pennington, "Poxviruses: Smallpox, molluscum contagiosum; parapoxvirus infections", in *Medical Microbiology: A Guide to Microbial Infections: Pathogenesis, Immunity, Laboratory, Diagnosis and Control,* eds. David Greenwood, Richard Slack, John Peutherer (New York: Churchill Livingstone, 1997, 15th edition), 426.

26. Pennington, "Poxviruses: Smallpox", 425.

27. Williams, *Angel of Death,* 20; Hopkins, *The Greatest Killer: Smallpox in History*, 3–4.

28. Pennington, "Poxviruses: Smallpox", 426. See also Williams, *Angel of Death,* 21 for an explanation of the medical terms in brackets used by Pennington.

29. Kelvin Jones and Graham Moon, *Health, Disease and Society: An Introduction to Medical Geography* (London and New York: Routledge, 1992), 146–150.

30. Jones and Moon, *Health, Disease and Society*, 148.

31. Jones and Moon, *Health, Disease and Society*, 148.

32. Williams, *Angel of Death*, 20.

33. Western Cape Archives and Records Service (WCARS), Verbatim Copies (hereafter VC) VC 20 *Dagh Register,* 6 May 1713, 121.

34. Johannes Van Steeland was born in 1659 in the city of Delft, The Netherlands. He died on 19 May 1717 aged fifty-seven in Delft. His entire career (more than thirty years) was served in various positions within VOC which began in 1679 as a salary accountant in Machilipatnam. He was promoted through the ranks and became the governor of Coromandel in 1705–1710, a strategic region on the east coast of India. Since November 1710, he was member of the Council of the Indies in Batavia until he returned to the Netherlands in 1713. See www.vocsite.nl and www.vocsite.nl /geschiedenis /biografie.html?id=505 (accessed on 15 February 2021).

35. Valentyn, *Description of the Cape of Good Hope,* 217.

36. www.resources.huygens.knaw.nl/das/detail/voyage/97167 (accessed on 15 February 2021); www.vocsite.nl and www.vocsite.nl/geschiedenis /biografie.html?id =505 (accessed on 15 February 2021).

37. www.resources.huygens.knaw.nl/das/detail/voyage/97167 (accessed on 15 February 2021).

38. Williams, *Angel of Death,* 18–19.

39. Valentyn, *Description of the Cape of Good Hope*, 217.

40. Williams, *Angel of Death,* 13.

41. Valentyn, *Description of the Cape of Good Hope*, 101.

42. WCARS VC 20 *Dagh Register*, 7 and 14 May 1713, 126.

43. Valentyn, *Description of the Cape of Good Hope*, 79.

44. See Daniel Sleigh, *Die Buiteposte: VOC-Buiteposte onder Kaapse bestuur 1652–1795* (Pretoria: Protea Boekhuis, 2007), 248, 282, 381, 498 and 499.

45. WCARS VC 20 *Dagh Register,* 18 April 1713, 109

46. WCARS VC 20 *Dagh Register,* 20 April 1713, 111.

47. WCARS VC 20 *Dagh Register*, 1 May 1713, 118. "*thans begint de sterfte door kinderpokjes onder de Africaense inboorlinge seer door te dringen*".

48. WCARS VC 20 *Dagh Register,* 3 May 1713, 119.

49. "*arme Hottentot niet zyn van ramspoedige dese siektes niet kennende*". WCARS VC 20 *Dagh Register*, 6 May 1713, 121.

50. WCARS VC 20 *Dagh Register*, 1 May 1713, 118; 3 May 1713, 119. "*gevolge deselven genesingh onkunding daarvoor seer jammerlijk worden weggeruk*".

51. WCARS VC 20 *Dagh Register*, May 1713, 118.

52. Russel Viljoen, "Medicine, Health and Medical Practice in Precolonial Khoikhoi society, An Anthropological and Historical Perspective", *History and Anthropology*, 11, no. 4 (1999):515–536.

53. Banister, et.al., *Contemporary Health Issues,* 11.

54. Wim van Damme and Wim van Lerberghe, W, "Editorial: Epidemics and Fear", *Tropical Medicine and International Health*, 5, no. 8 (August 2000): 511–514.

55. Philip D Curtin, "Killing Diseases of the Tropical World" in *Death by Migration. Europe's Encounter with the Tropical World in the Nineteenth Century,* ed. Philip D. Curtin (Cambridge: Cambridge University Press, 1989), 62–79.

56. WCARS VC 20 *Dagh Register*, 19 May 1713.

57. WCARS VC 20 *Dagh Register*, 28 November 1713.

58. WCARS VC 20 *Dagh Register*, 10 June 1713, 145, 23 June 1713, 157.

59. Travelling along the N7 from Cape Town to Piketberg, the distance is set to be about 130 kilometres. See WCARS VC 20 *Dagh Register*, 14 February 1714, 39, 45–46.

60. See WCARS VC 20 *Dagh Register*, 14 February 1714, 39, 45–46.

61. Hopkins, *The Greatest Killer*, 245.

62. TM, Zameer-Careem, "The History of Smallpox in Sri Lanka: Humanity's Triumph over a Global Scourge", *University of Colombo Review* (Series 111), 1, no. 1 (2020):21.

63. WCARS VC 27 *Dagh Register*, 12 and 20 May 1755.

64. WCARS C 492 *Letters Received*, 20 August 1755, 57–59.

65. WCARS VC 27 *Dagh Register*, 21 June 1755.

66. Viljoen, "Disease and Society", 29; WCARS VC 27 *Dagh Register*, 21 June 1755.

67. WCARS VC 27 *Dagh Register*, 24 June 1755.

68. In August 1755, the total death toll stood at 468, in September 1755, 107 and October 1755 it dropped to 35 deaths. Winter in South Africa began in May to August.

69. Viljoen, "Disease and Society", 36; WCARS VC 30, *Dagh Register*, 5 May 1767.

70. WCARS C 520 *Letters Received*, 22 February 1769, 58–59.

71. McNeill, *Plagues and Peoples*, 185ff.

72. S. L. Kotar and J. E. Gessler, *Smallpox: A History* (McFarland & Company Publishers, Jefferson, North Carolina and London, 2013), 5–6, 24, 26.

73. Moodie, *The Record,* 336.

74. Isaac Schapera, *The Khoisan Peoples of South Africa: Bushmen and Hottentots* (London: Routledge & Keegan Paul, 1963), 358–361.

75. WCARS VC 27 *Dagh Register,* 31 July 1755.

76. WCARS VC 27 *Dagh Register*, 10 July 1755.

77. WCARS VC 27 *Dagh Register* 8 July 1755: seventeen Europeans, twelve slaves died; 10 July 1755: fifteen slaves and fourteen burghers died; 11 July 1755: twelve burghers and twelve slaves died; 12 July 1755, twenty-three burghers and twelve slaves died; 13 July 1755: fourteen burghers died; 14 July 1755, fifteen burghers and nine slaves died.

78. WCARS VC 27 *Dagh Register*, 25 July 1755.

79. WCARS VC 27 *Dagh Register*, 4 and 9 August 1755.

80. Elphick, *Khoikhoi and the Founding of White South Africa*, 231.

81. Dorothy Fairbridge, *Lady Anne Barnard at the Cape of Good Hope 1797–1802* (Oxford: Clarendon Press, 1924), 68–69.

82. Carl Peter, Thunberg, *Carl Peter Thunberg Travels at the Cape of Good Hope 1772–1775* (VS Forbes (ed) Second Series no.17, (Cape Town: Van Riebeeck Society, 1986), 170.

83. Valentyn, *Description of the Cape of Good Hope,* 217.

84. Otto Friedrich, Mentzel, *A Geographical and Topographical Description of the Cape of Good Hope* (translated and edited by G.C. Marais, J. Hoge and H.J. Mandelbrote), Part 2, (Cape Town: Van Riebeeck Society, 1925), 127.

85. WCARS C 492 *Letters Received*, 20 August 1755, 57–59.

86. WCARS VC 30 *Dagh Register*, May 1767, 180ff. The monthly statistics of deaths among free blacks (freed slaves) Khoikhoi were recorded as follows: 30 June 1767, fifty-three Khoikhoi and free blacks died of smallpox; 31 August 1767, twenty-one Khoikhoi and freed slaves died; 30 September 1767, twenty-one Khoikhoi and free blacks died; 31 October 1767, fourteen Khoikhoi and free blacks died; November 1767, 31 December 1767, seven Khoikhoi and free blacks died.

87. WCARS VC 20 *Dagh Register*, 14 February 1714, 39, 45–46.

88. WCARS VC 20 *Dagh Register*, 14 February 1714, 39, 45–46.

89. WCARS VC 20 *Dagh Register*, 14 February 1714, 39, 45–46.

90. Elphick, *Khoikhoi and the Founding of White South Africa*, 191.

91. Elphick, *Khoikhoi and the Founding of White South Africa*, 233.

92. Sleigh, *Die Buiteposte*, 69,70.

93. Sleigh, *Die Buiteposte*, 68, 69,70.

94. Sleigh, *Die Buiteposte*, 70.

95. Elphick, *Khoikhoi and the Founding of White South Africa*, 230.

96. WCARS VC 27 *Dagh Register*, 31 October 1755.

97. Mark Harrison, "'The Tender Frame of Man': Disease, Climate, and Racial difference in India and West Indies, 1760–1860", *Bulletin of the History of Medicine*, 70, no. 1 (1996):68.

98. Leonard Guelke, "Freehold farmers and frontier settlers, 1657–1780", in *The Shaping South African Society, 1652–1840*, eds. Richard Elphick and Hermann Giliomee (Johannesburg: Maskew Miller Longman, 1989), 85.

99. EE Mossop, ed., *The Journals of Brink and Rhenius being The Journal of Carel Frederick Brink of the journey into Great Namaqualand (1761–2) Made by Captain Hendrik Hop and The Journal of Ensign Johannes Tobias Rhenius (1724)* (Cape Town: Van Riebeeck Society, no. 28, 1947), 57.

100. Part Two of Valentyn, *Description of the Cape of Good Hope with the Matters Concerning It*, eds. Raidt and Raven-Hart, 75.

101. See Inventories of the Orphan Chamber (MOOC) WCARS, MOOC 8/1/12, testator Jan Heijns, 12 August 1767; WCARS, MOOC 8/8/13 Testator Johanna Hanekom, 11 September 1755 for a two examples. See the website www.tanap.net

102. Thunberg, *Carl Peter Thunberg Travels at the Cape of Good Hope 1772–1775*, 97; Anders Sparrman, *A Voyage to the Cape of Good Hope towards the Antartic Polar Circle Round the World and the Country of the Hottentots and the Caffres from the year 1772–1776*, eds. V. Forbes and I. Rudner (Second Series no.6, Cape Town: Van Riebeeck Society, 1975), vol. 1, 283.

103. Allan Ingram, "How Small is Small?: Small Pox and Large Presence", in *Disease and Death in Eighteenth-Century Literature and Culture*, eds. Alan Ingram and Leigh Wetherall, Dickson (London: Palgrave Macmillan, 2016), 145–164.

BIBLIOGRAPHY

Banister, Eric W., Murray Allen, Samia Fadl, Gordon Bhakthan, and Dawn Howard. *Contemporary Health Issues*. London, Boston: Jones and Bartlett Publishers, 1988.

Boucher, Maurice. *The Cape of Good Hope and the Foreign Contacts 1735–1755*. Pretoria: University of South Africa Press, 1985.

Carrell, Jennifer Lee. *The Speckled Monster: A Historical Tale of Battling Smallpox*. New York: Dutton, 2003.

Curtin, Philip D. "Killing diseases of the tropical world", in *Death by Migration: Europe's Encounter with the Tropical World in the Nineteenth Century*, edited by Philip D Curtin. Cambridge: Cambridge University Press, 1989.

Davids, Achmat. "'The Revolt of the Malays': A Study of the reactions of the Cape Muslim to smallpox epidemics of nineteenth-century Cape Town", in *Studies in the History of Cape Town*, vol.5, edited by Christopher Saunders, 47–79. Cape Town, UCT, 1983.

Elphick, Richard. *Khoikhoi and the Founding of White South Africa*. Johannesburg: Ravan Press, 1985.

Fairbridge, Dorothy. *Lady Anne Barnard at the Cape of Good Hope 1797–1802*. Oxford: Clarendon Press, 1924.

Fauvelle-Aymar, Francois-Xavier and Karim Sadr. "Khoekhoe and the origins of herding in southern Africa", Special issue in *Southern African Humanities*, (December 2008):1–248.

Fenner, Frank, Donald Henderson, Isao Arita, Zdenek Jezek, and Ivan Ladnyi. *Smallpox and its Eradication.* Geneva: World Health Organization, 1988.

Guelke, Leonard. "Freehold farmers and frontier settlers, 1657–1780", in Richard Elphick and Hermann Giliomee, eds., *The Shaping South African Society, 1652–1840.* Johannesburg: Maskew Miller Longman, 1989.

Guelke, Leonard, and Robert Shell. "Landscape of Conquest: Frontier water alienation and Khoikhoi strategies of survival, 1652–1780", *Journal of Southern African Studies*, 18, no. 4 (1992):803–824.

Harrison, Mark. "'The Tender Frame of Man': Disease, Climate, and Racial difference in India and West Indies, 1760–1860", *Bulletin of the History of Medicine*, 70, no. 1 (1996):68.

Harrison, Mark. *Contagion: How Commerce Has Spread Disease*. New Haven and London: Yale University Press, 2012.

Hopkins, Donald R. *The Greatest Killer: Smallpox in History*. Chicago: The University of Chicago Press, 2002.

Ingram, Allan. "How Small is Small?: Small Pox and Large Presence", in *Disease and Death in Eighteenth-Century Literature and Culture,* edited by Alan Ingram and Leigh Wetherall, Dickson, 145–164. London: Palgrave Macmillan, 2016.

Jones, Kelvin, and Graham Moon. *Health, Disease and Society: An Introduction to Medical Geography*. London and New York: Routledge, 1992.

Kotar, S. L., and J. E. Gessler. *Smallpox: A History.* North Carolina and London: McFarland & Company Publishers, Jefferson, 2013.

La Croix, Sumner. "The Khoikhoi Population 1651–1780: A Review of the evidence and Two New Estimates", *Studies in Economics and Econometrics*, 42, no. 1 (2018):15–34.

McNeill, Willam H. *Plagues and Peoples*. London: Penguin, 1976.

Mentzel, Otto Friedrich. *A Geographical and Topographical Description of the Cape of Good Hope* (translated and edited by G.C. Marais, J. Hoge and H.J. Mandelbrote), Part 2, Cape Town: Van Riebeeck Society, 1925.

Moodie, Donald. *The Record Or Series of Official Papers Relative to the Condition and Treatment of the Native Tribes of South Africa.* Amsterdam and Cape Town: AA Balkema, 1960.

Mossop, E. E., ed. *The Journals of Brink and Rhenius being The Journal of Carel Frederick Brink of the Journey into Great Namaqualand (1761-2) Made by Captain Hendrik Hop and The Journal of Ensign Johannes Tobias Rhenius (1724),* no. 28, Cape Town: Van Riebeeck Society 1947.

Pennington, T. H. "Poxviruses: Smallpox, Molluscum Contagiosum; Parapoxvirus Infections", in *Medical Microbiology: A Guide to Microbial Infections: Pathogenesis, Immunity, Laboratory, Diagnosis and Control,* edited by David Greenwood, Richard Slack, and John Peutherer. New York: Churchill Livingstone, 1997, 15th edition.

Phillips, Howard. *Plague, Pox and Pandemics.* Auckland Park: Jacana, 2012.

Ross, Robert. "Smallpox at the Cape of Good Hope in the Eighteenth Century", in *African Historical Demography*, vol. 1, edited by C. Fyfe and D. McMasters. Centre for African Studies, University of Edinburgh, 1977.

Schapera, Isaac. *The Khoisan Peoples of South Africa: Bushmen and Hottentots.* London: Routledge & Keegan Paul, 1963.

Sleigh, Daniel. *Die Buiteposte: VOC-Buiteposte onder Kaapse bestuur 1652–1795.* Pretoria: Protea Boekhuis, 2007.

Smith, Andrew. "Khoikhoi Susceptibility to Virgin Soil Epidemics in the 18th Century", *South African Medical Journal,* 75, no. 7 (January 1989):25–26.

Smith, Andrew. "One Becoming Herders: Khoikhoi and San Ethnicity in Southern Africa", *African Studies*, 49, no. 2 (1990):51–73.

Smith, John R. *The Speckled Monster: Smallpox in England 1670–1970 with Particular Reference to Essex.* Chelmsford: Essex Record Office, 1987.

Sparrman, Anders. *A Voyage to the Cape of Good Hope towards the Antartic Polar Circle Round the World and the Country of the Hottentots and the Caffres from the Year 1772–1776,* vol. 1, V Forbes, J and I Rudner eds., Second Series no.6. Cape Town: Van Riebeeck Society, 1975.

Thom, H. B., ed. *Journal of Van Riebeeck Vol 2, 1656–1658.* Cape Town, Amsterdam: AA Balkema, 1954.

Thunberg, Carl Peter. *Carl Peter Thunberg Travels at the Cape of Good Hope 1772–1775,* VS Forbes, ed. Second Series no.17. Cape Town: Van Riebeeck Society, 1986.

Valentyn, François. *Description of the Cape of Good Hope with the Matters Concerning It.* Edited by P. Serton, R. Raven-Hart, and W.J. de Kock. Part 1, Second Series, no. 2. Cape Town: Van Riebeeck Society, 1971.

Van Damme, Wim, and Wim Van Lerberghe. "Editorial: Epidemics and Fear", *Tropical Medicine and International Health*, 5, no. 8 (August 2000):511–514.

Van Heyningen, Elizabeth. "Epidemics and Disease: Historical Writing on Health in South Africa", *South African Historical Journal*, 23 (1990):122–133.

Viljoen, Russel. "Debating and Debunking Some Myths surrounding the Decline of the Overberg Khoikhoi with reference to the smallpox epidemics of 1755 and 1767", Unpublished conference paper, South African Historical Society, Rhodes University, 1995.

Viljoen, Russel. "Disease and Society: VOC Cape Town, Its People and the Smallpox Epidemics of 1713, 1755 and 1767", *Kleio,* XXVII, (1995):22–45.

Viljoen, Russel. "Medicine, Health and Medical Practice in Precolonial Khoikhoi society, An Anthropological and Historical Perspective", *History and Anthropology*, 11, no. 4 (1999):515–536.

Williams, Gareth. *Angel of Death: The Story of Smallpox.* London: Palgrave Macmillan, 2010.

Zameer-Careem, T. M. "The History of Smallpox in Sri Lanka: Humanity's Triumph over a Global Scourge", *University of Colombo Review* (Series 111), 1, no. 1 (2020):21.

PRIMARY SOURCES

Western Cape Archives and Records Service (WCARS), Verbatim Copies (hereafter VC)

WCARS C 492 *Letters Received*, 20 August 1755.

WCARS C 520 *Letters Received*, 22 February 1769.

WCARS VC 20 *Dagh Register,* 18 April 1713.

WCARS VC 20 *Dagh Register*, 1, 3, 6, 7, 14, 19 May 1713.

WCARS VC 20 *Dagh Register*, 10, 23 June 1713.

WCARS VC 20 *Dagh Register*, 28 November 1713.

WCARS VC 20 *Dagh Register*, 14 February 1714.

WCARS VC 27 *Dagh Register*, 12 and 20 May 1755.

WCARS VC 27 *Dagh Register*, 21 and 24 June 1755.

WCARS VC 27 *Dagh Register,* 8, 10, 25, 31 July 1755.

WCARS VC 27 *Dagh Register*, 4 and 9 August 1755.

WCARS VC 27 *Dagh Register*, 31 October 1755.

WCARS VC 30 *Dagh Register*, 5 May 1767.

WCARS Inventories of the Orphan Chamber (MOOC) MOOC 8/1/12, 12 August 1767 MOOC 8//8/13, 11 September 1755.

WEBSITES

www.tanap.net

www.vocsite.nl and www.vocsite.nl/geschiedenis /biografie.html?id=505

www.resources.huygens.knaw.nl/das/detail/voyage/97167

Chapter 5

Measles

The Undercover Killer

Elizabeth van Heyningen

In the midst of the COVID-19 pandemic, we are all authorities on viral diseases. New words and their concepts have entered our vocabulary, such as 'cytokine storm'. But if one suggests that measles is a far more serious disease than COVID-19, one is met with blank incomprehension.

Measles arouses none of the fears associated with leprosy, smallpox or plague, to name only three of the infectious diseases that have ravaged human societies. Nor is it usually associated either with colonial conquest or with the social controls introduced into the colonized world under cover of public health. On the contrary, until 1963, when an effective vaccine was introduced and it was, briefly, eradicated from the Americas and parts of Europe, it was seen primarily as a minor childhood disease. Yet measles may be the single most infectious disease that has afflicted human beings. In the twentieth century, when populations were large enough to establish endemicity, it was very widespread. In most countries over 90% of children contracted it, conferring immunity for life.[1]

Such a view is misleading, for measles is a highly infectious and potentially lethal disease since it damages the immune system, often resulting in death from other ailments; on occasion its mortality rate has rivalled that of the Black Death. This is particularly true of communities that have not encountered the disease recently; where no 'herd immunity' has been achieved. Imperial expansion and conquest have played major roles in spreading measles to vulnerable indigenous societies. This chapter examines the way in which measles has impacted on the colonial world from the time of the Spanish conquest of South America in the fifteenth century to the twentieth century, arguing that measles was frequently introduced into societies whose health status was already eroded; in addition, this tendency of measles to suppress the immune system may have weakened further the ability of indigenous societies to resist other diseases introduced by colonial incursion.

While it is usually considered to be a childhood disease, measles could also be deadly to adults. In the American Civil War, about 20,000 cases were reported among Union soldiers, leading to at least 500 deaths and it was also severe among conscripts from the rural South in the United States, during the First World War.[2] The introduction of an effective vaccine, now in the form of the Mumps, Measles and Rubella (MMR) vaccine, has transformed the health of children, saving thousands of lives. Unfortunately, its efficacy has been eroded by the growth of the anti-vaccination (anti-vax) movement. The World Health Organisation (WHO) has reported that measles deaths have increased by 50% between 2016 and 2019, claiming 207,500 lives in 2019.[3]

MEASLES, THE DISEASE

Measles is caused by a virus, *Measles morbillivirus*, a member of a genus consisting of seven species, otherwise confined to cats and dogs. Its closest ancestor was rinderpest, a cattle disease, which is believed to have originated in Asia.[4] Historically rinderpest wrought havoc in cattle-based societies, but it was entirely eradicated in 2011, the second disease in history, after smallpox, to become extinct. It is thought that, when pastoralism developed, with close contact between cattle and people, the rinderpest virus passed to human beings where it transmuted, to become unique to the human species, transmitted directly from person to person. Measles is characterized by fever and respiratory inflammation, followed by a skin rash and small white spots in the mouth, known as Koplik's spots. While the disease itself may be serious, its repression of the immune system makes it far more dangerous. Most frequently, victims die of respiratory complications like bacterial pneumonia; the intestinal tract may be damaged, leading to ruptures and the inability to absorb food. Encephalitis occurs in one in 1,200–1,500 cases and there are also long-term consequences. A rare but fatal complication is *subacute sclerosing panencephalitis*, a neurological disease.[5]

It is not clear when the virus evolved to become a disease that was specific to human beings. Some writers have argued that it is ancient, appearing as early as the Neolithic revolution, 12,000 years ago. Authors drawing on written evidence have suggested that this transmutation had occurred by the ninth century CE, citing the work of the Persian physician al-Razi (890–923) who gave the first 'unambiguous' clinical description of this affliction. At this period it may have been rife in the Near East for some time.[6] More recent studies, drawing on modern scientific methodology, have challenged this opinion. Conclusions still vary widely, however. Some techniques have led to the hypothesis that measles diverged from rinderpest in the fourth century BCE.[7] Molecular clock analysis argues for a much later date of the eleventh to twelfth centuries.[8] Although measles is a fairly stable virus, changing little over time, it is considered that the current strain evolved at the beginning of the twentieth century – perhaps between 1908 and 1943.[9] Most researchers agree that the original divergence occurred in the Near or Middle East and it had certainly reached Europe by the thirteenth century. Measles was probably widespread by the time that the first European voyages of exploration began in 1419.

Unlike chickenpox which can remain latent in the human body for decades, measles depends on numbers to survive – somewhere somebody must be infected to pass the virus on. Like its close relation, rinderpest, then, measles is a candidate for complete eradication.[10] It has regularly disappeared completely from isolated communities and its reintroduction has often been the consequence of colonial trade, colonial conquest or the expansion of Christian missions.

In 1954, in the United States, John F. Enders and Thomas C. Peebles were able to isolate measles from the blood of a thirteen-year-old boy, David Edmonston, and an effective vaccine followed in 1963. From 1968 an improved strain enabled the Centers for Disease Control and Prevention (CDC) to eliminate measles from the United States and they achieved this in 2000.[11] While measles was not wholly eradicated in other countries, the use of the MMR vaccine reduced the incidence of measles considerably.

The recent resurgence of measles is largely the product of the anti-vax movement. As the Measles and Rubella Initiative points out, opposition to vaccination has a long history.[12] In the early days of vaccination there was good cause for suspicion since sanitary controls were limited; even the Salk vaccine against polio sometimes caused serious disease.[13] This is one reason for the careful controls that exist today in the production of new vaccines. The modern anti-vax movement was triggered by poor research and propagated by bad journalism. A paper published in *The Lancet* in 1998 fraudulently linked the MMR vaccine to autism. Although the study has now been discredited, and its author struck off the medical register in Britain, hostility to the practice of vaccination has continued to grow. The journalist, Julia Belluz, argues that journalists have been complicit in perpetuating Wakefield's claims. She cites Ben Goldacre:

> Even if it had been immaculately well conducted – and it certainly wasn't – Wakefield's 'case series report' of 12 children's clinical anecdotes would never have justified the conclusion that MMR causes autism, despite what journalists claimed: it simply didn't have big enough numbers to do so. But the media repeatedly reported the concerns of this one man, generally without giving

> methodological details of the research, either because they found it too complicated, inexplicably, or because to do so would have undermined their story.[14]

Tragically, it has been the less-developed countries which have suffered most from the anti-vax movement, for the severity of measles is exacerbated by poor nutrition and overcrowding. In Madagascar, between 2018 and 2019, there were over 50,000 cases and more than 300 deaths. In 2019, the Ukraine saw a surge of cases, while the Philippines has also suffered a major outbreak.[15] As one writer has observed: 'Will we still be writing about measles in present-day terms one hundred years from now? The odds are we will. . . . Measles outbreaks are turning out to be caused as much by the human condition as by the virus's "characteristics themselves"'.[16]

MEASLES IN THE POST-COLUMBIAN NEW WORLD

The easy victory of a handful of Spanish conquistadors over the sophisticated Aztec and Incan Empires has usually been ascribed partly to disease, often to smallpox.[17] In a substantial article David S. Jones has criticized this virgin soil hypothesis for its easy immunological determinism. It has, for instance, lent itself to racist assumptions that Europeans possessed an evolutionary superiority over the pristine societies of the New World. He urges that historians should acknowledge 'the complexity, the subtlety, and the contingency' of the process of the depopulation of the Americas. More heterogeneous analyses are needed to 'overcome the widespread public and academic appeal of immunologic determinism and do justice to the crucial events of the encounter between Europeans and Americans'.[18]

It remains extremely difficult to know precisely what diseases decimated the indigenous Americans. Modern research suggests that it may have been a type of enteric fever that was so lethal, rather than smallpox.[19] But, as Jones points out, the disease environment may have been much more complex than earlier scientists or historians have acknowledged. It is here that measles may have played its part. It is now recognized that some of the seeds of the downfall of the Aztec and Incan Empires lay in their very success. Their agricultural methods were remarkably productive, leading to dense settlement in some places. But, at the time of the arrival of the conquistadors, there was heavy ecological pressure on their lands, with serious erosion in Mexico and a salting of the coastal lands of Peru. 'Everything points to the conclusion that Amerindian populations were pressing hard against the limits set by available cultivable land in both Mexico and Peru when the Spaniards arrived'.[20] Possible malnutrition and overcrowding provided ideal conditions for measles to flourish while the fact that measles damaged the immune system may have contributed to the lowered resistance of the indigenous societies when they encountered Western diseases.

It is clear that the Spanish conquistadors brought a variety of ailments with them. They themselves were rarely healthy. Accounts of their voyages suggest that sickness was rampant on their ships. In 1494, Christopher Columbus himself was constantly ill, suffering from a number of uncertain afflictions.[21] Scurvy was probably widespread. The early Spanish settlers, and the indigenous people they encountered, died of malnutrition and epidemic disease in considerable numbers. For example, the town of Isabela on the island of Hispaniola in the present-day Dominican Republic, founded in 1494, was rapidly abandoned because of the high mortality of the Spanish settlers.[22] What is clear, then, is that the disease environment introduced by the Spanish was multifaceted. We can only surmise about the role measles might have played.

Measles is more readily identified later on. It is suggested that it spread through Mexico and Peru in 1530 and 1531, while the Pilgrim Fathers may have introduced it into New England.[23] English settlers brought the disease to the east coast of North America but Spanish missions played a significant part in its diffusion on the west coast. In California there were severe outbreaks of measles in many of the Spanish missions in 1806, in 1822–1823 and in 1828. Usually, measles was only one of the infectious diseases ravaging these communities, with epidemics of typhoid, diphtheria and smallpox as well. Living conditions on the mission stations were often poor and insanitary.[24] Briefly, measles, a highly infectious and common disease, which flourished in conditions of deprivation, to the detriment of the immune system, probably contributed to the decline of the indigenous populations of the Americas, but there is little unequivocal evidence for this. Under appropriate environmental conditions, human susceptibility to contract an array of diseases apart from measles in other parts of the globe proved fatal, often superseding class, culture and race (Ahmed, Dey, Steere-Williams and Viljoen in this volume).

MEASLES IN THE PACIFIC ISLANDS

The Pacific Islands provide the most vivid examples of the impact of measles on virgin communities. Broadly the islands comprise three groups, Melanesia (including the Solomon Islands, Vanuatu, New Caledonia and Fiji, which included Rotuma); Micronesia (Palau, Guam, the Northern Mariana Islands, the Marshall Islands and Kiribati are among the best known) and Polynesia (stretching from Hawaii to Easter Island (Rapa Nui), Samoa, the Cook Islands and Tahiti, among others). This vast and complex region was first occupied as far back as 2000 BCE. Early European mariners reached the Pacific in 1513, with the Dutch following on the heels of the Spanish. Sustained contact only occurred in the nineteenth century after the settlement of Australia and New Zealand provided a base for traders. The islands were vulnerable, however, to uncontrolled and often rapacious intrusions from whalers, roving seamen from a variety of countries and, occasionally, castaways. They contributed to the destabilization of local societies and encouraged the incursion of Christian missionaries who were appalled both by the lawlessness of the intruders and by some of the practices of the islanders. The London Missionary Society was one of the first to come, sending a party to Tahiti in 1797. Methodists reached Tonga in 1822 and Fiji in 1835, while Catholic missionaries began working in New Caledonia in the 1840s. Missionary activity further destabilized the island cultures, not only because their primary purpose was to 'reform' 'un-Christian' practices, but also because of conflict between different missionary groups. British Wesleyans and French Catholic missionaries, as representatives of imperial societies, that were already in conflict over control of indigenous peoples, fell out with one another politically and doctrinally. The Pacific Islands were a microcosm of Victorian imperialism. But epidemics followed in their wake, 'some of them serious'.[25] After the 1850s Europeans introduced plantation agriculture, first cotton and then sugar. Both products are associated with a grasping desire for high profits and the exploitation of labour, inevitably conducive to poor nutrition and living conditions.

The great distances and the slow voyages of sailing ships probably prevented diseases like measles from reaching the Pacific Islands until the nineteenth century, for any cases on board would have burnt out long before the ships reached the Pacific. Increased contact with Australia and the shorter voyages that followed the arrival of steam altered the situation just at a time when the destruction of indigenous cultures, followed by malnutrition and poor living conditions on the plantations, made the Island populations more vulnerable to infectious disease. A series of devastating epidemics decimated Pacific Island populations and often destroyed their ruling structures, driving the people further into the arms of the colonial powers. In 1848 in Hawaii about 10,000 people, 10% of the population died; in 1861 on Aneityum in the New Hebrides (Vanuatu) about 60% of the population died of measles; in 1875 between 20 and 25% of the population again died of measles and a severe epidemic followed once more in 1907; in 1911, 16% of the population of Rotuma (a dependency of Fiji) also died of measles.[26]

Hawaii was one of the first islands to lose its traditional rulers to disease. In 1823, King Kamehameha II voyaged to England, partly to negotiate an alliance with England to protect his country from Russia. In London, he and his entourage were feted by society and made a number of public appearances. One such occasion was a visit to the Royal Military Asylum, actually an orphanage for the children of soldiers who had died in service. The king and queen probably contracted measles on this visit, on 5 June 1834, and they both died not long after, the queen on 8 July and the king on 14 July, in both cases from pulmonary complications. The British king, George IV, did undertake to protect the Hawaiian kingdom from external forces and to maintain a consul general there, without interfering in their internal affairs, but he could not protect Hawaii from epidemic disease. In 1848, the territories were laid waste by measles, whooping cough, dysentery and influenza. Medical missionaries estimated that between 10,000 and 30,000 people died, 10–30% of the population. This epidemic was probably introduced into Hawaii by an American naval frigate, *Independence*. A report in the *Missionary Herald* of 5 May 1849 noted that the impact was so great that 'whole villages, were prostrate with this disease, there not being persons enough in health to prepare food for the sick'. Several members of the royal family died as well. For the rest of the nineteenth century, periodic epidemics of measles further devastated the population.[27]

In Fiji, measles was introduced in 1875. Fiji consists of over 800 islands but the majority of the population live on the island of Viti Levu. At the time of European contact Fijians had a vigorous and complex culture and a rich spiritual life. The history of Western colonization is too complicated to relate in any detail but the belief that the Fijians were cannibals provided a moral imperative for colonization. Consequently, the imposition of Christianity was particularly vicious, giving rise also to intertribal warfare between those who accepted conversion and those who did not. The increase in the price of cotton as a result of the American Civil War (1861–1865) led Australians and Americans to seize land on the Fijian islands to grow cotton on plantations. Cotton is a labour-intensive crop and the new settlers brought in workers under atrocious conditions that were closely allied to slavery (known as blackbirding). Fijian leaders tried to steer a course through this impossible maze of land grabbling, exploitation of labour and loss of spiritual identity. Finally the leading chief, Ratu Cakobau, agreed to annexation by Britain in order to establish some kind of stability. In 1874, Sir Hercules Robinson was appointed the new governor. He persuaded Cakobau, to visit Sydney, Australia, to sign the new Deed of Cession.

In Sydney, Cakobau and his sons contracted measles but, with careful nursing, neither Cakobau nor his entourage died. On the return journey on HMS *Dido*, however, the medical personnel failed to place the ship or its passengers in quarantine for they were unaware of the effect of measles on a virgin population. The leaders arrived home to a large meeting of high chiefs, in order to explain the new arrangements. The delegations then scattered to their homes, carrying measles with them. Within a week islanders took sick and began to die. The onslaught was so severe that perhaps one-third of the Fijian population expired. At the time 'death drums sounded incessantly in seemingly deserted villages' and 'graves were only half dug because no one had the strength to dig'.[28] A more careless version suggests that the malignancy of the disease was increased by cultural practices.

> The increasingly hostile islanders refused all conventional measles treatment and attempted to allay their fever by bathing in icy rivers, laying themselves open to the all-too-common secondary complications of a disease against which they had in any case no natural immunity. The outbreak coincided with a spell of appalling weather: howling gales did nothing to help weakened immune systems stave off serious illness.[29]

Between 36,000 and 40,000, a third of the Fijian population died.[30]

Isolated Pacific Islands continued to be devastated by measles into the twentieth century. Rotuma, 'one of the most isolated places on earth' was one such example. The island was inhabited by a Polynesian people, intermixed with other Pacific Islanders and a handful of European seamen. Their subsistence economy was based on root crops and coconuts, with pigs and fish supplying protein. It fell under British control after rival British Wesleyan and French Catholic missionaries took up arms against one another in 1878. The Rotuma chiefs ceded the island to Britain in an effort to preclude further French intervention. From 1881 Rotuma was governed by Britain as part of the Colony of Fiji, some 500 miles away. A resident commissioner was appointed, usually a medical officer. Oral evidence suggested that the island had been ravaged by an epidemic early in the nineteenth century and, by the twentieth century, there was growing concern about the decline in the Polynesian population and particularly about the high infant mortality rate. Tuberculosis was common, suggesting that the health of the islanders was compromised well before 1911. But both its remoteness, and controls introduced after the 1875 epidemic in Fiji, protected Rotuma from infectious disease until 1911. In January of that year a ship arrived with two women on board, infected with measles. The medical officer was absent at the time and, without informed medical intervention, the disease spread rapidly, ultimately killing nearly 13% of the population. Good population and mortality registers have survived, enabling historians to analyse the details of the disaster unusually fully. An analysis of these sources has led some academics to conclude that the genetic homogeneity of the population, combined with their limited exposure to microbes, made them particularly vulnerable.

In all, there were about 2,200 people living on the island in 1911. In that year 491 Rotumans died, two-thirds from measles. Measles deaths started in February, peaked in April and decreased rapidly in May, with a trickle of deaths after that. The greatest number of deaths occurred among children under the age of six and young adults (16–35 years). The great majority (75%) of measles-associated deaths occurred from gastrointestinal illnesses rather than from the respiratory diseases that were more common elsewhere.

Shanks and his associates believe that malnutrition and dehydration may explain this phenomenon. They speculate that, because an entire village would be affected at one time, care providers could not supply enough food, water or nursing care. But this measles epidemic occurred in a larger disease environment, with widespread tuberculosis for example. In an effort to explain the high mortality in Rotuma, Shanks and his associates compared the Rotuma outbreak with those of the Danish Faroe Islands, where Peter Panum had conducted the first modern scientific study of measles, and with an outbreak among an isolated Inuit population in southern Greenland. They note that the mortality in both these cases was far lower than that of Rotuma; they speculate that there could be a genetic component to the mortality risk, although they doubt that it was a predominant factor.[31]

THE CONCENTRATION CAMPS OF THE SOUTH AFRICAN WAR (1899–1902)

The measles epidemic that ravaged the concentration camps of the South African War provides much fuller data than most other accounts of the disease before the twentieth century.[32] This measles epidemic occurred in different circumstances from that of 'island' societies; it broke out in states that, although the populations were widely scattered on farms, had larger populations than existed on the Pacific islands and occurred in places that had been exposed to measles before. The South African War started on 12 October 1899, between Great Britain on the one side and the two Boer Republics of the South African Republic (Transvaal) and the Orange Free State (OFS) on the other. Underlying the hostilities was Britain's desire to control the production of the gold that had been discovered on the Witwatersrand in the Transvaal in 1884. The two republics had been established by settlers of Dutch origin who had trekked north in 1834, after the British annexation of the Cape in 1813. In the process of settlement the Boers conquered and displaced existing African societies. By 1900, some indigenous people had been forced into ever-smaller areas of partial independence but many black people now resided on white-owned farms, on mission stations or enjoyed some other form of partial economic independence.[33] While black people were not officially combatants in the war, in one way or another they were also drawn into the conflict. Many men found fairly lucrative employment with the British army, while others remained bound to their Boer employees as servants. Their wives and families were left adrift in the veld or found refuge in nearby town 'locations'.[34]

The concentration camps were the product of a 'scorched earth' policy that was introduced primarily by the British commander-in-chief, General Lord Kitchener, in the second part of the war. After the capitals of Bloemfontein and Pretoria fell in March and June 1900, respectively, the British thought that the war was over. The Boers, however, fought on. Boer tactics altered from the conventional pattern of set battles as they took to the veld in a guerrilla war that the British found extremely difficult to quell. In desperation the British resorted to a 'scorched earth' policy in which the veld was cleared of any means of support for the Boer commandoes. Farms were burnt, livestock were killed or captured and farming families were rounded up and brought into 'concentration' camps. Although the camps were established as part of a military strategy, in February 1902 their administration passed, in theory, to civilians, although many of the camp staff were seconded from the military.

Black people were left, at first, to fend for themselves but, in time, black concentration camps were also established. The rationale for these camps was different from those of the white camps; they were entirely under military control, the intention being to create farm colonies where the families could grow their own food while their men were serving the British – concentration on the cheap. In actual fact, their living conditions were far worse than those of the Boer families.

Prior to the war, relatively little is known about the disease environment of the Boers. There was no registration of births and deaths and, apart from the gold-mining area of Johannesburg, there were very few doctors. For many generations the Boers had been accustomed to doctor themselves and they had developed a medical culture based partly on a dimly remembered Galenic philosophy of medicine (sweating out of fevers, for example) and a pharmacopeia that was a mix of remedies learnt from indigenous people, traditional remedies brought from Europe and a reliance on a limited number of patent medicines (*Huis Apotheek*).[35] Afrikaners long believed that the Boers were a tough and healthy people. While there is an element of truth to this, an analysis of the census records suggests that they had a classic pre-industrial pattern of mortality and life expectancy, with large families, a high infant mortality rate and a restricted lifespan.

The Boers were not unfamiliar with epidemics of infectious diseases and scattered evidence suggests that they had encountered measles before. *Volksgeneeskuns in Suid-Afrika* lists seventy remedies for measles, about twenty of them based on goat dung (*bokmis*).[36] Bloemfontein's local holiday resort is called 'Maselspoort'. Above all, the pattern of measles mortality in the camps indicates that this was a partly immunized population, for few adults in the camps died of the disease and the same was true of children under the age of a year. Prior to the war infectious diseases were probably spread through the practice of *nagmaal* (communion) when, every three months, farming families congregated in the local towns for church meetings. We know almost nothing about the health of the black communities but it seems possible that the health of conquered indigenous communities was inferior to that of the

Boers. None of the wartime sources makes any reference to measles among black families but it is very unlikely that they had better immunity to the disease. What is probable is that in the first part of the war, for which there is evidence only for the OFS, when living conditions for black refugees from the farms were appalling, their children died in substantial numbers from pneumonia, before the measles epidemic started.[37]

Statistical sources for mortality in the white camps are quite full. This is no accident. One of Britain's great achievements in the nineteenth century had been a revolution in public health. Statistics are the basis of epidemiology and it was through the collection of data that, for instance, Dr John Snow was able to demonstrate that cholera was a waterborne disease, and it was statistical data that proved that good public health reform rested on clean water, decent housing and adequate nutrition. Men like Alfred, Lord Milner, high commissioner for South Africa, understood this. For a man of the modern world, like Milner, the object of conquest, of the imposition of imperial control, was not only to acquire economic assets but to spread the message of the superiority of British 'civilization'.

Between December 1900 and May 1901, five of the OFS camps were visited by the English philanthropist and reformer, Emily Hobhouse. Her report on these camps, about which Kitchener had been secretive, was published in Britain in June 1901. It resulted in an outcry that led to questions in the House of Commons and a hasty effort at reform on the part of the War Office. St John Brodrick, the secretary of state for war, recruited a 'Committee of Ladies' to investigate camp conditions. In addition, camp reports, ration scales and other information were published in a 'Blue Book', Cd 819, in November 1901. Full control of the camps passed to the Colonial Office, of whom the secretary of state was Joseph Chamberlain. In effect, management of the camps passed to Milner, who acted with vigorous decision. He insisted that the reports of the Ladies' Committee be acted upon promptly and fully; he brought in personnel from the Indian Civil Service who had dealt with plague and famine camps in India and he insisted on the accurate collection of statistical data.[38]

Underlying the actions of Chamberlain and Milner was a very different motivation from that of the military. Conquered Boers would become British citizens and Milner understood that these new colonies of the Transvaal and the Orange River Colony (ORC) would only function successfully if these new white citizens embraced the values of the British Empire. In some respects the British Empire was a laboratory for the study and implementation of modernization and control; India was the laboratory par excellence.[39] In the controlled conditions of camps such as the Indian famine and plague camps, modern hygiene practices could be inculcated and colonized societies could be measured and managed. The South African camps were no different; in the brief space of about a year the British attempted to 'civilize' their Boer subjects: to educate the children, to train young Boer women as nurses and to 'learn' about their new citizens through the collection of statistical data. It is hardly surprising that enlightened British administrators floundered as they tried to impose control over an embittered rural population of white Christians, the like of which they had encountered before only in French-speaking Canada.[40]

The concentration camps started about September 1900. The military kept few records so it was only after February 1901 that camp registers were opened and the collection of statistics began. It is clear that the authorities took some care to ensure accuracy. In the Free State records there was a regular correspondence between the Chief Superintendent Refugee Camps and the camp superintendents and medical officers, checking and rechecking names and numbers. When the recruits from India replaced the original chief superintendents in 1902, they imposed a greater degree of uniformity on the camps.

Over time there were about forty-five white camps and sixty-four black camps. There was some mobility in the numbers as camps were opened and closed and there were a handful of places, like Ladybrand in the ORC, where groups of 'refugees' were rationed but they never formed part of the official structures. The war ended on 31 May 1902, with the signing of the Treaty of Vereeniging. Over the next six months the camps were gradually closed, the last few remaining until about February 1903.

In the early months conditions were appalling as the number of Boers brought into the camps overwhelmed the resources. Tents were worn and overcrowded. The original ration scales, probably drawn up by military medical officers, were inadequate and unsuitable for small children. It consisted only of flour, salt, coffee and meat. There were no fresh vegetables and the quality of the meat deteriorated rapidly under wartime conditions. Eventually the authorities resorted to tinned meat and, towards the end of the war, to frozen meat. The one ameliorating factor was that shops were opened in the camps from which the camp families could supplement their rations with such items as tinned sardines. Since a number of the camp inmates were paid for work in the camps – men for a variety of tasks, women as nurse-aids in the hospitals – there was a substantial camp economy.

The ration scales and the quality of the food only improved after Milner took control in November 1901. Food gardens were established and milk was made available to children. In time, too, the number and quality of the tents improved and solid brick buildings began to be constructed. At the height of the measles epidemic, however, the living conditions of the camp families were conducive to serious illness.

Measles was probably introduced into the republics from Cape Town which suffered annual epidemics of the disease. The population of Cape

Town was far too small to sustain endemicity but the weekly mailships from Britain ensured that the disease was introduced regularly into the town.[41] By February 1900, measles was probably already spreading in the Boer republics. In the old Paardeberg Museum, for instance, a jacket was displayed of a man who was reputed to have died of measles.[42] The first child known to have succumbed to measles was the son of General J. B. M. Hertzog, later prime minister of South Africa. The child probably contracted the disease in Jagersfontein in 1900, as his mother and family were being transferred to East London camp.[43]

At first, camp doctors were not concerned about the arrival of measles. In British cities they were familiar with this minor childhood ailment and they were taken aback at its virulence in the camps. Their focus was elsewhere for they were much more concerned about typhoid fever (enteric). Typhoid, a waterborne bacterial disease, was the soldiers' disease par excellence. By 1900, the necessity of a clean water supply was fully understood and the fact that the disease killed 964 soldiers in Bloemfontein alone, and was not contained, was an indictment of the negligence of the British military authorities and their lack of concern for their common soldiers.[44] The Modder (Mud) river, which ran through the Paardeberg battlefield and onto Bloemfontein, was heavily contaminated and a large number of Bloemfontein residents also contracted the disease. A distressing feature of the camps was the extreme emaciation of some children. The single most famous image of the camps, that of Lizzie van Zyl, who probably died of typhoid, illustrates this phenomenon, and it occurred with measles cases as well.[45] Children whose digestive tracts were damaged were unable to absorb nutrition; slowly they wasted away and died. Although the phenomenon was known elsewhere, for the Boer mothers it was terrifying; many were convinced that their children were being deliberately starved by the British doctors whom they distrusted. Equally disturbing was the phenomenon of 'cancrum oris' or 'noma', when an abscess developed on the jaw and gradually ate away the face; it was invariably fatal.[46]

The epidemic that is most fully recorded occurred in Mafeking camp. Mafeking town, which, famously, had already endured a seven-month siege, was located in the northern Cape, on the banks of the Molopo River. By 1901, the camp was extensive, scattered for a mile along the banks of the river. When the Ladies' Committee arrived in South Africa in August 1901, Mafeking was the first camp they visited. Perhaps because they were still inexperienced, they found little to criticize. The superintendent seemed competent and the camp was healthy. However, shortly after they left, a family from Taung, a remote mining village, was brought in and with them came measles. The disease spread like wildfire through the camp and, in the classic fashion of epidemics, it revealed all the hidden failings of the management.

In October 1901, Mafeking recorded the highest mortality of all the camps. It was so great that the Ladies' Committee returned in November and, now more experienced, their comments reveal a number of the administrative shortcomings. Subsequently, there was a second inquiry into the cause of the high mortality rate.

In the face of disaster, the camp superintendent, R. L. McCowat, proved apathetic. Both the doctors were foreigners, German speaking and they had been intimidated by the authoritarian management of the camps. Although they knew that they needed more staff and medical supplies, they did not press for them and the camp was woefully understaffed. The Mafeking camp records include a death register which indicates clearly that the medical officers failed to visit the sickest children regularly – many had not seen a doctor for a week or more before they died. The impression that one gains is that this was a camp in which the senior staff were both exhausted and passive in the face of disaster. What the investigations also revealed was the larger disease environment. Typhoid was widespread and the children suffered from a host of other complaints, with whooping cough being another significant killer, while babies died, not of measles, but of diarrhoea-related ailments. Unusually in these South African camps, meningitis (perhaps in fact, encephalitis) was also a significant cause of mortality.

From the end of 1901, the epidemic, and mortality, declined rapidly. The virus may have burnt itself out but the reforms introduced by the British undoubtedly improved conditions as well. The hospitals were enlarged and better supplied and large numbers of doctors and nurses were recruited from as far afield as New Zealand. New ration scales were introduced and food gardens started. The children were given milk and, although it was not popular with the Boers, frozen meat meant that the supply of protein was greater. Sports, music, schools and other activities helped to improve the morale of the families.

Few historical studies explore the long-term medical consequences of measles. In the case of South Africa, however, it is possible to speculate a little. Post-war studies on 'poor whites' suggest that the health status of many Afrikaner families was not good. The 1918 influenza epidemic was particularly lethal in South Africa and it is, perhaps, possible that their weakened immune systems left black and white residents of the old Boer republics particularly vulnerable to this flu.

CONCLUSION

Several points emerge from these case studies. Epidemics of measles rarely occurred in isolation. Measles, introduced from the European-Asian world, was usually only one of a number of diseases infecting invaded societies, others ranging from smallpox to tuberculosis. Uniquely, however, the damage that measles wrought on the immune system almost certainly increased the lethality of other ailments. Frequently, also, measles broke out in communities in which the environment had been degraded before colonizers arrived, where indigenous societies were already suffering from malnutrition and poor housing. Colonial conquest tended to damage living conditions further, once more providing an environment in which measles flourished.

Measles continues to be a significant killer of children, mainly in the developing world. This is the result of a combination of factors – poverty and deprived living conditions, poor governance and a lack of trust in medical science. The long hand of colonial conquest still lies heavily on indigenous societies.

NOTES

1. W.H. McNeill, *Plagues and Peoples* (London: Penguin, 1976), 62–63; A. Cliff, P. Haggett, and M. Smallman-Raynor, *Measles. An Historical Geography of a Major Human Viral Disease from Global Expansion to Local Retreat, 1840–1900* (Oxford: Blackwell, 1993), 4–34.
2. M.B.A. Oldstone, *Viruses, Plagues, & History* (Oxford: Oxford University Press, 2009), 146–47; G.D Shanks, Z. Hu, M. Waller, S. Lee, D. Terfa, A. Howard, E. Van Heyningen, & J.F. Brundage, "Measles epidemics of variable lethality in the early 20th century," *American Journal of Epidemiology* 179, no. 4 (2013), 413–422.
3. World Health Organization (WHO), "Worldwide measles deaths climb 50% from so16 to 2019 claiming over 207,5000 lives in 2019." Accessed 27 November 2020 from https://www.who.int/news/item/12-11-2020-worldwide-measles-deaths-climb-50-from- 2016-to-2019-claiming-over-207-500-lives-in-2019.
4. R. da F. Budaszewski and V. Von Messling, "Morbillivirus experimental animal models. Measles virus pathogenesis insights from Canine Distemper Virus" *Viruses*, 2016. Accessed 1 February 2021 from https://www.ncbi.nlm.nih.gov/pmc/articles/PMC5086610/; J. Ball, "Could relatives of measles virus jump from animals to us?" *BBC News*. 2020. Accessed 1 February 2021 from https://www.ncbi.nlm.nih.gov/pmc/articles/PMC5086610/.
5. B. Gastel, "Measles: a potentially finite history," *Journal of the History of Medicine and Allied Sciences* 28, no. 1 (1973), 34–44.
6. McNeill, *Plagues and Peoples*, 114; Gastel, Measles, 35.
7. A. Düx et al., "The history of measles from a 1912 genome to an antique origin," *bioRxiv*, (2019). Posted 30 December 2019 from https://doi.org/10.1101/2019.12.29.889667.
8. Y. Furuse, A. Suzuki, & H. Oshitani, H. "Origin of measles virus: divergence from rinderpest virus between the 11th and 12th centuries." *Virology Journal* 7

(2010). Accessed 15 July 2021 from https://virologyj.biomedcentral.com/articles/10.1186/1743-422X-7-52.

9. S.M. Beaty and B. Lee, "Constraints on the genetic and antigenic variability of measles virus," *Viruses* 8, no. 4 (2016), https://doi.org/10.3390/v8040109, 109.

10. McNeill, *Plagues and Peoples*, 54.

11. Centres for Disease Control and Prevention (CDC). "Measles (Rubeola)." Accessed on 27 November 2020 from https://www.cdc.gov/measles/about/history.html; E. Conis, "Measles and the modern history of vaccination," *Public Health Reports* 134, no. 2 (2019), 118–25; T. Haelle, (2019). "Why it took so long to eliminate measles," *History* (2019). Accessed on 27 November 2020 from https://www.history.com/news/measles- vaccine-disease.

12. S. Blume, "Anti-vaccination movements and their interpretations," *Social Science & Medicine*, 62, no. 3 (2006), 628–42; Measles and Rubella Initiative, "The anti-vaccination movement." Accessed 27 November 2020 from https://measlesrubellainitiative.org/anti-vaccination-movement/.

13. P.A. Offit, *The Cutter Incident: How America's First Polio Vaccine Led to a Growing Vaccine Crisis* (New Haven & London: Yale University Press, 2006); M. Fitzpatrick, "The Cutter incident: how America's first polio vaccine led to a growing vaccine crisis," *Journal of the Royal Society of Medicine* 99, no. 3 (2006), 155–56.

14. A.J. Wakefield, S.H. Murch, A. Anthony, J. Linnell, D.M. Casson, M. Malik, M. Berelowitz, A.P. Dhillon, M.A.Thomson, P. Harvey, A. Valentine, S.E. Davies, & J.A. Walker-Smith, "Ileal-lymphoid-nodular hyperplasia, non-specific colitis, and pervasive developmental disorder in children," *The Lancet* 351, no. 9103 (1998), 637–41. Accessed 13 November 2020 from https://briandeer.com/mmr/lancet-paper.htm; J. Belluz, "Research fraud catalyzed the anti-vaccination movement. Let's not repeat history." *Vox* (2019). Accessed 13 November 2020 from https://www.vox.com/2018/2/27/17057990/andrew-wakefield- vaccines-autism-study.

15. D. McKenzie, & B. Swails, "Tens of thousands infected in measles outbreak in Madagascar," *CNN Health* (2019). Accessed 27 November 2020 from https://edition.cnn.com/2019/02/07/health/madagascar-measles-outbreak/index.html; M. Wadman, (2019). "Measles cases have tripled in Europe, fueled by Ukraine outbreak," *Science* (2019). Accessed 27 November 2020 from https://www.sciencemag.org/news/2019/02/measles-cases-have-tripled-europe-fueled- ukrainian-outbreak; "Philippines: Measles outbreak kills more than 130," *Aljazeera* (2019). Accessed 27 November 2020 from https://www.aljazeera.com/news/2019/02/19/philippines-measles-outbreak-kills-more-than-130/; N. McCarthy, "The countries with the most reported measles cases in 2019," *Forbes* (2019). Accessed on 27 November 2020 from https://www.forbes.com/sites/niallmccarthy/2019/04/16/the-countries-with-the-most- reported-measles-cases-in-2019-infographic/?sh=5d330579164c.

16. R.F. Najera, "A brief history of measles," *The History of Vaccines* (2019). Retrieved on 27 November 2020 from https://www.historyofvaccines.org/content/blog/brief-history-measles.

17. A.W. Crosby, *The Columbian Exchange: Biological and Cultural Responses to 1492* (Westport, CT: Greenwood Press, 1972); McNeill, *Plagues and Peoples*; J.

Diamond, *Guns, Germs and Steel: A Short History of Everybody for the Last 13,000 Years* (London: Vintage, 1997).

18. D.S. Jones, "Virgin soils revisited," *The William and Mary Quarterly* 60, no. 4 (2003), 703–42; R.J. Wolfe, "Alaska's great sickness, 1900: an epidemic of measles and influenza in a virgin soil population," *Proceedings of the American Philosophical Society* 126, no. 2 (1982), 92–93.

19. "500 years later, scientists discover what probably killed the Aztecs." Accessed 19 November 2020 from *The Guardian,* https://www.theguardian.com/world/2018/jan/16/mexico-500-years-later-scientists-discover-what-killed-the-aztecs.

20. McNeill, *Plagues and Peoples*, 188–89.

21. N.D. Cook, *Born to Die: Disease and New World Conquest, 1492–1650* (Cambridge: Cambridge University Press, 1998), 33–34.

22. V. Tiesler, et al., "Scurvy-related morbidity and death among Christopher Columbus' crew at La Isabela, the first European town in the New World (1494–1498): an assessment of the skeletal and historical information," *International Journal of Osteoarchaeology* 26, no. 2 (2016), 191–202.

23. McNeill, *Plagues and Peoples*, 194; Gastell, Measles, 36–37.

24. 24C.M. Orbann, "Traditional kinship structures and European-derived diseases at Mission San Diego, California: a study of the 1805–1806 measles epidemic" (PhD thesis, University of Missouri, 2014), 63–75.

25. J.N. Hays, *Epidemics and Pandemics: Their Impacts on Human History* (Santa Barbara, CA: ABC-CUO, 2005), 298.

26. K.L. Gould, K.L. Herrman, & J.J. Witte, "The epidemiology of measles in the U.S. Trust Territory of the Pacific Islands," *A.J.P.H.* 61, no. 8 (1971), 1602.

27. S.T. Shulman, D.H. Shulman & R.H. Sims, "The Tragic 1824 journey of the Hawaiian King and Queen to London. A history of measles in Hawaii," *The Pediatric Infectious Diseases Journal* 28, no. 8 (2009), 728–33.

28. Measles and Rubella Initiative, "Fiji and measles: from devastation to elimination" (2012). Accessed 27 November 2020 from https://measlesrubellainitiative.org/fiji-and-measles- from-devastation-to-elimination/.

29. Devastating Disasters, "Fiji: A tragic epidemic – 1875," Accessed 8 December 2020 from https:// devastatingdisasters.com/fiji-a-tragic-epidemic-1875/.

30. Hays, *Epidemics and Pandemics*, 297–301; G.D. Shanks, "Pacific Island societies destabilised by infectious diseases," *Journal of Military and Veterans Health* 24, no. 8 (2016), 71–74.

31. Ibid.; Shanks et al, "Measles epidemics of variable lethality."

32. E. van Heyningen, "Lies, damned lies and statistics: Statistics and the British concentration camps database" in R.J. Constantine (ed.), *New Perspectives on the Anglo-Boer War* (Bloemfontein: War Museum of the Boer Republics, 2013), 121–36.

33. E. van Heyningen, *The Concentration Camps of the South African War. A Social History* (Auckland Park: Jacana, 2013) ch. 2.

34. Ibid. 150–78; S.V. Kessler, *The Black Concentration Camps of the Anglo-Boer War 1899- 1902* (Bloemfontein: War Museum of the Boer Republics, 2012).

35. E. van Heyningen, "Medical history and Afrikaner society in the Boer republics at the end of the nineteenth century," *Kleio* 37 (2005), 16–23; Suid-Afrikaanse

Akademie vir Wetenskap en Kuns (ed.), *Volksgeneeskuns in Suid-Afrika. 'n Kultuurhistoriese Oorsig, Benewens 'n Uitgebreide Versameling Boererate* (Pretoria: Protea Boekhuis, 2010). [Folk Medicine in South Africa. A Cultural-Historical Overview, In addition to an Extensive Collection of Home Remedies].

36. Ibid.

37. Van Heyningen, *Concentration Camps*, 154–58.

38. Ibid., ch. 8.

39. A. Forth, *Barbed-Wire Imperialism. Britain's Empire of Camps, 1876–1903* (Oakland, CA: University of California Press, 2017).

40. Van Heyningen, *Concentration Camps*, 256–83; Forth, *Barbed-Wire Imperialism*, ch. 7.

41. Van Heyningen, *Concentration Camps*, 142.

42. The Battle of Paardeberg, the last major battle of the war, took place between 17 and 27 February 1900. This museum has now been moved to the War Museum of the Boer Republics in Bloemfontein.

43. Van Heyningen, *Concentration Camps*, 142–43.

44. J.C. de Villiers, *Healers, Helpers and Hospitals: A History of Military Medicine in the Anglo- Boer War*. Volume 2 (Pretoria: Protea, 2008), 106–12.

45. Van Heyningen, *Concentration Camps*, 137–40.

46. Ibid., 143.

BIBLIOGRAPHY

"500 years later, scientists discover what probably killed the Aztecs." Accessed 19 November 2020 from *The Guardian*, https://www.theguardian.com/world/2018/jan/16/mexico-500-years-later-scientists-discover-what-killed-the-aztecs

Ball, J. "Could relatives of measles virus jump from animals to us?" *BBC News*. 2020. Accessed 1 February 2021 from https://www.ncbi.nlm.nih.gov/pmc/articles/PMC5086610/

Beaty, S. M., and B. Lee. "Constraints on the genetic and antigenic variability of measles virus", *Viruses*, 8, no. 4 (2016), https://doi.org/10.3390/v8040109

Belluz, J. "Research fraud catalyzed the anti-vaccination movement. Let's not repeat history." *Vox* (2019). Accessed 13 November 2020 from https://www.vox.com/2018/2/27/17057990/andrew-wakefield-vaccines-autism-study

Blume, S. "Anti-vaccination movements and their interpretations." *Social Science & Medicine*, 62, no. 3 (2006), 628–42.

Budaszewski, R. da F., and V. Von Messling. "Morbillivirus experimental animal models. Measles virus pathogenesis insights from Canine Distemper Virus", *Viruses*, 2016. Accessed 1 February 2021 from https://www.ncbi.nlm.nih.gov/pmc/articles/PMC5086610/

Centres for Disease Control and Prevention. "Measles (Rubeola)." Accessed on 27 November 2020 from https://www.cdc.gov/measles/about/history.html

Cliff, A., P. Haggett, and M. Smallman-Raynor. *Measles. An Historical Geography of a Major Human Viral Disease from Global Expansion to Local Retreat, 1840–1900* (Oxford: Blackwell, 1993).

Conis, A. E. "Measles and the modern history of vaccination," *Public Health Reports*, 134, no. 2 (2019), 118–25.

Cook, N. D. *Born to Die: Disease and New World Conquest, 1492-1650* (Cambridge: Cambridge University Press, 1998).

Crosby, A. W. *The Columbian Exchange: Biological and Cultural Responses to 1492* (Westport, CT: Greenwood Press, 1972).

de Villiers, J. C. *Healers, Helpers and Hospitals: A History of Military Medicine in the Anglo-Boer War* (Pretoria: Protea, 2008).

Devastating Disasters. "Fiji: A tragic epidemic – 1875," Accessed 8 December 2020 from https://devastatingdisasters.com/fiji-a-tragic-epidemic-1875/

Diamond, J. *Guns, Germs and Steel: A Short History of Everybody for the Last 13,000 Years* (London: Vintage, 1997).

Düx, A., et al. "The history of measles from a 1912 genome to an antique origin," *bioRxiv*, (2019). Posted 30 December 2019 from https://doi.org/10.1101/2019.12.29.889667

Fitzpatrick, M. "The Cutter incident: how America's first polio vaccine led to a growing vaccine crisis," *Journal of the Royal Society of Medicine*, 99, no. 3 (2006), 156.

Forth, A. *Barbed-Wire Imperialism. Britain's Empire of Camps, 1876-1903* (Oakland, CA: University of California Press, 2017).

Furuse, Y., A. Suzuki, and H. Oshitani. "Origin of measles virus: divergence from rinderpest virus between the 11th and 12th centuries," *Virology Journal*, 7 (2010). Accessed 15 July 2021 from https://virologyj.biomedcentral.com/articles/10.1186/1743-422X-7-52

Gastel, B. "Measles: A potentially finite history" *Journal of the History of Medicine and Allied Sciences*, 28, no. 1 (1973).

Gould, K. L., K. L. Herrman, and J. J. Witte. "The epidemiology of measles in the U.S. Trust Territory of the Pacific Islands," *A.J.P.H.* 61, no. 8 (1971), 1602.

Haelle, T. "Why it took so long to eliminate measles," *History* (2019). Accessed on 27 November 2020 from https://www.history.com/news/measles-vaccine-disease

Hays, J. N. *Epidemics and Pandemics: Their Impacts on Human History* (Santa Barbara, CA: ABC-CUO, 2005).

Jones, D. S. "Virgin soils revisited," *The William and Mary Quarterly* 60, no. 4 (2003), 703–42.

Kessler, S. V. *The Black Concentration Camps of the Anglo-Boer War 1899-1902* (Bloemfontein: War Museum of the Boer Republics, 2012).

McCarthy, N. "The countries with the most reported measles cases in 2019" *Forbes* (2019). Accessed on 27 November 2020 from https://www.forbes.com/sites/niallmccarthy/2019/04/16/the-countries-with-the-most-reported-measles-cases-in-2019-infographic/?sh=5d330579164c

McKenzie, D., and B. Swails. "Tens of thousands infected in measles outbreak in Madagascar," *CNN Health* (2019). Accessed 27 November 2020 from https://edition.cnn.com/2019/02/07/health/madagascar-measles-outbreak/index.html

McNeill, W. H. *Plagues and Peoples* (London: Penguin, 1976).

Measles and Rubella Initiative. "The antivaccination movement." Accessed 27 November 2020 from https://measlesrubellainitiative.org/anti-vaccination-movement

Measles and Rubella Initiative. "Fiji and measles: from devastation to elimination" (2012). Accessed 27 November 2020 from https://measlesrubellainitiative.org/fiji-and-measles-from-devastation-to-elimination/

Najera, R. F. "A brief history of measles," *The History of Vaccines* (2019). Retrieved on 27 November 2020 from https://www.historyofvaccines.org/content/blog/brief-history-measles

Offit, P. A. *The Cutter Incident: How America's First Polio Vaccine Led to a Growing Vaccine Crisis* (New Haven and London: Yale University Press, 2006).

Oldstone, M. B. A. *Viruses, Plagues, & History* (Oxford: Oxford University Press, 2009).

Orbann, C. M. "Traditional kinship structures and European-derived diseases at Mission San Diego, California: a study of the 1805-1806 measles epidemic" (PhD thesis, University of Missouri, 2014); "Philippines: Measles outbreak kills more than 130," *Aljazeera* (2019). Accessed 27 November 2020 from https://www.aljazeera.com/news/2019/02/19/philippines-measles-outbreak-kills-more-than-130/

Shanks, G. D. "Pacific Island societies destabilised by infectious diseases," *Journal of Military and Veterans Health*, 24, no. 8 (2016), 71–74.

Shanks, G. D., Z. Hu, M. Waller, S. Lee, D. Terfa, A. Howard, E. Van Heyningen, and J.F. Brundage. "Measles epidemics of variable lethality in the early 20th century," *American Journal of Epidemiology*, 179, no. 4, (2013), 413–22.

Shulman, S. T., D. H. Shulman, and R. H. Sims. "The Tragic 1824 journey of the Hawaiian King and Queen to London. A history of measles in Hawaii," *The Pediatric Infectious Diseases Journal*, 28, no. 8 (2009), 728–33.

Suid-Afrikaanse Akademie vir Wetenskap en Kuns, ed. *Volksgeneeskuns in Suid-Afrika. 'n Kultuurhistoriese Oorsig, Benewens 'n Uitgebreide Versameling Boererate* (Pretoria: Protea Boekhuis, 2010). [Folk Medicine in South Africa. A Cultural-Historical Overview, In addition to an Extensive Collection of Home Remedies]

Tiesler, V., et al. "Scurvy-related morbidity and death among Christopher Columbus 'crew at La Isabela, the first European town in the New World (1494-1498): an assessment of the skeletal and historical information," *International Journal of Osteoarchaeology*, 26, no. 2 (2016), 191–202.

van Heyningen, E. *The Concentration Camps of the South African War. A Social History* (Auckland Park: Jacana, 2013).

van Heyningen, E. "Lies, damned lies and statistics: Statistics and the British concentration camps database," in R.J. Constantine (ed.), *New Perspectives on the Anglo-Boer War* (Bloemfontein: War Museum of the Boer Republics, 2013).

van Heyningen, E. "Medical history and Afrikaner society in the Boer republics at the end of the nineteenth century," *Kleio*, 37 (2005), 16–23.

Wadman, M. "Measles cases have tripled in Europe, fueled by Ukraine outbreak," *Science* (2019). Accessed 27 November 2020 from https://www.sciencemag.org/news/2019/02/measles-cases-have-tripled-europe-fueled-ukrainian-outbreak

Wakefield, A. J., S. H. Murch, A. Anthony, J. Linnell, D. M. Casson, M. Malik, M. Berelowitz, A. P. Dhillon, M. A.Thomson, P. Harvey, A. Valentine, S. E. Davies, and J. A. Walker-Smith. "Ileal-lymphoid-nodular hyperplasia, non-specific colitis, and pervasive developmental disorder in children," *The Lancet*, 351, no. 9103 (1998), 637–41. Accessed 13 November 2020 from https://briandeer.com/mmr/lancet-paper.htm

Wolfe, R. J. "Alaska's great sickness, 1900: An epidemic of measles and influenza in a virgin soil population," *Proceedings of the American Philosophical Society* 126, no. 2 (1982), 92–93.

World Health Organization. "Worldwide measles deaths climb 50% from so16 to 2019 claiming over 207,5000 lives in 2019." Accessed 27 November 2020 from https://www.who.int/news/item/12-11-2020-worldwide-measles-deaths-climb-50-from-2016-to-2019-claiming-over-207-500-lives-in-2019

Chapter 6

Merchants, Explorers and Academicians

Scientific Travel from the Seventeenth to Nineteenth Centuries

Matthew E. Franco

The early modern period was one of novelty and discovery. Early modern Europeans travelled to New Worlds, inhabited by new people and filled with new flora and fauna to be collected, studied, displayed and admired. Historians of science have reflected at length on European travel from the fourteenth century onwards and, more recently, on how that travel was understood by and fit into the chronologies of extra-European cultures. While these early voyages were concerned with discovery and exploration, by the nineteenth century, scientific travel could be described as a series of expeditions. This shift reflected the increasing professionalization of the sciences and the role of science as a tool for imperial control. Nineteenth-century expeditions were increasingly seen not as modes of discovery, but as 'civilizing mission[s]' to deliver European values and solidify European political and economic supremacy.[1]

This chapter will survey scholarship on the history of scientific travel, focusing on developments between the seventeenth and nineteenth centuries. Focusing in on this time frame allows us to reflect on not only the changing nature of scientific travel during this period, but also the changing ways historians of science have studied scientific travel. Whether controlled by 'centres of calculation' in the metropole or the methodology of 'science in the field', historians of science have been fascinated by the sites where knowledge is made.[2] These studies have also reinforced the observation that knowledge is both socially and culturally embedded. While previous studies championed the heroic figure of the scientific traveller or scientific practice within a specific national or imperial context, recent studies have focused on the community of scholars and global exchange of ideas. This shift reflects a change from studies asking how knowledge is created to asking instead how ideas circulate.

DESTINATIONS

Scientific travel in the Atlantic world began in the north Atlantic in the fourteenth century with increasing mercantile activity along Atlantic Africa by the Iberian fisherman.[3] Spanish and Portuguese imperial science dominated the early Atlantic world, mapping its contours and encountering its people.[4] Nicolás Wey Gómez and Ricardo Padrón have described how these early Iberian travellers worked to render legible to European eyes the Atlantic space and its people.[5] By the seventeenth century, European engagement in Atlantic scientific travel had expanded beyond the Iberian monarchies.[6] It was also during the seventeenth century that newly formed scientific societies – the Royal Society of London and the Académie des sciences – began to dispatch natural philosophers to collect, observe and study the natural world.[7] Nicholas Dew has described how during the seventeenth century scientific travellers might experience difficulty reaching their desired destinations, sometimes travelling aboard slave ships or merchant vessels.[8] English gentlemen, such as Hans Sloane, were able to cross the Atlantic and collect natural specimen to satisfy their curiosities while contributing to the growth of scientific culture in the Atlantic world.[9] The British Atlantic has been the subject of tremendous scholarly interest and is representative of broader shifts in how scholars have framed the growth of Atlantic science.[10]

During the eighteenth century, European colonial powers turned to scientific travel as a tool to reform their empires, reinvigorate their imperial economies and inspire loyalty from colonial subjects. Spanish scientific travel increased under the Bourbon monarchs, reaching its apex during the reign of Charles III of Spain.[11] Graham Burnett shows how British exploration of its South American colony of Guyana similarly used the mastery of modern science to imply mastery of its imperial space.[12]

The Pacific was also the subject of tremendous interest by European travellers between the seventeenth and nineteenth centuries.[13] Iberian travellers entered the Pacific in the mid-sixteenth century.[14] Spanish merchants soon established strong commercial connections to Asia through their Pacific colonies, especially the Philippines and its associated Manila galleon. The eighteenth century saw rapid expansion of European interest in the Pacific.[15] The heroic voyages of James Cook, Alejandro Malaspina and Louis Antoine de Bougainville characterized the increasing European interest in the Pacific during the eighteenth century and were the subject of an emerging genre of travel literature that captivated European readers.[16] In the nineteenth century, the United States and Great Britain competed with Imperial Russia to chart the Pacific and control its resources.[17]

Entering the Pacific, European travellers remapped a space that had been well documented in indigenous geographic systems. David Chang has challenged us to think of indigenous people as active agents of exploration, not merely passive subjects of the imperial gaze.[18] Chang's detailed study of Native Hawaiian spatial methodologies adds necessary context to the existing literature on how Europeans experienced the Pacific. Likewise, Joshua L. Reid has produced an intricate study of the spatial history of the Makahs in the Pacific Northwest.[19] By telling the Makahs's history from their indigenous point of view, Reid reveals how the Makahs engaged European actors and shaped the experience of contact.

Portuguese travellers entered the Indian Ocean world in the late fifteenth century.[20] Once there, they encountered a robust culture of travel and knowledge circulation in the Indo-Persian world.[21] Travel through the Indian Ocean world followed the Spice Route before the arrival of European explorers and merchants.[22] Even after Portuguese and Dutch merchants entered the Indian Ocean world, Ottoman merchants still brought spices to European markets via the Persian Gulf.[23] As travellers moved within the Indian Ocean world, they encountered enslaved peoples. Pier Larsen has shown how colonial travel and enslavement contributed to creolization as part of the African diaspora in the Indian Ocean.[24] The development of new mercantile relationships accelerated travel in the Indian Ocean.[25] Dutch merchants' engagement with the Indian Ocean also contributed to ongoing epistemological debates.[26] The British Empire also left indelible marks on its colonies in the Indian Ocean world. Matthew Edney has shown how the British triangulation survey worked to both spatially define its colonial realm and legitimate its colonial control.[27] This imperial science not only served as an instrument of empire, but also allowed subaltern peoples to imagine their independence in a modern world.[28]

In addition to these three theatres of scientific travel – the Atlantic, the Pacific and the Indian Ocean world – a fourth grouping of scientific travel must be recognized, circumnavigation.[29] The first circumnavigation was organized by Ferdinand Magellan and completed by Juan Sebastián Elcano during the early sixteenth century.[30] Sir Francis Drake and Henry Cavendish also completed circumnavigations for the English monarchy in the later sixteenth century. However, such expeditions were impractical for commercial and imperial interests. In the eighteenth century, three famous voyages would be undertaken that exemplify the heroic style of scientific traveller described in the next section.

AGENTS OF SCIENTIFIC PRODUCTION

Scientific travel steadily increased during the eighteenth century to all three destinations described in the previous section. Rob Iliffe's summary of scientific travel in the eighteenth century connects the major explorations of the period to the strategic concerns of imperial governance.[31] Great Britain, France, Spain and Russia were all major forces in this century, competing for territorial sovereignty, commercial resources and philosophical supremacy. More importantly, these interests were not in competition, but were overlapping. Examining eighteenth-century scientific travel, in particular, is useful for outlining three different ways scholars have studied participation in scientific travel, namely, heroic voyages, international collaborative expeditions, and enslaved or indigenous collaborators.

A major characteristic of the eighteenth century was the imperial voyage, exemplified by 'heroic' voyagers such as James Cook; Louis Antoine de Bougainville; Jean François de Galaup, comte de Lapérouse; and Alejandro Malaspina. Originally motivated by sending observers to disparate locations for isolated scientific observations, these expeditions morphed into highly competitive endeavours to secure territorial rights and navigational supremacy through the prestige of circumnavigation. Key questions posed by these missions included the charting and documenting the southernmost and northernmost seas (i.e. Northwest passage and Australian continent). Louis Antoine de Bougainville completed the first eighteenth-century scientific circumnavigation in 1763, which was also the first French circumnavigation of the globe.[32]

Undoubtedly, the most studied eighteenth-century scientific circumnavigations were three voyages to the Pacific between 1768 and 1779 led by James Cook.[33] Cook was already an experienced hydrographer and officer in the Royal Navy before his voyages to the Pacific. The first, aboard the HMS *Endeavour*, was dispatched to observe the Transit of Venus in 1769 and, secretly, to search in the South Pacific for future opportunities for British colonization. Accompanying Cook on his first voyage were Daniel Carl Solander, a botanist associated with the global efforts of Carl Linnaeus; Sydney Parkinson, a Scottish botanical illustrator; and the botanist Joseph Banks.[34] The success of Cook's first voyage led to two more voyages to the Pacific, before he was killed in Hawaii on his third voyage.[35]

In the global Spanish monarchy, this style of scientific travel is associated with the 1789–1794 expedition of Alejandro Malaspina.[36] The Malaspina expedition explored and mapped the Spanish Pacific, focusing on the American coast from Cape Horn to the Gulf of Alaska. His voyage, modelled after the heroic styles of James Cook and Louis Antoine de Bougainville, was both a high and low point for Spanish science in the eighteenth century. His politic sympathies (arguing for the independence of the American colonies) eventually had him exiled to Italy, where he died.

The figure of the heroic voyager would change slightly in the nineteenth century, when two of the most recognizable examples would be the missionary and geographer David Livingstone and the colonial administrator Henry Morgan Stanley.[37] The Scramble for Africa and associated mystique of the African interior popularized the narrative of the heroic voyager, moving their exploits from travel literature to popular journalism.

Early in the eighteenth century, we see the rise of 'international' models of science.[38] The most well known of these would be the 1735 expeditions to measure the global meridian and the Linnaean botanical machine. Such internationalism returned at mid-century, inspired by the transits of Venus in the 1760s. Internationalism came both in the form of granting access to foreign scientists and multinational teams of observers. Controversy arose early in the eighteenth century between Cartesians and Newtonians concerning the true shape of the earth. Was it a perfect sphere, as Rene Descartes argued, or a compressed ellipsoid owing to gravitational magnetism, as Isaac Newton suggested? The Paris Academy of Arts and Sciences attempted to settle the debate by dispatching expeditions to measure the length of one degree of latitude at the pole and one at the equator. Two teams of academicians were dispatched on voyages to Lapland and to Quito. The arctic expedition was led by Pierre Louis Maupertuis, who was accompanied by Alexis Claude Clairaut and Pierre Charles Le Monnier.[39] Meanwhile a team of observers including Louis Godin, Pierre Bouguer, Charles Marie de La Condamine and two young Spanish scientists, Jorge Juan and Antonio de Ulloa, travelled to the equatorial region to measure the length of an arc degree.[40] The 1735 Spanish-French expedition to Peru to measure the global meridian had been required to take Spanish agents as a condition for travel through Spanish America.

International cooperation also shaped botanical expeditions in the eighteenth century.

From Sweden, Carl Linnaeus oversaw a global network of scholars – whom he called his 'Apostles' – who collected, described, and drew samples to be added to his collections.[41] Global botanical expeditions served to both quench scientific curiosity and stimulate commercial interest.[42] No eighteenth-century botanical sparked quite as much interest as the antimalarial drug quinine and its source, cinchona bark.[43] Spain dispatched three major botanical expeditions to the Americas during the reign of Charles III.[44] These expeditions build upon the impressive earlier botanical surveys, including the work of Francisco Hernández in the early sixteenth century.[45]

Importantly, botany also engaged a variety of populations including European travellers, local botanists, and indigenous and enslaved collaborators.[46] These diverse categories of actors reflect growing research on the impact of non-European artists and naturalists on European natural philosophy. They also indicate the noticeable changes in the social and cultural environment of the place as a result of the knowledge of indigenous plants and their specific uses (Sohini Das in this volume). As Daniela Bleichmar has observed regarding the Americas, "indigenous peoples were not only informants, they were also knowledge makers in their own right".[47] Londa Schiebinger balances the contributions of these different actors in describing knowledge of the 'peacock flower' in the Atlantic world, both as medicine for European subjects and as an abortive tool for indigenous and enslaved women in Dutch Surinam.[48] A more recent example of this focus is Pablo Gómez, who has elucidated the healing practices of free and enslaved Caribbean communities.[49]

SPACES OF SCIENCE

Scientific travellers practiced knowledge production in a variety of spaces. For some, observations were collected abroad but knowledge was created in the metropole. For others, the field was the site of knowledge creation. As described previously, indigenous and enslaved actors also produced knowledge about the natural world that was appropriated or mimicked by European scientific travellers. As scholars have studied scientific travel, they have increasingly examined not only who practiced science, as described in the previous section, but also where science was understood to happen. Daniela Bleichmar describes this global era as a moment when the "learned and the curious flocked to the places where they could experience the things of the world: marketplaces, pharmacies, gardens, and the virtual space offered by book".[50]

One site of particular interest to scholars has been the ship. Knowledge was constructed aboard ships, but, as Richard Sorrenson has argued, ships also created knowledge.[51] Writing about British hydrographic surveys of the Pacific, Sorrenson argues that the ship's trace on the survey map demonstrates that the ship, itself, was the key instrument that measured the ocean floor. Other scholars have argued that it was the naval background of hydrographic voyagers that shaped knowledge creation aboard the ship.[52] Across Europe, military officers trained in surveying became a leading class of scientific agents. In Spain, in particular, naval officers trained at the Naval Observatory in Cádiz were dispatched on many of the key Spanish scientific expeditions of the long eighteenth century, often bringing instruments from the observatory collection, such as theodolites, chronometers and sextants.[53] The rhythm of naval observation also penetrated the 'land-based ship' according to Fabian Locher.[54] Locher examines the role of naval observation practices in informing the observational methodology of meteorological and geomagnetic observers during the nineteenth-century geomagnetism crusades. Larrie Ferreiro has written extensively about the science of naval architecture during the early modern and modern eras, showing how the ship was purposefully constructed to accommodate the needs of scientists, their equipment and their samples.[55]

Ships might also house another important tool for scientific travellers – a library. Scientific travellers referred to previous accounts of travel through a specific region or employed comparative methodologies when assessing the novelty of new botanical or mineral samples.[56] Safier describes an Amazonian observational regimen where books were trunked downriver and fact-checking occurred in real time. This immediate consultation changes the expedition from a fact-gathering to a knowledge-creating endeavour.

Lastly, when the European scientific traveller did return from their expedition, knowledge production was practiced in a variety of repositories in the metropole: museums, gardens and menageries.[57] Paula Findlen has written extensively about cabinets of curiosity and the creation of museum culture in early modern Italy.[58] The assembling of a collection allowed curators to 'travel' in their minds by assembling an order in nature, exposing the connections and differences between samples from across the globe. The most famous of these early modern Italian collections was the one housed at the Collegio Romano and organized by Athanasius Kircher.[59] Jesuits departed from Rome to evangelize globally and they brought back items to be added to the impressive collection that Kircher organized.[60] The garden was another institution intimately tied to the fruits of scientific travel, including Joseph Banks' samples in Key Garden and the Royal Botanical Garden in Madrid.[61] By the nineteenth century, these early collecting institutions had diverged into a series of distinct spaces for the ordering and displaying of samples. The singular space of the museum or cabinet of curiosity became multiple spaces that reflected the establishment of distinct scientific disciplines, such as anthropology, zoology and pharmacology.[62]

MAKING KNOWLEDGE

Scientific travel was an act itself, but the production of new natural knowledge engaged a variety of epistemologies from tactical to visual knowledges.[63] As European natural philosophers received personal accounts of America and of its natural wonder, the primacy of eye witnessing first augmented and then replaced ancient authorities such as Pliny and Ptolemy. The changes brought about by European engagement with nature in the Atlantic, Pacific and Indian Ocean worlds were profound, even if the shifts were gradual and uneven. It was at this time that early modern scholars turned from texts to reading the 'Book of

Nature' through lived experience and images of the natural world.[64] Hugh Cagle has written about how Portuguese agents were forced to construct the tropics as a legible, global category to explain both medicine and natural history gathered within their global empire as arising from a single cohesive region.[65]

In addition to expanding descriptive and analytical categories, scientific travellers also developed new epistemologies based upon their observations and specimens. Alexander von Humboldt, for example, has been credited with ushering in a new style of science that viewed nature as an interconnected system.[66] Humboldt's travels through South America between 1799 and 1804 have been credited with inspiring his unity, most famously his cross-sectional map of the Chimborazo that associated plant distribution with altitude.[67] Humboldt encapsulates all the themes described here: he was a 'heroic' voyager, he collaborated with local and international communities and he relied on local and indigenous knowledge.[68]

Perhaps no scientific traveller has received quite as much scholarly attention as Charles Darwin.[69] As is well known, a young Darwin accompanied the HMS *Beagle*, and its captain, Robert FitzRoy, on its hydrographic survey expedition from 1831 to 1836. Both Darwin's notebooks from the *Beagle* voyage and his personal correspondence have been made available in scholarly editions by Cambridge University Press.[70] Scholars have argued that the experience of voyaging aboard a naval vessel influenced Darwin's observations.[71] Darwin's later works on evolution would be indebted to the fieldwork he conducted during this voyage, especially his observational notes and specimens from the Galapagos Islands.[72]

Foremost in debates on how knowledge was constructed in relation to scientific travel have been studies regarding scientific observation.[73] Scholars have focused in on the question of whether the observer or the scientific instrument created knowledge.[74] Proponents of the actor-network theory have argued that facts and observations were collected by scientific travellers and easily transported along networks of information exchange to 'centres of calculations', where they could be analysed and transformed into knowledge.[75] This narrative has been challenged recently, as scholars have identified polycentric networks of knowledge creation and examined the role of intermediaries in the circulation of knowledge and knowledge products.[76]

DISEASES AND THERAPEUTICS

Medical knowledge was particularly impacted by developments in scientific travel between the seventeenth and nineteenth centuries. Just as scientific travel, generally, served as a tool of imperial control, medical knowledge served to control and categorize non-European bodies.[77] European medicine developed in concert with colonial conquest from the seventeenth century onwards, constructing new systems to categorize disease and its spread such as Germ theory or a focus on sanitation. As nineteenth-century scientific expeditions were recategorized as 'civilizing missions', the growing field of public health and concerns about sanitation furthered the othering of colonial bodies. As Warwick Anderson has shown, colonizers struggled to adapt their bodies to 'tropical' climes while also claiming racial superiority over local populations.[78] The nineteenth century also saw the growing association of Christian missionaries with medical agents, who sought to bring Western medicine to the colonial clinic.[79] A central function of government authority in all contexts was the control of epidemic disease and the organization of meaningful responses to death, famine and hunger.[80] Hygiene, eugenics and public health all functioned in overlapping ways as tools of colonial power into the twentieth century during the emergence of global health.[81]

While medicine was employed as a tool of empire by scientific travellers, disease categories and novel therapeutics were also utilized by affluent non-European members of society to carve out spaces of resistance, adaptation and pluralism.[82] While medical missions sought, in part, to disrupt indigenous practices, traditional medicine persisted or was adapted in the wake of Western exploration and colonization.[83] Marginalized health practitioners – indigenous, enslaved, creole and subaltern – thrived in the 'grey zones of medicine', maintaining traditional therapeutics while also mediating their healing practices with the influence of Western medicine.[84] Conversely, the introduction of new materia medica to the European medical marketplace as a result of scientific travel altered Western therapeutic regimens.[85] The discovery of quinine as an antimalarial agent and associated growth of a vibrant market for cinchona bark is one example of this phenomenon.[86] Additionally, the description of extra-European medical techniques by travellers led to their appropriation and adoption. Lady Mary Montagu's advocacy for smallpox inoculation is a well-known example of this phenomenon, but, as Mary Lindemann has shown, the role of Montagu in the widespread adoption of inoculation should not be overstated.[87] This all serves to underscore the false dichotomy drawn between Western and non-Western medicine as separate and independently developing fields in the era of scientific travel. Instead, from the moment of contact onwards, the exchange of ideas, therapeutics, techniques and instrumentation functioned bidirectionally.[88]

CONCLUSION

What happens when you encounter new worlds, new continents, new people, new plants and animals? How does that change your understanding of the world? Early modern European engagement with extra-European societies and their natural philosophies dislodged the dominant Aristotelian epistemology in Europe. What replaced it were new systems of astronomy, physics, medicine and geography influenced by the discovery of new flora, fauna and civilizations of the Atlantic, Pacific and Indian Ocean worlds. European colonization expanded globally between the seventeenth century and the nineteenth century to accommodate both economic interests and philosophical questions. Slave traders and merchants joined natural philosophers in traveling throughout the Atlantic, Pacific and Indian Ocean worlds, circulating goods and collecting natural resources for commodification and classification. Aided by indigenous collaborators, these actors sought to produce new knowledge to add to the European understanding of global nature and new materia medica to treat disease. Their economic and scientific gazes each served to further travel, as the act of collection promoted a new objectivity in Europe which inspired fresh expeditions. While scholars traditionally excluded the contributions of non-European actors to these scientific voyages, the last thirty years of scholarship has seen a re-evaluation of the contributions non-European actors made to knowledge production during early modern and modern scientific voyages. Likewise, a critical re-evaluation of the contributions of merchants to scientific expeditions has illustrated the important role of economic enterprise played in knowledge production. The history of scientific travel is a robust literature that reflects the diverse actors and cultures that influenced science and medicine between the seventeenth and nineteenth centuries.

NOTES

1. I borrow this terminology from Lewis Pyenson, *Civilizing Mission: Exact Sciences and French Overseas Expansion, 1830–1940* (Baltimore: Johns Hopkins University Press, 1993). For more on nineteenth-century scientific travel as a tool of imperial power, see Felix Driver, *Geography Militant: Cultures of Exploration in the Age of Empire* (Oxford: Blackwell, 2001).

2. For 'centres of calculation', see Bruno Latour, *Science in Action: How to Follow Scientists and Engineers Through Society* (Cambridge, MA: Harvard University Press, 2002). For a reflection on science in the field, see Hernika Kuklick and Robert E. Kohler, eds., *Science in the Field*, *Osiris* 11 (1996).

3. For one recent reflections on the role of Iberian fisherman in early colonization, see Gabriel de Avilez Rocha, "The Pinzones and the coup of the *acedares*: fishing and colonization in the fifteenth-century Atlantic," *Colonial Latin American Review*, 28:4 (2019), 427–449. doi: 10.1080/10609164.2019.1681146; Juan Manuel Bello León, *La pesca en Andalucía y Canarias en el tránsito de la Edad Media a la moderna (siglos XV y XVI)* (Santa Cruz de Tenerife: Ediciones Idea, 2008). For the role of

Africa and Africans in the shaping of the Atlantic world, see John Thornton, *Africa and Africans in the Making of the Atlantic World, 1400–1800* (New York: Cambridge University Press, 2017).

4. For good overviews of Iberian science in Atlantic history, see Daniela Bleichmar, Paula De Vos, Kristin Huffine, and Kevin Sheehan, eds., *Science in the Spanish and Portuguese Empires, 1500–1800* (Stanford, CA: Stanford University Press, 2009); Jorge Cañizares-Esguerra, *Nature, Empire, and Nation: Explorations of the History of Science in the Iberian World* (Stanford, CA: Stanford University Press, 2006). For Spanish attempts to both collect and control knowledge of the New World, see María M. Portuondo, *Secret Science: Spanish Cosmography and the New World* (Chicago: University of Chicago Press, 2009).

5. Nicolás Wey Gómez, *The Tropics of Empire: Why Columbus Sailed South to the Indies* (Cambridge, MA: MIT Press, 2008); Ricardo Padrón, "Mapping Plus Ultra: Cartography, Space, and Hispanic Modernity," *Representations* 79, no. 1 (2002): 28–60.

6. James Delbourgo and Nicholas Dew, *Science and Empire in the Atlantic World* (New York: Routledge, 2008); Anthony Pagden, *European Encounters with the New World: From Renaissance to Romanticism* (New Haven: Yale Univ. Press, 1998).

7. For classic histories of these institutions, see Robert Hahn, *The Anatomy of a Scientific Institution: The Paris Academy of Sciences, 1666–1803* (Berkeley: University of California Press, 1971); Michael Hunter, *Establishing the New Science: The Experience of the Early Royal Society* (Woodbridge: Boydell, 1989).

8. Nicholas Dew, "Scientific Travel in the Atlantic World: The French Expedition to Gorée and the Antilles, 1681–1683," *British Journal for the History of Science* 43 (2010): 1–17.

9. For a biography of Hans Sloane and his role in the creation of the British Museum, see James Delbourgo, *Collecting the World Hans Sloane and the Origins of the British Museum* (Cambridge, MA: Belknap Press of Harvard University Press, 2017). For science in the British Atlantic, see James Delbourgo, "Science," in *The British Atlantic World, 1500–1800*, ed. David Armitage and Michael J. Braddick (London: Palgrave Macmillan, 2009), 92–110.

10. For an excellent historiographical review of science in the British Atlantic, see Joyce E. Chaplin, "The Curious Case of Science and Empire," *Reviews in American History* 34, no. 4 (2006): 434–40. For another perspective on the state of Atlantic science, see Neil Safier, "Itineraries of Atlantic Science: New Questions, New Approaches, New Directions," *Atlantic* Studies 7, no. 4 (2010), 357–64. doi: 10.1080/14788810.2010.540873

11. Antonio Lafuente and Leoncio López-Ocón, "Scientific Traditions and Enlightenment Expeditions in Eighteenth-century Hispanic America," in *Science in Latin America*, edited by Juan José Saldaña, translated by Madrigal Bernabé (Austin: University of Texas Press, 2006), 123–50; Alejandro R. Díez Torre, Tomás Mallo, and Daniel Pacheco Fernández, eds., *De la ciencia ilustrada a la ciencia romántica: actas de las II Jornadas sobre "España y las expediciones científicas en America y Filipinas"* (Madrid: Doce Calles, 1995). For Spanish science during the reign of

Charles III, see Manuel A. Sellés, José Luis Peset Reig, and Antonio Lafuente. *Carlos III y la ciencia de la ilustración*. Madrid: Alianza, 1989.

12. D. Graham Burnett, *Masters of All They Surveyed: Exploration, Geography, and a British El Dorado* (Chicago: University of Chicago Press, 2000).

13. For synthetic overviews of European encounters with the Pacific, see Tony Ballantyne, ed., *Science, Empire and the European Exploration of the Pacific* (Florence: Routledge, 2018); Matt K. Matsuda, *Pacific Worlds: A History of Seas, Peoples, and Cultures* (New York: Cambridge University Press, 2012).

14. Ricardo Padrón, *The Indies of the Setting Sun: How Early Modern Spain Mapped the Far East As the Transpacific West* (Chicago: University of Chicago Press, 2020); Rainer F. Buschmann, Edward R. Slack, and James B. Tueller, *Navigating the Spanish Lake: The Pacific in the Iberian World, 1521–1898* (Honolulu: University of Hawai'i Press, 2014).

15. Margarette Lincoln, ed., *Science and Exploration in the Pacific European Voyages to the Southern Oceans in the Eighteenth Century* (Woodbridge: Boydell Press, 2001); John Gascoigne, *Encountering the Pacific in the Age of Enlightenment* (Cambridge: Cambridge University Press, 2014).

16. Juan Pimentel, *Testigos del mundo: ciencia, literatura y viajes en la Ilustración* (Madrid: Marcial Pons/ Ediciones de Historia, 2003). For literary analysis of eighteenth-century travel writing, see Michelle Burnham, "Trade, Time, and the Calculus of Risk in Early Pacific Travel Writing," *Early American Literature* 46, no. 3 (2011), 425–47.

17. D. Graham Burnett, "Hydrographic Discipline among the Navigators Charting an 'Empire of Commerce and Science' in the Nineteenth-Century Pacific," in *The Imperial Map: Cartography and the Mastery of* Empire, James Akerman, ed. (Chicago: University of Chicago Press, 2009), 185–260; Ilya Vinkovetsky, *Russian America: An Overseas Colony of a Continental Empire, 1804–1867* (Oxford, Oxford University Press, 2014); Gwenn A. Miller, *Kodiak Kreol: Communities of Empire in Early Russian America* (Ithaca, NY: Cornell University Press, 2015).

18. David A. Chang, *The World and All the Things Upon It: Native Hawaiian Geographies of Exploration* (Minneapolis: University of Minnesota Press, 2016).

19. Joshua L. Reid, *The Sea Is My Country: The Maritime World of the Makahs, an Indigenous Borderlands People* (New Haven: Yale University Press, 2018).

20. For Portuguese expansion into the Indian Ocean, see Kirti N. Chaudhuri, "The Portuguese Maritime Empire, Trade, and Society in the Indian Ocean During the Sixteenth Century," *Portuguese Studies* 8 (1992): 57–70. For the Portuguese empire in Asia, see Sanjay Subrahmanyam, *The Portuguese Empire in Asia, 1500–1700: A Political and Economic History* (Chichester, UK: John Wiley & Sons, 2012). For a synthetic introduction to the Indian Ocean world, see Kenneth McPherson, *The Indian Ocean: A History of People and the Sea* (New Delhi: Oxford University Press, 2006).

21. Muzaffar Alam and Sanjay Subrahmanyam, *Indo-Persian Travels in the Age of Discoveries, 1400–1800* (Cambridge: Cambridge University Press, 2010); Sinnappah Arasaratnam, *Maritime India in the Seventeenth Century* (New Delhi: Oxford University Press, 1994).

22. For a good introduction to the *longue duree* history of the Spice Route, see John Keay, *The Spice Route: A History* (Berkeley: University of California Press, 2006).

23. Giancarlo Casale, "The Ottoman Administration of the Spice Trade in the Sixteenth-Century Red Sea and Persian Gulf," *Journal of the Economic and Social History of the Orient* 49/2 (2006), 170–98. Casale has argued that the Ottoman Empire was an active participant in the European Age of Exploration, see Giancarlo Casale, *The Ottoman Age of Exploration* (Oxford: Oxford University Press, 2012).

24. Pier Martin Larson, *Ocean of Letters: Language and Creolization in an Indian Ocean Diaspora* (Cambridge, UK: Cambridge University Press, 2009). For the circulation of enslaved people in the Indian Ocean through the lens of the lived experience of one individual, see Omar H. Ali, *Malik Ambar: Power and Slavery Across the Indian Ocean* (New York: Oxford University Press, 2016).

25. Eric Tagliacozzo, "Trade, Production and Incorporation. The Indian Ocean in Flux, 1600–1900," *Itinerario.* 26, no. 1 (2002), 75–106.

26. For analysis of how merchants with the Dutch East Indies Company (VOC) shaped emerging conceptions of facts and observational epistemologies, see Harold J. Cook, *Matters of Exchange: Commerce, Medicine, and Science in the Dutch Golden Age* (New Haven: Yale University Press, 2008).

27. Matthew H. Edney, *Mapping an Empire: The Geographical Construction of British India, 1765–1843* (Chicago: University of Chicago Press, 1999).

28. Gyan Prakash, *Another Reason: Science and the Imagination of Modern India* (Princeton: Princeton University Press, 2007).

29. For an overview of the topic of circumnavigation, see Joyce E. Chaplin, *Round About the Earth: Circumnavigation from Magellan to Orbit* (New York: Simon & Schuster, 2014).

30. For one account of their voyage, see Antonio Pigafetta, *Magellan's Voyage: A Narrative Account of the First Circumnavigation,* R. A. Skelton, trans. (New Haven: Yale University Press, 1969).

31. Rob Iliffe, "Science and Voyages of Discovery," in *The Cambridge History of Science*, edited by Roy Porter (Cambridge: Cambridge University Press, 2003), 4, 618–46.

32. For an overview of Bougainville, his voyage and its importance, see Etienne Taillemite, ed., *Bougainville Et Ses Compagnons Autour Du Monde: 1766–1769, Journaux De Navigation* (Paris: Imprimerie nationale, 1977).

33. For a scholarly biography of Cook, see John Cawte Beaglehole, *The Life of Captain James Cook* (Stanford, CA: Stanford Univ. Press, 1998).

34. For more on the significance of botany and Joseph Banks to the *Endeavour* voyage, see David Mackay, "A Presiding Genius of Exploration: Banks, Cook, and Empire, 1767–1805," in Robin Fisher and Hugh Johnston, eds., *Captain Cook and His Times* (Seattle: University of Washington Press, 1979), 21–39.

35. For botany on the three Cook voyages, see Phyllis I. Edwards, "Sir Joseph Banks and the Botany of Captain Cook's Three Voyages of Exploration," *Pacific Studies* 2, no.1 (1978): 20–43. For zoology on the Cook voyages, see P.J.P.

Whitehead, "A Guide to the Dispersal of Zoological Material from Captain Cook's Voyages," *Pacific Studies* 2, no. 1 (1978), 52–93.

36. For an introduction to the Malaspina expedition, see Juan Pimentel Igea, *La física de la monarquía: ciencia y política en el pensamiento colonial de Alejandro Malaspina (1754–1810)* (Aranjuez: Doce Calles, 1998); Alessandro Malaspina, *The Malaspina Expedition, 1789–1794: Journal of the Voyage by Alejandro Malaspina*, 3 vols., Works issued by the Hakluyt Society 3rd ser., no. 8 (London: Hakluyt Society in association with the Museo Naval, Madrid, 2001).

37. For entries into the Livingstone and Stanley exploits, see Driver, *Geography* Militant, 68–89; Felix Driver, "Henry Morton Stanley & His Critics: Geography, Exploration & Empire," *Past and Present* 133 (1991): 134–66; John Stuart, "David Livingstone, British Protestant missions, memory and empire," in Dominik Geppert and Frank Lorenz Müller, eds., *Sites of Imperial Memory* (Manchester: Manchester University Press, 2016), 153–69; Felix Driver, "Missionary Travels: Livingstone, Africa and the book," *Scottish Geographical Journal* 129, no. 3–4 (2013):164–78.

38. Sverker Sörlin, "National and International Aspects of Cross-Boundary Science: Scientific Travel in the 18th Century," in Elisabeth Crawford, Terry Shinn, and Sverker Sörlin, eds., *Denationalizing Science: The Contexts of International Scientific Practice* (Dordrecht: Springer Netherlands, 1993), 43–72.

39. For an account of the Lapland expedition and Maupertuis's role, see Mary Terrall, *The Man Who Flattened the Earth: Maupertuis and the Sciences in the Enlightenment* (Chicago: University of Chicago Press, 2002).

40. The Spanish-French expedition has received extensive scholarly focus; for one informative account, see Neil Safier, *Measuring the New World: Enlightenment Science and South America* (Chicago: University of Chicago Press, 2008).

41. For one account of the eighteenth-century botanical revolution, see Patricia Fara, *Sex, Botany and Empire: The Story of Carl Linnaeus and Joseph Banks* (London: Icon Books, 2017). For a biography of Carl Linnaeus, see Lisbet Koerner, *Linnaeus: Nature and Narration* (Cambridge, MA: Harvard University Press, 1999).

42. For a survey of colonial botany and botanical expeditions, see Londa L. Schiebinger and Claudia Swan, eds., *Colonial Botany: Science, Commerce, and Politics in the Early Modern World* (Philadelphia, PA: University of Pennsylvania Press, 2007); David Philip Miller and Peter Hanns Reill, eds., *Visions of Empire: Voyages, Botany, and Representations of Nature* (Cambridge: Cambridge University Press, 1996). For an example of the international market for local botanical knowledge, see Hugh Cagle, "Cultures of Inquiry, Myths of Empire: Natural History in Colonial Goa," in *Medicine, Trade, and Empire: Garcia de Orta's* Colloquies on the Simples and Drugs of India *(1563) in Context*, Andrew Cunningham and Palmira Fontes da Costa, eds. (Burlington, VT: Ashgate, 2015), 107–28.

43. For a recent summary of the early cinchona market, see Matthew James Crawford, *The Andean Wonder Drug: Cinchona Bark and Imperial Science in the Spanish Atlantic, 1630–1800* (Pittsburgh: University of Pittsburgh Press, 2016). For later attempts to cultivate cinchona outside Latin America, see Arjo Roersch van der Hoogte and Toine Pieters, "Science in the service of colonial agro-industrialism: the case of cinchona cultivation in the Dutch and British East Indies, 1852–1900," *Studies*

in history and philosophy of biological and biomedical sciences, 47 Pt A (2014), 12–22.

44. For overviews of these expeditions, see Daniela Bleichmar, "Botanical Conquistadors: Plants and Empire in the Hispanic Enlightenment," in Yota Batsaki, Sarah Burke Cahalane, and Anatole Tchikine (eds.), *The Botany of Empire in the Long Eighteenth Century* (Washington, DC: Dumbarton Oaks/Harvard University Press, 2017), 35–60; Daniela Bleichmar, *Visible Empire: Botanical Expeditions and Visual Culture in the Hispanic Enlightenment* (University of Chicago Press, 2012).

45. For earlier Spanish botanical surveys, see José Pardo Tomás and María Luz López Terrada. *Las primeras noticias sobre plantas americanas en las relaciones de viajes y crónicas de Indias, 1493–1553* (València: Instituto de estudios documentales e históricos sobre la ciencia, Universitat de València-CSIC, 1993); Antonio Barrera-Osorio, "Local Herbs, Global Medicines: Commerce, Knowledge, and Commodities in Spanish America" in Pamela Smith and Paula Findlen, eds., *Merchants and Marvels: Commerce, Science, and Art in Early Modern Europe* (New York: Routledge, 2002), 163–82; Jose Maria Lopez Piñero and Maria Luz Lopez Terrada. *La influencia española en la introducion en Europa de las plantas americanas (1493–1623)* (Valencia: Universitat de Valencia, Instituto de Estudios Documentales e Historicos sobre la Ciencia, 1998).

46. Kathleen Murphy, "Translating the vernacular: Indigenous and African knowledge in the eighteenth-century British Atlantic," *Atlantic Studies,* 8, no. 1 (2011), 29–48; Alex Calder, Jonathan Lamb, and Bridget Orr, eds., *Voyages and Beaches: Pacific Encounters, 1769–1840* (Honolulu: University of Hawai'i Press, 1999).

47. Bleichmar, *Visual Voyages*, 26.

48. Londa L. Schiebinger, *Plants and Empire: Colonial Bioprospecting in the Atlantic World* (Cambridge: Harvard University Press, 2004).

49. Pablo F. Gómez, *The Experiential Caribbean: Creating Knowledge and Healing in the Early Modern Atlantic* (Chapin Hill: University of North Carolina Press, 2017).

50. Daniela Bleichmar, *Visual Voyages: Images of Latin American Nature from Columbus to Darwin* (New Haven: Yale University Press in association with The Huntington Library, Art Collections, and Botanical Gardens, 2017), 91.

51. Richard Sorrenson, "The Ship as a Scientific Instrument in the Eighteenth Century," *Osiris* 11 (1996), 221–36.

52. Randolph Cock, "Scientific Servicemen in the Royal Navy and the Professionalisation of Science, 1816–55," in *Science and beliefs: from natural philosophy to natural science, 1700–1900*, David Knight and Matthew Eddy, eds. (Aldershot: Ashgate, 2005), 95–112; Penelope K. Hardy, "Every Ship a Floating Observatory: Matthew Fontaine Maury and the Acquisition of Knowledge at Sea," in *Soundings and Crossings: Doing Science at Sea 1800–1970*, edited by Katharine Anderson and Helen M. Rozwadowski (Sagamore Beach, MA: Science History Publications/Watson Publishing International, 2016), 17–48; D. Graham Burnett, "Hydrographic Discipline among the Navigators Charting an 'Empire of Commerce and Science' in the Nineteenth-Century Pacific," in *The Imperial Map: Cartography and the Mastery*

of Empire, James Akerman, ed. (Chicago: University of Chicago Press, 2009), 185–260.

53. For a history of the Spanish naval academy and observatory in Cádiz, see Antonio Lafuente, *El Observatorio de Cádiz (1753–1831)* (Madrid: Ministerio de Defensa; Instituto de Historia y Cultura Naval, 1988); María Dolores González-Ripoll Navarro, "La formación académica y práctica de los marinos del siglo XVIII Cosme de Churruca (1761–1805), un oficial científico," in Alejandro R. Díez Torre, Tomás Mallo, and Daniel Pacheco Fernández, eds., *De la ciencia ilustrada a la ciencia romántica: actas de las II Jornadas sobre "España y las expediciones científicas en America y Filipinas"* (Madrid: Doce Calles, 1995), 313–24. For a detailed accounting of the naval instrument collection and it use on scientific expeditions, see Francisco González González, *Instrumentos Científicos del Observatorio de San Fernando: (siglos XVIII, XIX, XX)* (Madrid: Instituto de Historia y Cultura Naval, 1995).

54. Fabien Locher, "The Observatory, the Land-Based Ship and the Crusades: Earth Sciences in European Context, 1830–50," *British Journal for the History of Science* 40 (2007), 491–504.

55. Larrie D. Ferreiro, *Ships and Science: The Birth of Naval Architecture in the Scientific Revolution, 1600–1800* (Cambridge: MIT Press, 2014); Larrie D. Ferreiro, *Bridging the Seas: The Rise of Naval Architecture in the Industrial Age, 1800–2000* (Cambridge: MIT Press, 2020). For how the sea, itself, became an object of study, see the classic Margaret Deacon, *Scientists and the Sea, 1650–1900: A Study of Marine Science* (Aldershot, Hampshire, Great Britain: Ashgate, 1997).

56. Neil Safier, "'Every day that I travel . . . is a page that I turn': Reading and Observing in Eighteenth-Century Amazonia," *Huntington Library Quarterly* 70, no. 1 (2007), 103–28; Daniela Bleichmar, "Exploration in Print: Books and Botanical Travel from Spain to the Americas in the Late Eighteenth Century," *Huntington Library Quarterly* 70, no. 1 (2007), 129–52.

57. For a summary of the history of museum collections as producers of new knowledge, see Eilean Hooper-Greenhill, *Museums and the Shaping of Knowledge* (London: Routledge, 2009). For the movement of objects from the expedition to the museum, see Kurt Schmutzer, "Metamorphosis between field and museum: collections in the making," *Journal of the History of Science Technology* 5 (2012), 68–83. For how museums have informed social and political cultures, see the informative essays in Sheila E. R. Watson, Suzanne Macleod, and Simon J. Knell, eds., *Museum Revolutions: how museums change and are changed* (London: Routledge, 2007).

58. Paula Findlen, *Possessing Nature: Museums, Collecting and Scientific Culture in Early Modern Italy* (Berkeley: University of California Press, 1994).

59. For Kircher and the Colegio Romano, see Daniel Stolzenberg, ed., *The Great Art of Knowing: The Baroque Encyclopedia of Athanasius Kircher* (Stanford: Stanford University Libraries, 2001); Paula Findlen, ed., *Athanasius Kircher: The Last Man Who Knew Everything* (New York: Routledge, 2004).

60. For the global Jesuit scientific production, see, for example, Florence C. Hsia, *Sojourners in a Strange Land: Jesuits and Their Scientific Missions in Late Imperial China* (University of Chicago Press, 2009); Andrés I. Prieto, *Missionary Scientists:*

Jesuit science in Spanish South America, 1570–1810 (Nashville: Vanderbilt University Press, 2011).

61. For one account of the imperial botanical garden, see Zaheer Baber "The Plants of Empire: Botanic Gardens, Colonial Power and Botanical Knowledge," *Journal of Contemporary Asia*, 46, no. 4 (2016), 659–79. doi: 10.1080/00472336.2016.1185796

62. For more on the establishment of distinct museum spaces that reflected scientific disciplinary distinctions, see Caroline Cornish, "Nineteenth-Century Museums and the Shaping of Disciplines: Potentialities and Limitations at Kew's Museum of Economic Botany," *Museum History Journal* 8, no. 1 (2015), 8–27. doi: 10.1179/1936981614Z.00000000042. For how objects are shaped by curatorial choice, see Samuel J. M. M. Alberti, "Objects and the Museum", *Isis,* 96, no. 4 (2005), 559–71.

63. The history of knowledge and knowledge production has gained increasing interest in the past few years. For an informative introduction to this reframing of interconnected historiographies, see Peter Burke, *What Is the History of Knowledge?* (Cambridge: Polity Press, 2016). Reflecting the growing interest in this subfield, a *Journal for the History of Knowledge* was established in 2020. For more on the promise of this new field, see their inaugural issue forum, especially Philipp Sarasin, "More Than Just Another Specialty: On the Prospects for the History of Knowledge," *Journal for the History of Knowledge* 1, no. 1 (2020), 1–5. doi: 10.5334/jhk.25

64. For scientific travel and changes to natural history, see the essays in section three of Nicholas Jardine, J. A. Secord, and Emma C. Spary, eds., *Cultures of Natural History* (Cambridge: Cambridge University Press, 1996).

65. For the creation of the tropics in the global Portuguese empire and its scientific travels, see Hugh Cagle, *Assembling the Tropics: Science and Medicine in Portugal's Empire, 1450–1700* (Cambridge: Cambridge University Press, 2020). For another perspective on the legibility of the tropics, see Nicolás Wey Gómez, *The Tropics of Empire: Why Columbus Sailed South to the Indies* (Cambridge, MA: MIT Press, 2008); Surekha Davies, *Renaissance Ethnography and the Invention of the Human: New Worlds, Maps and Monsters* (New York: Cambridge University Press, 2017), 23–48.

66. For a recent argument about the Humboldtian synthesis, see Andrea Wulf, *The Invention of Nature: Alexander Von Humboldt's New World* (New York: Alfred A. Knopf, 2015). For the differences between Humboldt and Humboldtians, see Michael Dettelbach, "Humboldtian Science," in Nicholas Jardine, J. A. Secord, and Emma C. Spary, eds., *Cultures of Natural History* (Cambridge: Cambridge University Press 1996), 287–304. For a reassessment of the unity of Humboldt's thought, see Michael Dettelbach, "Alexander Von Humboldt between Enlightenment and Romanticism," *Northeastern Naturalist* 8 (2001), 9–20.

67. Malcolm Nicolson, "Alexander von Humboldt, Humboldtian Science and the Origins of the Study of Vegetation", *History of Science* 25, no. 2 (June 1987): 167–94; Michael Dettelbach, "The Face of Nature: Precise Measurement, Mapping, and Sensibility in the Work of Alexander von Humboldt," *Studies in History and Philosophy of Biological and Biomedical Sciences* 30, no. 4 (1999), 473–504. Humboldt's

works are the subject of a new series of critical editions from the University of Chicago Press, see, for example, Alexander von Humboldt, *Views of the Cordilleras and monuments of the indigenous peoples of the Americas: a critical edition*, edited and translated by Vera M. Kutzinski and Ottmar Ette (Chicago: University of Chicago Press, 2013).

68. For questions regarding Humboldt's reliance on local collaborators and the originality of his synthesis, see Jorge Cañizares-Esguerra, "How Derivative Was Humboldt? Microcosmic Narratives in Early Modern Spanish America and the (Other) Origins of Humboldt's Ecological Sensibilities," in *Nature, Empire, and Nation: Explorations of the History of Science in the Iberian World* (Stanford: Stanford University Press, 2006), 112–28; Gregory T. Cushman, "Humboldtian Science, Creole Meteorology, and the Discovery of Human-Caused Climate Change in South America," *Osiris,* 26, no. 1 (2011): 16–44.

69. The literature on Darwin is voluminous, but for an excellent overview of Darwin's career and writing see the two-volume authoritative biography by Janet Browne: Janet Browne, *Charles Darwin: Voyaging, vol. 1* (Princeton: Princeton Univ. Press, 1996); Janet Brown, *Charles Darwin: the Power of Place, vol. 2* (Princeton: Princeton Univ. Press, 2003).

70. Gordon Chancellor and John Van Wyhe, eds., *Charles Darwin's Notebooks from the Voyage of the "Beagle,"* (New York: Cambridge University Press, 2009); Richard Darwin Keynes, ed., *Charles Darwin's "Beagle" Diary* (Cambridge: Cambridge University Press, 2004).

71. See, for example, Alistair Sponsel, "An Amphibious Being: How Maritime Surveying Reshaped Darwin's Approach to Natural History," *Isis,* 107, no. 2 (2016), 254–281.

72. For two representative articles on Darwin's experiences in the Galapagos, see Frank J. Sulloway, "Darwin and his finches: The evolution of a legend," *Journal of the History of Biology,* 15 (1982), 1–53; Janet Browne, "Darwin's Botanical Arithmetic and the 'Principle of Divergence,' 1854–1858," *Journal of the History of Biology,* 13 (1980), 53–89.

73. Lorraine Daston, "On Scientific Observation", *Isis.* 99, no. 1 (2008), 97–110; Lorraine Daston and Elizabeth Lunbeck, eds. *Histories of Scientific Observation* (Chicago and London: University of Chicago Press, 2011).

74. For representative views of the debate, see Simon Schaffer, "Astronomers Mark Time: Discipline and the Personal Equation," *Science in Context* 2, no. 1 (1988), 115–45; Charles W. J. Withers, "Science, Scientific Instruments and Questions of Method in Nineteenth-Century British Geography," *Transactions of the Institute of British Geographers* 38, no. 1 (2013), 167–79.

75. For Latour's conception of actor-network theory in the history of science, see Bruno Latour, *Science in Action: How to Follow Scientists and Engineers Through Society* (Cambridge, MA: Harvard University Press, 2002). For a recent assessment, see Matthew Sargent, "Recentering Centers of Calculation: Reconfiguring Knowledge Networks Within Global Empires of Trade," in Paula Findlen ed, *Empires of Knowledge: Scientific Networks in the Early Modern World* (London: Routledge, 2019), 297–316.

76. Kapil Raj, *Relocating Modern Science: Circulation and the Construction of Knowledge in South Asia and Europe, 1650–1900* (New York: Palgrave Macmillan, 2010); Simon Schaffer, Lissa Roberts, Kapil Raj, James Delbourgo, eds., *The Brokered World: Go-Betweens and Global Intelligence, 1770–1820* (Sagamore Beach, MA: Science History, 2009).

77. For excellent summaries of the intersection of medical travel and imperial expansion, see Pratik Chakrabarti, *Medicine and Empire: 1600–1960* (Basingstoke: Palgrave Macmillan, 2014); Roy M. MacLeod and Milton James Lewis, eds., *Disease, Medicine, and Empire: Perspectives on Western Medicine and the Experience of European Expansion* (London: Routledge, 1988); Davies, *Renaissance Ethnography and the Invention of the Human.*

78. Warwick Anderson, *Colonial Pathologies American Tropical Medicine, Race, and Hygiene in the Philippines* (Durham: Duke University Press, 2008). For more on the development of tropical medicine as a legible category, see Philip D. Curtin, *Death by Migration: Europe's Encounter with the Tropical World in the Nineteenth Century* (New York: Cambridge University Press, 2003); David Arnold, ed. *Warm Climates and Western Medicine: The Emergence of Tropical Medicine, 1500–1900*, Clio Medica 35 (Amsterdam: Rodopi, 1996).

79. For more on medical missionaries in Asia and Africa, see David Hardiman, ed., *Healing Bodies, Saving Souls*, Clio Medica 80 (Leiden, The Netherlands: Brill Rodopi, 2006) doi: 10.1163/9789401203630

80. Gyan Prakash, *Another Reason: Science and the Imagination of Modern India* (Princeton, N.J.: Princeton University Press, 1999), 123–58; Paul Ramírez, "'Like Herod's Massacre': Quarantines, Bourbon Reform, and Popular Protest in Oaxaca's Smallpox Epidemic, 1796–1797," *The Americas* 69, no. 2 (2012): 203–35; Martha Few, "Circulating Smallpox Knowledge: Guatemalan Doctors, Maya Indians and Designing Spain's Smallpox Vaccination Expedition, 1780–1803," *The British Journal for the History of Science* 43, no. 4 (2010): 519–37; Mike Davis, *Late Victorian Holocausts: El Niño Famines and the Making of the Third World* (London: Verso, 2001).

81. For more on the emergence of global health as a field and its growth out of colonial medicine, see Randall M. Packard, *A History of Global Health: Interventions into the Lives of Other Peoples* (Baltimore: Johns Hopkins University Press, 2016).

82. Andrew Cunningham and Bridie Andrews, eds., *Western Medicine as Contested Knowledge* (Manchester, UK: Manchester University Press, 1997); Poonam Bala, ed., *Biomedicine as a Contested Site: Some Revelations in Imperial Contexts* (Lanham: Lexington Books, 2009).

83. Kent Maynard, "European Preoccupations and Indigenous Culture in Cameroon: British Rule and the Transformation of Kedjom Medicine," *Canadian Journal of African Studies* 36 (2002), 79–117; William Gallois, "Local Responses to French Medical Imperialism in Late Nineteenth-Century Algeria," *Social History of Medicine* 20 (2007), 315–31.

84. Pablo F. Gómez and Diego Armus, eds., *The Gray Zones of Medicine: Healers and History in Latin America* (Pittsburg: University of Pittsburgh Press, 2021).

85. Shigehisa Kuriyama, "The Geography of Ginseng and the Strange Alchemy of Needs," in *The Botany of Empire in the Long Eighteenth Century*, ed. Yota Batsaki, Sarah Burke Cahalan, and Anatole Tchikine, Dumbarton Oaks Symposia and Colloquia (Washington, DC: Dumbarton Oaks/Harvard University Press, 2017), 61–72; James Beattie, "Thomas McDonnell's Opium: Circulating Plants, Patronage, and Power in Britain, China, and New Zealand, 1830s-50s," in *The Botany of Empire in the Long Eighteenth Century*, ed. Yota Batsaki, Sarah Burke Cahalan, and Anatole Tchikine, Dumbarton Oaks Symposia and Colloquia (Washington, DC: Dumbarton Oaks/Harvard University Press, 2017), 165–92.

86. For a recent summary of the early cinchona market, see Matthew James Crawford, *The Andean Wonder Drug: Cinchona Bark and Imperial Science in the Spanish Atlantic, 1630–1800* (Pittsburgh: University of Pittsburgh Press, 2016).

87. Mary Lindemann, *Medicine and Society in Early Modern Europe* (Cambridge: Cambridge University Press, 2013), 74–76.

88. Waltraud Ernst, "Beyond East and West: From the History of Colonial Medicine to a Social History of Medicine(s) in South Asia," *Social History of Medicine* 20 (2007), 505–524. For a particularly passionate rebuttal to the "theoretical fallacies and ambiguous dualisms" of bifurcating colonial science in Western and non-Western categories, see Helen Tilley, *Africa as a Living Laboratory: Empire, Development and the Problem of Scientific Knowledge, 1870–1950* (Chicago: The University of Chicago Press, 2016), quote on 10.

BIBLIOGRAPHY

Alam, Muẓaffar, and Sanjay Subrahmanyam. *Indo-Persian Travels in the Age of Discoveries, 1400–1800*. Cambridge: Cambridge University Press, 2010.

Alberti, Samuel J. M. M. "Objects and the Museum." *Isis* 96, no. 4 (December 2005): 559–71.

Ali, Omar H. *Malik Ambar: Power and Slavery Across the Indian Ocean*. New York: Oxford University Press, 2016.

Anderson, Warwick. *Colonial Pathologies American Tropical Medicine, Race, and Hygiene in the Philippines*. Durham: Duke University Press, 2008.

Arasaratnam, Sinnappah. *Maritime India in the Seventeenth Century*. New Delhi: Oxford University Press, 1994.

Armus, Diego, and Pablo F. Gómez, eds. *The Gray Zones of Medicine: Healers and History in Latin America*. Pittsburgh: University of Pittsburgh Press, 2021.

Arnold, David, ed. *Warm Climates and Western Medicine: The Emergence of Tropical Medicine, 1500–1900*. Clio Medica 35. Amsterdam: Rodopi, 1996.

Avilez Rocha, Gabriel de. "The Pinzones and the Coup of the *Acedares*: Fishing and Colonization in the Fifteenth-Century Atlantic." *Colonial Latin American Review* 28, no. 4 (October 2, 2019): 427–49.

Baber, Zaheer. "The Plants of Empire: Botanic Gardens, Colonial Power and Botanical Knowledge." *Journal of Contemporary Asia* 46, no. 4 (October 2016): 659–79.

Bala, Poonam, ed. *Biomedicine as a Contested Site: Some Revelations in Imperial Contexts*. Lanham: Lexington Books, 2009.

Ballantyne, Tony, ed. *Science, Empire and the European Exploration of the Pacific*. Florence: Routledge, 2018.

Barrera-Osorio, Antonio. "Local Herbs, Global Medicines: Commerce, Knowledge, and Commodities in Spanish America." In *Merchants & Marvels: Commerce, Science, and Art in Early Modern Europe*, edited by Pamela H Smith and Paula Findlen, 163–82. New York: Routledge, 2002.

Beaglehole, John Cawte. *The Life of Captain James Cook*. Stanford, CA: Stanford University Press, 1998.

Beattie, James. "Thomas McDonnell's Opium: Circulating Plants, Patronage, and Power in Britain, China, and New Zealand, 1830s-50s." In *The Botany of Empire in the Long Eighteenth Century*, edited by Yota Batsaki, Sarah Burke Cahalan, and Anatole Tchikine, 165–92. Dumbarton Oaks Symposia and Colloquia. Washington, DC: Dumbarton Oaks/Harvard University Press, 2017.

Bello Léon, Juan Manuel. *La pesca en Andalucía y Canarias en el tránsito de la Edad Media a la moderna, siglos XV y XVI*. Biblioteca económica canaria. Santa Cruz de Tenerife: Ediciones Idea, 2008.

Bleichmar, Daniela. "Botanical Conquistadors: Plants and Empire in the Hispanic Enlightenment." In *The Botany of Empire in the Long Eighteenth Century*, edited by Yota Batsaki, Sarah Burke Cahalan, and Anatole Tchikine, 35–60. Dumbarton Oaks Symposia and Colloquia. Washington, DC: Dumbarton Oaks/Harvard University Press, 2017.

———. "Exploration in Print: Books and Botanical Travel from Spain to the Americas in the Late Eighteenth Century." *Huntington Library Quarterly* 70, no. 1 (March 1, 2007): 129–51.

———. *Visible Empire. Colonial Botany and Visual Culture in the Eighteenth-Century Hispanic World*. Chicago: University of Chicago Press, 2012.

———. *Visual Voyages: Images of Latin American Nature from Columbus to Darwin*. New Haven: Yale University Press in association with The Huntington Library, Art Collections, and Botanical Gardens, 2017.

Bleichmar, Daniela, Paula De Vos, Kevin Sheehan, and Krisitin Huffine, eds. *Science in the Spanish and Portuguese Empires, 1500–1800*. Stanford, CA: Stanford University Press, 2009.

Browne, Janet. *Charles Darwin: The Power of Place, Vol. 2*. Princeton, NJ: Princeton University Press, 2003.

———. *Charles Darwin: Voyaging, Vol. 1*. Princeton, NJ: Princeton University Press, 1996.

———. "Darwin's Botanical Arithmetic and the 'Principle of Divergence,' 1854–1858." *Journal of the History of Biology* 13, no. 1 (1980): 53–89.

Burke, Peter. *What Is the History of Knowledge?* What Is History. Cambridge, UK: Polity Press, 2016.

Burnett, D. Graham. "Hydrographic Discipline among the Navigators: Charting an 'Empire of Commerce and Science' in the Nineteenth-Century Pacific." In *The*

Imperial Map: Cartography and the Mastery of Empire, edited by James Akerman, 185–259. Chicago: University of Chicago Press, 2009.

———. *Masters of All They Surveyed: Exploration, Geography, and a British El Dorado*. Chicago: University of Chicago Press, 2000.

Burnham, Michelle. "Trade, Time, and the Calculus of Risk in Early Pacific Travel Writing." *Early American Literature* 46, no. 3 (2011): 425–47.

Buschmann, Rainer F., James B. Tueller, and Edward R. Slack. *Navigating the Spanish Lake: The Pacific in the Iberian World, 1521–1898*. Honolulu: University of Hawai'i Press, 2014.

Cagle, Hugh. *Assembling the Tropics: Science and Medicine in Portugal's Empire, 1450–1700*, 2020.

———. "Cultures of Inquiry, Myths of Empire: Natural History in Colonial Goa." In *Medicine, Trade, and Empire: Garcia de Orta's Colloquies on the Simples and Drugs of India (1563) in Context*, edited by Palmira Fontes da Costa and Andrew Cunningham, 107–28. Burlington, VT: Ashgate, 2015.

Calder, Alex, Jonathan Lamb, and Bridget Orr, eds. *Voyages and Beaches: Pacific Encounters, 1769–1840*. Honolulu: University of Hawai'i Press, 1999.

Cañizares-Esguerra, Jorge. "How Derivative Was Humboldt? Microcosmic Narratives in Early Modern Spanish America and the (Other) Origins of Humboldt's Ecological Sensibilties." In *Nature, Empire, and Nation: Explorations of the History of Science in the Iberian World*, 112–28. Stanford, CA: Stanford University Press, 2006.

———. *Nature, Empire, and Nation: Explorations of the History of Science in the Iberian World*. Stanford, CA: Stanford University Press, 2006.

Casale, Giancarlo. "The Ottoman Administration of the Spice Trade in the Sixteenth-Century Red Sea and Persian Gulf." *Journal of the Economic and Social History of the Orient* 49, no. 2 (2006): 170–98.

———. *The Ottoman Age of Exploration*. Oxford: Oxford University Press, 2012. Chakrabarti, Pratik. *Medicine and Empire, 1600–1960*. Houndmills, Basingstoke, Hampshire, New York, NY: Palgrave Macmillan Division of St Martin's Press LLC, 2014.

Chancellor, Gordon Chancellor, and John Van Wyhe, eds. *Charles Darwin's Notebooks from the Voyage of the "Beagle."* Cambridge: Cambridge University Press, 2009.

Chang, David A. *The World and All the Things Upon It: Native Hawaiian Geographies of Exploration*. Minneapolis: University of Minnesota Press, 2016.

Chaplin, Joyce E. *Round About the Earth: Circumnavigation from Magellan to Orbit*. New York: Simon & Schuster, 2014.

———. "The Curious Case of Science and Empire." *Reviews in American History* 34, no. 4 (2006): 434–40.

Chaudhuri, Kirti N. "The Portuguese Maritime Empire, Trade, and Society in the Indian Ocean During the Sixteenth Century." *Portuguese Studies* 8 (1992): 57–70.

Cock, Randolph. "Scientific Servicemen in the Royal Navy and the Professionalisation of Science, 1816–55." In *Science and Beliefs: From Natural Philosophy to*

Natural Science, 1700–1900, edited by David M Knight and Matthew Eddy, 95–112. Aldershot: Ashgate, 2005.

Cook, Harold John. *Matters of Exchange: Commerce, Medicine, and Science in the Dutch Golden Age*. New Haven: Yale University Press, 2007.

Cornish, Caroline. "Nineteenth-Century Museums and the Shaping of Disciplines: Potentialities and Limitations at Kew's Museum of Economic Botany." *Museum History Journal* 8, no. 1 (January 2015): 8–27.

Crawford, Matthew James. *The Andean Wonder Drug: Cinchona Bark and Imperial Science in the Spanish Atlantic, 1630–1800*. Pittsburgh, PA: University of Pittsburgh Press, 2016.

Cunningham, Andrew, and Bridie Andrews, eds. *Western Medicine as Contested Knowledge*. Manchester, UK: Manchester University Press, 1997.

Curtin, Philip D. *Death by Migration: Europe's Encounter with the Tropical World in the Nineteenth Century*. New York: Cambridge University Press, 2003.

Cushman, Gregory T. "Humboldtian Science, Creole Meteorology, and the Discovery of Human-Caused Climate Change in South America." *Osiris* 26, no. 1 (January 2011): 16–44.

Daston, Lorraine. "On Scientific Observation." *Isis* 99, no. 1 (2008): 97–110.

Daston, Lorraine, and Elizabeth Lunbeck, eds. *Histories of Scientific Observation*. Chicago and London: The University of Chicago Press, 2011.

Davis, Mike. *Late Victorian Holocausts: El Niño Famines and the Making of the Third World*. New York: Verso, 2001.

Davies, Surekha. *Renaissance Ethnography and the Invention of the Human: New Worlds, Maps and Monsters*. New York: Cambridge University Press, 2017.

Deacon, Margaret. *Scientists and the Sea, 1650–1900: A Study of Marine Science*. New York: Academic Press, 1971.

Delbourgo, James. *Collecting the World: Hans Sloane and the Origins of the British Museum*. Cambridge, Massachusetts: The Belknap Press of Harvard University Press, 2017.

———. "Science." In *The British Atlantic World, 1500–1800*, edited by David Armitage and Michael J. Braddick, 92–110. New York: Palgrave Macmillan, 2009.

Delbourgo, James, and Nicholas Dew, eds. *Science and Empire in the Atlantic World*. New York: Routledge, 2008.

Dettelbach, Michael. "Alexander Von Humboldt between Enlightenment and Romanticism." *Northeastern Naturalist* 8, no. sp1 (November 2001): 9–20.

———. "Humboltdian Science." In *Cultures of Natural History*, edited by Nicholas Jardine, James A. Secord, and Emma C. Spary, 287–304. Cambridge: Cambridge University Press, 1996.

———. "The Face of Nature: Precise Measurement, Mapping, and Sensibility in the Work of Alexander von Humboldt." *Studies in History and Philosophy of Biological and Biomedical Sciences,* 30, no. 4 (1999): 473–504.

Dew, Nicholas. "Scientific Travel in the Atlantic World: The French Expedition to Gorée and the Antilles, 1681–1683." *British Journal for the History of Science* 43, no. 156 (2010): 1–18.

Díez Torre, Alejandro, Tomás Mallo, and Daniel Pacheco Fernández, eds. *De La Ciencia Ilustrada a La Ciencia Romántica: Actas de Los II Jornadas Sobre "España y Las Expediciones En América y Filipinas."* Madrid: Ed. Doce Calles, 1995.

Driver, Felix. *Geography Militant: Cultures of Exploration and Empire*. Malden, MA: Blackwell Publishers, 2001.

———. "Henry Morton Stanley & His Critics: Geography, Exploration & Empire." *Past and Present* 133 (1991): 134–66.

———. "*Missionary Travels*: Livingstone, Africa and the Book." *Scottish Geographical Journal* 129, no. 3–4 (December 2013): 164–78.

Edney, Matthew H. *Mapping an Empire: The Geographical Construction of British India, 1765–1843*. Chicago: University of Chicago Press, 1997.

Edwards, Phyllis I. "Sir Joseph Banks and the Botany of Captain Cook's Three Voyages of Exploration." *Pacific Studies* 2, no. 1 (1978): 20–43.

Ernst, Waltraud. "Beyond East and West. From the History of Colonial Medicine to a Social History of Medicine(s) in South Asia." *Social History of Medicine* 20, no. 3 (October 9, 2007): 505–24.

Fara, Patricia. *Sex, Botany and Empire: The Story of Carl Linnaeus and Joseph Banks*. London: Icon Books Ltd, 2017.

Ferreiro, Larrie D. *Bridging the Seas: The Rise of Naval Architecture in the Industrial Age, 1800–2000*. Transformations: Studies in the History of Science and Technology. Cambridge, MA: The MIT Press, 2020.

———. *Ships and Science: The Birth of Naval Architecture in the Scientific Revolution, 1600–1800*. Cambridge, MA: MIT Press, 2007.

Few, Martha. "Circulating Smallpox Knowledge: Guatemalan Doctors, Maya Indians and Designing Spain's Smallpox Vaccination Expedition, 1780–1803." *The British Journal for the History of Science* 43, no. 4 (December 2010): 519–37.

Findlen, Paula, ed. *Athanasius Kircher: The Last Man Who Knew Everything*. New York: Routledge, 2004.

———. *Possessing Nature: Museums, Collecting, and Scientific Culture in Early Modern Italy*. Berkeley: University of California Press, 1994.

Gallois, William. "Local Responses to French Medical Imperialism in Late Nineteenth-Century Algeria." *Social History of Medicine* 20, no. 2 (August 1, 2007): 315–31.

Gascoigne, John. *Encountering the Pacific in the Age of the Enlightenment*. Cambridge: Cambridge University Press, 2014.

Gómez, Pablo F. *The Experiential Caribbean: Creating Knowledge and Healing in the Early Modern Atlantic*. Chapel Hill: University of North Carolina Press, 2017.

González González, Francisco. *Instrumentos Científicos Del Observatorio de San Fernando: (Siglos XVIII, XIX, XX)*. Madrid: Instituto de Historia y Cultura Naval, 1995.

González-Ripoll Navarro, María Dolores. "La Formación Académica y Práctica de Los Marinos Del Siglo XVIII: Cosme de Churruca (1761–1805), Un Oficial Científico." In *De La Ciencia Ilustrada a La Ciencia Romántica: Actas de Los II Jornadas Sobre "España y Las Expediciones En América y Filipinas,"* edited by Alejandro Díez Torre, Tomás Mallo, and Daniel Pacheco Fernández, 312–23. Madrid: Ed. Doce Calles, 1995.

Hahn, Roger. *The Anatomy of a Scientific Institution: The Paris Academy of Sciences, 1666–1803*. Berkeley: University of California Press, 1971.

Hardiman, David. *Healing Bodies, Saving Souls: Medical Missions in Asia and Africa*. Clio Medica 80. Leiden, Netherlands: Rodopi, 2006.

Hardy, Penelope K. "Every Ship a Floating Observatory: Matthew Fontaine Maury and the Acquisition of Knowledge at Sea." In *Soundings and Crossings: Doing Science at Sea 1800–1970*, edited by Katharine Anderson and Helen M. Rozwadowski, 17–48. Sagamore Beach, MA: Science History Publications/Watson Publishing International, 2016.

Hooper-Greenhill, Eilean. *Museums and the Shaping of Knowledge*. Heritage. London: Routledge, 2009.

Hsia, Florence C. *Sojourners in a Strange Land: Jesuits and Their Scientific Missions in Late Imperial China*. Chicago: University of Chicago Press, 2009.

Humboldt, Alexander von. *Views of the Cordilleras and Monuments of the Indigenous Peoples of the Americas: A Critical Edition*. Edited by Vera M Kutzinski and Ottmar Ette. Translated by J. Ryan Poynter. Chicago: University of Chicago Press, 2012.

Hunter, Michael Cyril William. *Establishing the New Science: The Experience of the Early Royal Society*. Woodbridge: The Boydell Press, 1989.

Iliffe, R. "Science and Voyages of Discovery." In *The Cambridge History of Science, Vol. 4: Eighteenth-Century Science*, edited by Roy Porter, 618–45. Cambridge, UK: Cambridge University Press, 2003.

Jardine, Nicholas, James A. Secord, and Emma C. Spary, eds. *Cultures of Natural History*. Cambridge: Cambridge University Press, 1996.

Keay, John. *The Spice Route: A History*. Berkeley: University of California Press, 2006.

Keynes, Richard Darwin, ed. *Charles Darwin's "Beagle" Diary*. Cambridge: Cambridge University Press, 2004.

Knell, Simon J., Suzanne Macleod, and Sheila E. R. Watson, eds. *Museum Revolutions: How Museums Change and Are Changed*. London: Routledge, 2007.

Koerner, Lisbet. *Linnaeus: Nature and Nation*. Cambridge, MA: Harvard University Press, 1999.

Kuklick, Henrika, and Robert E. Kohler, eds. *Science in the Field*. Osiris, Ser. 2, Vol. 11. Chicago, IL: The Univ. of Chicago Press, 1996.

Kuriyama, Shigehisa. "The Geography of Ginseng and the Strange Alchemy of Needs." In *The Botany of Empire in the Long Eighteenth Century*, edited by Yota Batsaki, Sarah Burke Cahalan, and Anatole Tchikine, 61–72. Dumbarton Oaks Symposia and Colloquia. Washington, DC: Dumbarton Oaks/Harvard University Press, 2017.

Lafuente, Antonio, and Leoncio López-Ocón. "Scientific Traditions and Enlightenment Expeditions in Eighteenth-Century Hispanic America." In *Science in Latin America: A History*, edited by Juan José Saldaña, translated by Bernabé Madrigal, 123–50. Austin: University of Texas Press, 2006.

Lafuente, Antonio, and Manuel Sellés. *El Observatorio de Cádiz (1753–1831)*. Madrid: Ministerio de Defensa; Instituto de Historia y Cultura Naval, 1988.

Larson, Pier Martin. *Ocean of Letters: Language and Creolization in an Indian Ocean Diaspora*. Critical Perspectives on Empire. Cambridge, UK: Cambridge University Press, 2009. Latour, Bruno. *Science in Action: How to Follow Scientists and Engineers Through Society*. Cambridge, Mass: Harvard University Press, 1987.

Lincoln, Margarette, ed. *Science and Exploration in the Pacific: European Voyages to the Southern Oceans in the Eighteenth Century*. Woodbridge: Boydell Press, 2001.

Lindemann, Mary. *Medicine and Society in Early Modern Europe. New Approaches to European History*. Cambridge: Cambridge University Press, 2013.

Locher, Fabian. "The Observatory, the Land-Based Ship and the Crusades: Earth Sciences in European Context, 1830–50." *The British Journal for the History of Science* 40, no. 4 (December 1, 2007): 491–504.

López Piñero, José María, and María Luz López Terrada. *La influencia española en la introducción en Europa de las plantas americanas (1493–1623)*. Valencia: Valencia Instituto de Estudios Documentales e Históricos sobre la Ciencia, 1998.

Mackay, David. "A Presiding Genius of Exploration: Banks, Cook, and Empire, 1767–1805." In *Captain James Cook and His Times*, edited by Robin Fisher and Hugh Johnston, 21–39. Seattle: University of Washington Press, 1979.

MacLeod, Roy M., and Milton James Lewis, eds. *Disease, Medicine, and Empire: Perspectives on Western Medicine and the Experience of European Expansion*. London: Routledge, 1988.

Malaspina, Alessandro. *The Malaspina Expedition, 1789–1794: Journal of the Voyage by Alejandro Malaspina*. 3 vols. Works Issued by the Hakluyt Society, 3rd ser., no. 8. London: Hakluyt Society in association with the Museo Naval, Madrid, 2001.

Matsuda, Matt K. *Pacific Worlds: A History of Seas, Peoples, and Cultures*. Cambridge: Cambridge University Press, 2012.

Maynard, Kent. "European Preoccupations and Indigenous Culture in Cameroon: British Rule and the Transformation of Kedjom Medicine." *Canadian Journal of African Studies / Revue Canadienne Des Études Africaines* 36, no. 1 (January 2002): 79–117.

McPherson, Kenneth. *The Indian Ocean: A History of People and the Sea*. New Delhi, India: Oxford University Press, 2006.

Miller, David Philip, and Peter Hanns Reill, eds. *Visions of Empire: Voyages, Botany, and Representations of Nature*. Cambridge: Cambridge University Press, 1996.

Miller, Gwenn A. *Kodiak Kreol: Communities of Empire in Early Russian America*. Ithaca, NY: Cornell University Press, 2015.

Murphy, Kathleen S. "Translating the Vernacular: Indigenous and African Knowledge in the Eighteenth-Century British Atlantic." *Atlantic Studies* 8, no. 1 (March 2011): 29–48.

Nicolson, Malcolm. "Alexander von Humboldt, Humboldtian Science and the Origins of the Study of Vegetation." *History of Science* 25, no. 2 (June 1987): 167–94.

Packard, Randall M. *A History of Global Health: Interventions into the Lives of Other Peoples*. Baltimore: Johns Hopkins University Press, 2016.

Padrón, Ricardo. "Mapping Plus Ultra: Cartography, Space, and Hispanic Modernity." *Representations* 79, no. 1 (August 1, 2002): 28–60.

———. *The Indies of the Setting Sun: How Early Modern Spain Mapped the Far East as the Transpacific West*. Chicago: The University of Chicago Press, 2020.

Pagden, Anthony. *European Encounters with the New World: From Renaissance to Romanticism*. New Haven: Yale University Press, 1993.

Pardo Tomás, José, and María Luz López Terrada. *Las Primeras Noticias Sobre Plantas Americanas En Las Relaciones de Viajes y Crónicas de Indias, 1493–1553*. Cuadernos Valencianos de Historia de La Medicina y de La Ciencia ; Serie A, Monografías 40. Valencia: Instituto de Estudios Documentales e Históricos sobre la Ciencia, Universitat de València, C.S.I.C, 1993.

Pigafetta, Antonio. *Magellan's Voyage: A Narrative Account of the First Circumnavigation*. Translated by R.A. Skelton. New Haven: Yale University Press, 1969.

Pimentel, Juan. *Testigos Del Mundo: Ciencia, Literatura y Viajes En La Ilustración*. Estudios. Madrid: Marcial Pons Historia, 2003.

Pimentel Igea, Juan. *La Física de La Monarquía: Ciencia y Política En El Pensamiento Colonial de Alejandro Malaspina (1754–1810)*. Aranjuez: Doce Calles, 1998.

Portuondo, María M. *Secret Science: Spanish Cosmography and the New World*. Chicago: University of Chicago Press, 2009.

Prakash, Gyan. *Another Reason: Science and the Imagination of Modern India*. Princeton, NJ: Princeton University Press, 2007.

Prieto, Andrés I. *Missionary Scientists: Jesuit Science in Spanish South America, 1570–1810*. Nashville: Vanderbilt University Press, 2011.

Pyenson, Lewis. *Civilizing Mission: Exact Sciences and French Overseas Expansion, 1830–1940*. Baltimore: Johns Hopkins University Press, 1993.

Raj, Kapil. *Relocating Modern Science: Circulation and the Construction of Knowledge in South Asia and Europe, 1650–1900*. Houndmills, Basingstoke, Hampshire: Palgrave Macmillan, 2007.

Ramírez, Paul. "'Like Herod's Massacre': Quarantines, Bourbon Reform, and Popular Protest in Oaxaca's Smallpox Epidemic, 1796–1797." *The Americas* 69, no. 2 (October 2012): 203–35.

Reid, Joshua L. *The Sea Is My Country: The Maritime World of the Makahs, an Indigenous Borderlands People*. New Haven: Yale University Press, 2018.

Roersch van der Hoogte, Arjo, and Toine Pieters. "Science in the Service of Colonial Agro-Industrialism: The Case of Cinchona Cultivation in the Dutch and British East Indies, 1852–1900." *Studies in History and Philosophy of Science Part C: Studies in History and Philosophy of Biological and Biomedical Sciences* 47 (September 2014): 12–22.

Safier, Neil. "'Every Day That I Travel . . . Is a Page That I Turn': Reading and Observing in Eighteenth-Century Amazonia." *Huntington Library Quarterly* 70, no. 1 (March 2007): 103–28.

———. "Itineraries of Atlantic Science: New Questions, New Approaches, New Directions." *Atlantic Studies* 7, no. 4 (December 1, 2010): 357–64.

———. *Measuring the New World: Enlightenment Science and South America*. Chicago: University of Chicago Press, 2008.

Sarasin, Philipp. "More Than Just Another Specialty: On the Prospects for the History of Knowledge." *Journal for the History of Knowledge* 1, no. 1 (July 15, 2020): 1–5.

Sargent, Matthew. "Recentering Centers of Calculation: Reconfiguring Knowledge Networks Within Global Empires of Trade." In *Empires of Knowledge: Scientific Networks in the Early Modern World*, edited by Paula Findlen, 297–316. London: Routledge, 2019.

Schaffer, Simon. "Astronomers Mark Time: Discipline and the Personal Equation." *Science in Context* 2, no. 1 (1988): 115–45.

Schaffer, Simon, James Delbourgo, Kapil Raj, and Lissa Roberts, eds. *The Brokered World: Go-Betweens and Global Intelligence, 1770–1820*. Sagamore Beach, MA: Science History Publications, 2009.

Schiebinger, Londa L. *Plants and Empire: Colonial Bioprospecting in the Atlantic World.* Cambridge, MA: Harvard University Press, 2004.

Schiebinger, Londa L, and Claudia Swan, eds. *Colonial Botany: Science, Commerce, and Politics in the Early Modern World.* Philadelphia: University of Pennsylvania Press, 2005.

Schmutzer, Kurt. "Metamorphosis between Field and Museum: Collections in the Making." *Journal of the History of Science Technology* 5 (2012): 68–83.

Sellés, Manuel, José Luis Peset, and Antonio Lafuente, eds. *Carlos III y La Ciencia de La Ilustración*. Madrid: Alianza Editorial, 1988.

Sörlin, Sverker. "National and International Aspects of Cross-Boundary Science: Scientific Travel in the 18th Century." In *Denationalizing Science: The Contexts of International Scientific Practice*, edited by Elisabeth Crawford, Terry Shinn, and Sverker Sörlin, 16:43–72. Sociology of the Sciences A Yearbook. Dordrecht: Springer Netherlands, 1993.

Sorrenson, Richard. "The Ship as a Scientific Instrument in the Eighteenth Century." *Osiris* 11 (1996): 221–36.

Sponsel, Alistair. "An Amphibious Being: How Maritime Surveying Reshaped Darwin's Approach to Natural History." *Isis* 107, no. 2 (June 1, 2016): 254–81.

Stolzenberg, Daniel, ed. *The Great Art of Knowing: The Baroque Encyclopedia of Athanasius Kircher*. Stanford: Stanford University Press, 2001.

Stuart, John. "David Livingstone, British Protestant Missions, Memory and Empire." In *Sites of Imperial Memory: Commemorating Colonial Rule in the Nineteenth and Twentieth Centuries*, edited by Dominik Geppert and Frank Lorenz Müller, 153–69. Manchester: Manchester University Press, 2016.

Subrahmanyam, Sanjay. *The Portuguese Empire in Asia, 1500–1700: A Political and Economic History*. Chichester, UK: John Wiley & Sons, 2012.

Sulloway, Frank J. "Darwin and His Finches: The Evolution of a Legend." *Journal of the History of Biology* 15, no. 1 (1982): 1–53.

Tagliacozzo, Eric. "Trade, Production, and Incorporation. The Indian Ocean in Flux, 1600–1900." *Itinerario* 26, no. 1 (March 2002): 75–106.

Taillemite, Etienne, ed. *Bougainville et Ses Compagnons Autour Du Monde: 1766–1769, Journaux de Navigation*. Voyages et Découvertes. Paris: Imprimerie nationale, 1977.

Terrall, Mary. *The Man Who Flattened the Earth: Maupertuis and the Sciences in the Enlightenment*. Chicago: University of Chicago Press, 2002.
Thornton, John K. *Africa and Africans in the Making of the Atlantic World, 1400–1800*. 2nd ed. Cambridge; New York: Cambridge University Press, 1998.
Tilley, Helen. *Africa as a Living Laboratory: Empire, Development and the Problem of Scientific Knowledge, 1870–1950*. Chicago: University of Chicago Press, 2016.
Vinkovetsky, Ilya. *Russian America: An Overseas Colony of a Continental Empire; 1804–1867*. Paperback ed. Oxford: Oxford University Press, 2014.
Wey Gómez, Nicolás. *The Tropics of Empire: Why Columbus Sailed South to the Indies*. Cambridge, MA: MIT Press, 2008.
Whitehead, P.J.P. "A Guide to the Dispersal of Zoological Material from Captain Cook's Voyages." *Pacific Studies* 2, no. 1 (1978): 52–93.
Withers, Charles W.J. "Science, Scientific Instruments and Questions of Method in Nineteenth-Century British Geography." *Transactions of the Institute of British Geographers* 38, no. 1 (January 2013): 167–79.
Wulf, Andrea. *The Invention of Nature: Alexander von Humboldt's New World*. New York: Alfred A. Knopf, 2015.

Chapter 7

The Continuing Search for Green Gold

Quest for Medical Plants in the Colonial Period

Sohini Das

Pluralism not only in the form of medical practices but also in structure has been identified as a chief characteristic of South Asian medical tradition.[1] This pluralism has led Charles Leslie to describe it as 'Cosmopolitan'.[2] Within this broad rubric of South Asian medicine, medicinal plants constitute only a segment. South Asian medicine unlike its Greek counterpart developed a sound pharmacology.[3] This chapter attempts to focus upon the circulation of herbal remedies during the colonial period. It is never contended at any point that such exchanges and circulation were not conducted prior to the arrival of the Europeans. In fact, even in pre-modern period, people travelled across the Indian Ocean looking for treatment as well as to procure items prescribed in materia medica. The lists of ingredients one finds in the pre-modern pharmacopoeias include *Egyptian Opium, Socotra aloes, the ambergris of Azania, Syrian sumac, Armenian bole, Persian sweetmeats, Indian aloeswood and cinnamon* from Sri Lanka.[4] Such exchanges have been briefly discussed by economic historians largely as an item of commerce without delving deep into the associated medical practices. Any discussion on such botanical transfer is constricted largely either within the trope of 'Ecological Nationalism' or 'Ecological Imperialism', both of which suffer from Eurocentrism that tends to obscure the fact that plant transfer had been integral to human history.[5] The early plant transfers and exchanges on Indian Ocean date back to at least 8,000 years and were crucial in shaping the environment and society of that terrain. The earliest transfers and exchanges may not have followed the logic of imperialism but they were crucial in shaping the environmental and social history of the place.[6] In this regard, an interesting observation has been made by Michael Pearson. He points out how for a substantial point of time maritime history has been in a dilemma whether to include the history of the terrain and to what extent.[7] According to him, the greatest link that binds the vast geographical expanse of Indian Ocean is disease which has been discussed by David Arnold in his article.[8] Medical knowledge spread through the travels of the Hadhramis who were referred by the Portuguese as 'cacizes' who were shaf'i Muslim religious specialists. Gradually, this spread of medical knowledge increased with the advent of the steamships during the nineteenth century.[9] This chapter will focus on the spread of indigenous knowledge about materia medica with expansion of the trade routes and also how such transfer of knowledge was facilitated by various intermediaries. This quest for knowledge however started fading away and selective appropriation of knowledge began to gain dominance as will be highlighted in the following sections, with particular focus on India.

LONG-DISTANCE TRADE AND CIRCULATION OF KNOWLEDGE

Expansion of long-distance trade during the fifteenth century also developed an increasing tendency towards facts gathering and experimentation with newer drugs. Reassessment of the classical texts like Pliny the elder's work of *Natural History*, Greek naturalist Theophrastus's *Enquiry into the plants* and *De Materia Medica of Dioscordies* also commenced around this time.[10] As Richard Grove points out, apothecary gardens were first developed in the universities of Portugal and later these gardens became the repository of the earliest plant transfers. The three dominant countries in the field of plant transfer were the Netherlands, Italy and Portugal. Universities even developed curriculums and pioneered in preparation of books of dried plants known as *Hortus Sicci*.[11] In this process of expansion of the knowledge system, the European travellers played a crucial role as they were advised to observe indigenous practices and collect materials so as to extend the European materia medica.[12] Thus, Garcia da Orta in case of Goa, Hendrick van Rheede in case of Malabar, J. G. Koenig in case of Tranquebar and Robert Wight in case of Madras devoted themselves in the study of local plants and their medicinal usages.[13]

But the fundamental nature of European ascendancy was different in Indian Ocean than Atlantic Ocean. Unlike the Atlantic there was no biological imperialism that paved the way for cultural and political dominance; instead, it was the European constitution that felt threatened.[14] Additionally, during this period, it was commonly believed since Indian environment was different from that of Europe, India was afflicted with very different types of diseases. Hence many of the European remedies might not be efficient here.

Similar rationale was also applied in case of West Indies. Londa Schiebinger traces how before the onset of racism in the nineteenth century the indigenous knowledge of the Americans, Africans, East Indies and Indian subcontinent was much valued for. The search for valuable medicinal herbs, as Nicolas-Louis Bourgeois, secretary of Chamber of Agriculture during his twenty-eight years of residence in Haiti, considered, was not a curiosity but a requisite.[15] The need was of course protection of European lives against the unknown diseases. Hans Sloane (1660–1753), the future president of Jamaica, collated data about various types of plants that he encountered at the tropics with the help of the local informants. Often many Carib remedies were sought because when the Europeans first came to America the diseases that confronted them could only be cured through local remedies. In the third volume of *Histories Des Maladies de Saint Dominigue*, Pouppe Desportes presented an 'American pharmacopoeia' which contained a list of Caribbean remedies. It was one of the first books to have compiled the Amerindian remedies; yet the Latin names were used instead of Amerindian names.[16]

Another authoritative text was *Historia medicinal de las cosas que se traen de nuestras Indias Occidentales* (Medical study of the products imported from our West Indian possessions) by Nicolas Monardes composed around 1565. This text was compiled by Monardes without setting his foot in the New World.[17] A trained physician, Monardes learnt about New World through his partnership with a businessman named Herrera who had contact with the New World. He also kept regular contact with apothecaries, travellers and administrators. He dealt with the products from the New World and often added those in his medical practice after years of experimentation.[18] For instance, he was quite sceptical about the use of the 'Michoacán root' at first but after hearing about the advantages of the plant repeatedly from those returning from New World he was convinced of its benefit.[19] His work was widely read all over Europe as the only available source of New World materia medica. The greatest drawback of the text was that it never did encompass the vast world of New World materia medica and understanding of the plants by the locals. In the process it even undermines the contributions of the Amerindians. A particular instance proves the fact. The use of balsam for treating war wounds was learnt by the Spaniards from Amerindians but the herb was named after the Spanish soldier who popularized it.[20] Whether it was complete ignorance or prejudice, the New World theories were never taken into account. Daniela Bleichmar points out that since the healing theories have a religious element it would put the Christian beliefs and practices to question. Thus, these new world products were stripped of their cultural connotations before being shipped to Europe.

In case of Dutch East Indies, Jacobus Bonitus might have been appreciative of the local knowledge prevalent among the women especially but he like his contemporaries never took into account the cultural context and connotations. He, as Harold Cook points it out, 'universalized and objectified it, making it a kind of commodity'.[21] This search for herbal remedies continued even at a later period and even then, it was the Indo-European women who were seen to perform the task of mediation.[22] Even in case of New Zealand we see women playing an important role in preservation of the herbal knowledge, despite facing much resistance from patent medicine. The newly arrived European women integrated the Maori medical knowledge in their sphere of domestic medicine.[23] But often such medical exchanges were blinded by racial prejudices which prevented the Europeans to adopt the native medical practices. Jonathan Roberts illustrates this aspect in respect to Gold Coast, widely regarded as the 'Whiteman's Grave'. He shows despite the success of native herbal remedies against several diseases, racial supremacy impeded its inclusion in European medicine.[24]

This attempt at compiling the indigenous herbal remedies was widespread across all the colonies. Knowledge of indigenous herbs continued alongside travels that were ordained for other scientific knowledge as part of imperial curiosities (Matthew Franco in this volume). The epithet of the earliest chronicler of the knowledge of medicinal plants of India can be attributed to Garcia da Orta. He along with Hendrik von Tot Drakenstein Rheede compiled the vast knowledge about the medicinal plants of South Asia. With the opening of trade routes in 1498, the Portuguese were soon followed by the Dutch, English and the French. This initiated a process of transfer that involved not only commodities but also knowledge, men, flora and fauna. Since the focus of the chapter is medical botany the rest of the factors will be discussed in relation to it. It should be mentioned at the outset that such process of plant transfers was not unilateral. The Europeans too introduced several plants that have been gradually incorporated into Indian pharmacopoeias. The move to investigate the local materia medica was conducted globally. In case of India, this attempt of cataloguing the plants as well as enlisting their medicinal properties finds its first manifestation in the work of Garcia da Orta.

Garcia da Orta intended to compile descriptions of the plants in the East and particularly that of India from which drugs were extracted. His book *Colloquies dos simples e drogas he consas medicinas da Indica* (Colloquies on the simple drugs of India by Garcia da Orta) was written in 1563 in Goa. Orta personifies the contradiction prevalent among the European practitioners of the time which often leads to a form of eclecticism that can be used to describe his preference for Islamic system of medicine, when confronted with a choice between the Galenic system and Islamic system. Such a preference could also have been as a result of wide practice of Islamic medicine along the western coast as well. But this eclecticism can never be equated with uncritical acceptance of the system; rather, it involved proper investigation and examination of the prevalent practices. For instance, he was not convinced about the therapeutic value of an Indian variety of purgative aloe until he was able to achieve it through experiment.[25]

Orta's book, a compilation of field observation and indigenous knowledge, never privileged the European preconceptions and learning over indigenous knowledge. It is evident from his work that Orta was much reliant on the Malayali doctors for procuring information. But there remains much doubt to the extent he was able to acquire knowledge from them[26] as such information seldom flowed outside caste barriers.[27]

Another pioneer in this regard was Hendrik Van Rheede tot Drakenstein. His work *Hortus Malabaricus* was organized essentially on 'non-European precepts'; in his study he shows how in studies of colonized societies Brahmanical knowledge might have been privileged but in case of diffusion of medico-botanical knowledge, the non-Brahmanical knowledge found favour. Though there lie certain structural and organizational differences between the two works (*Hortus Malabaricus* and *Colloquies . . .*) both these books are very similar in their approach. The most important similarity and perhaps the most pertinent one in our discussion is the rejection of the Arabic and European nomenclature in favour of the indigenous system.[28] Van Rheede soon came to the conclusion that the knowledge of Brahmins was restricted only to the texts only. For greater part of field collection, they relied more on the knowledge of the lower castes. *Hortus Malabaricus* was actually much more influenced by Ezhava knowledge. They identified the plants, talked about their virtues and their methods of classification. Seven hundred and eighty species of most important plants of Malabar were described in *Hortus Malabaricus*, supported by 794 illustrations. This Ezhava categorization of the plants was later even included in the works of Roxburgh, Linnaeus. Thus, these texts were much instrumental in successful survival and co-option of this indigenous knowledge.

A lesser-known text in this respect is L'Empereur's *Jardin de Lorixa*. Nicolas L'Empereur who joined the Compagnie des Indes as a surgeon major undertook the project around 1690s with an aim to extend the rather limited traditional European knowledge on herbs. Another important rationale behind this project was that the herbs so thus carried lost its efficacy at the end of the journey. So, with an aim to translate the Indian books on medicine L'Empereur took this project. Much like Orta and Van Rheede he too did not rely on the Brahmanical knowledge. The actual source of his information as he confesses was the fakirs. Though a rough translation of the book suggests it to be based on the flora of Orissa but some of the names thus so available in the book were written in Tamil such as *chinamalli* which in fact is small jasmine in Tamil.[29] Much similarity lay between *Hortus Malabaricus* and *Jardin de Lorixa* in terms of illustrations. But there lies a basic difference between the two texts – unlike Van Rheede who transcribes the local names in Roman script along with their Malayali and Konkani names, L'Empereur only provides such names he gathers in Latin scripts.[30] Despite his hard work and toil, *Jardin de Lorixa* was never acknowledged in contemporary French academia and did not receive its due acknowledgement.

Anna Winterbottom in her article focuses upon the collaboration with the native apothecaries and botanists in Madras, an important settlement in the Coromandel Coast. Her article emphasizes upon the works undertaken by two medical surgeons Samuel Browne (1668) and Edward Bulkley (1692) within the backdrop of the exchange networks centred around court rulers of Arcot and Golconda, East India Company, Maratha armies, city hospital and bazaar. They collected specimens of dried plants and sent them to England along with the Tamil names. But unlike *Hortus Malabaricus*, the names of the collaborators are not mentioned.[31]

By the eighteenth century, the English East India Company was able to oust other European companies from the subcontinent. Interest in tropical science, technology, medicine and religion resulted in the growth of the Asiatic Society (1784), Calcutta Botanical Garden (1787), Agri-Horticultural Society (1820) and Serampore Mission (1799).[32] Botanical and geographical investigation drew young explorers and botanists to the subcontinent. In the initial period, amateur colonial officials assumed the role of botanists. However, at a later stage they were replaced by trained botanists. In the period post-1750, the new group of explorers who came to India received greater support from their peers in England. In 1759, James Anderson joined the English East India Company and in 1778 obtained a large land near fort of St George from the Madras government where he conducted experiments. He introduced insects and various commercial plants such as coffee, sugarcane, European apples and American cotton.[33] By the middle of seventeenth century, the English East India Company, in its quest of actively cultivating medicinal plant, set up botanical gardens at Samalkot in Carnatic and Calcutta.

A crucial role in this respect was played by William Roxburgh. His greatest achievement lay in bringing 2,200 species of plants and 800 species of medicinal plants to the Calcutta Botanical Garden.[34] William Roxburgh's correspondences with the Danish Moravian Mission in Tranquebar and the French made him aware about the medicinal remedies employed by them. William Roxburgh's work was published in *Asiatic Researches*, sample of which was also sent to Europe for further examination.[35] Roxburgh's work reflected a shift towards more systematic study of Indian materia medica. According to Mark Harrison, the introduction of the Linnaean system in European Botany and the economic and military imperative contributed to such a shift.[36] There was a deeper impulse of Colonial Botany towards the discursive framing of Indian botanical material which in turn enabled its easy dissociation from their sociocultural milieu.[37]

A contemporary of William Roxburgh, William Jones's treatise 'Botanical Observations on Select Indian Plants' emphasized on the uses of Indian medicinal plants (*Asiatic Researches*, no. 4, 1793–1794, 231–303). Jones was not in favour of the Linnaean system and thus collected the Sanskrit names of the plants and sought their medicinal properties. Nathaniel Wallich, who succeeded Roxburgh as the superintendent of the Calcutta Botanical Garden, was in favour of preserving the Linnaean model of the garden.[38]

Mark Harrison has pointed out that during this time specific remedies were highlighted upon rather than Indian medicine in totality. Even those interested in Indian medicine could only appreciate certain aspects of Indian medicine. With the development of the knowledge of physiology and anatomy, this gulf widened even further.[39] Poonam Bala too agrees that the initial years of colonial rule saw accommodation of the indigenous medicine which gradually diminished in the later years. Thus, in 1813, the Court of Directors of the English East India Company recommended that the government must go through Indian tracts on medicine which might prove valuable to Indian doctors. It stated that, 'There are also many tracts of merits, we are told, on the virtues of plants and drugs, and on the application of them in medicine, the knowledge of which might prove desirable to the European practitioners'.[40] Thus, there was transformation in the European attitude towards such indigenous knowledge. What began as an eclectic pursuit gradually paved way for selective assimilation backed by racial arrogance.

1820–1850

One of the first writings on Indian medicinal plants was 'A catalogue of Indian Medicinal Plants and Drugs' written by John Fleming in 1820. He wanted the book to guide the medical professionals arriving in India regarding the materia medica of the country.[41] Another important work in this regard was undertaken by Whitelaw Ainslie's *Materia Medica of Hindoosthan.* After having joined East India Company as an assistant surgeon on 17 June 1788, Whitelaw Ainslie served subsequent years in different parts of Madras. After serving in army as a medical surgeon, he retired in 26 February 1815.[42] He collected data from indigenous people. His most acclaimed work *Materia Medica of Hindoosthan* was a catalogue of such medicine, which were either produced in India or were procured from Asian market. Many of the drugs belonged to Tamil, Telugu and Persian materia medica.[43] It also contained short descriptions of medicine which were commonly practiced by Hindus and people in Eastern part. He also provided the reader with a catalogue of books on medicine and science.[44]

From 1820s to 1830s onwards a more assertive attitude was observed among the colonial officials such as James Mill and Ranald Martin who were in unison when they agreed that ancient Indian texts had very little to offer.[45] This shift to particular selective remedy is reflected even in Whitelaw Ainslie's 'Materia Medica' (1826). It was a collection of remedies he had found through translation of Indian texts.[46] The continued interest in the indigenous drugs was evident in Sir William Brooke O'Shaughnessy's compilation of *Bengal Pharmacopoeia* (1844). It dealt with the medicinal plants available in Bengal. O'Shaughnessy while working with the government even proposed for an inquiry of the Indian material medica for knowing certain remedies. After this, cannabis was included in British Pharmacopeia.[47] Chittabrata Palit argues that the British pharmacopoeia continued to appropriate indigenous medicine. O'Shaughnessy compiled the *Bengal Pharmacopeia* in 1837 dealing exclusively with the properties of medicinal plants in Bengal. A medical lab was even set up in Calcutta to process the drugs which were used in various charitable hospitals.[48]

R. H. Irvine wrote *Pharmacopoeia of the City of Patna* in 1848. It was a compendium of names of plants, which is reproduced in English, Devanagari and Urdu manuscripts along with illness that may be used for. John Forbes Royle in 1832 wrote *List of Articles of Materia Medica Obtained in the Bazaars of Western and Northern Provinces of India*. The necessity of these manuals was to procure drugs from bazaar by using their local names. But the descriptions so provided often did not match the reality.[49] John Forbes Royle in 1837 published an account of the Indian remedies in *Essays on the Antiquity of Hindoo Medicine*. Royle was the professor of Materia Medica at King's College, London. He admitted to have relied on native assistance for its compilation.[50] The government also was eager to minimize the supplies from Britain and replace them with indigenous produces, and Deepak Kumar considers that Forbes Royle's *Manual of Materia Medica* was driven by such motive.[51] From 1830s onwards, dependence on indigenous sources for procuring indigenous drugs came to be increasingly resented. Another significant concern of the administrators was the need to reduce expenses of importing drug. Thus, the Medical Board of all the three presidencies were keen to look for an alternative. Hence various studies were conducted. In 1837, the *Quarterly Journal of the Medical and Physical Society* stated that the official materia medica of Bombay consists of ninety European medicines and seventy locally procured drugs. During this time much trial and experimentation was conducted before making a drug available in the market.[52] In 1841, certain indigenous remedies such as kala dana, kut kelija and opium were used by the Western medical men.[53] Perhaps due to no mortality, these country medicines were continued to be used in the state dispensaries.[54]

Irschick in *History and Dialogue* writes that this study of Indian medicinal plants and minerals was rather appropriation than a thirst for knowledge.[55] These remedies however were not accepted without any scientific testing. Even during compilation of Medical Topographies between 1825 and 1860, folk medicine and folk knowledge on health and disease were also taken into account.[56] The period between 1820 and 1850 can be considered as crucial in moulding the European attitude towards indigenous medicinal herbs. While on the one hand, there was continued interest in finding such indigenous remedies, at the same time there was growing resentment towards procurement of indigenous drugs. This distance between Western and indigenous medicine kept on further increasing in the 1840s. Moreover, after the 1857 Mutiny the authorities were cautious so as not to hurt native sensibilities. Another problem that plagued such writings on medicinal plants was the dilemma surrounding identification of the herbs and native nomenclature, which was a perennial problem for the medical authorities. C. B. Clarke in reprint of William Roxburgh's *Flora Indica* complains about the non-sustainability of vernacular names.[57] Major Crawford of Madras Indigenous Drug Committee had tried to argue how among the lower classes of natives, gardeners, there is accurate knowledge of many drugs which have a vernacular nomenclature. Despite the vast literature produced to organize the vast chaotic mass of botanical products, there remained much confusion well into the end of the nineteenth century.[58]

INDIGENOUS DRUGS AND DRUG SUBSTITUTION POLICY

From 1850s, with the standardization of Western pharmacopeia, Indian remedies were being critically looked upon.[59] Many of the local remedies were excluded from Western materia medica. Thus in 1868, the *Pharmacopoeia of India* was written by E. J. Waring. Apart from continued interest in Indian flora and fauna during the nineteenth century, an important development took place. In order to reduce the cost of drug importing, government encouraged the use of local remedies. From this time onwards the government started upholding the 'Drug Substitution Policy'. The obvious reason cited for the Drug Substitution Policy was cutting down the import expenses.[60] In the First Medical Congress held in December 1894 at Calcutta the issue of drug substitution was emphasized. Kanai Lal Dey presided over the Pharmacology Department and talked about development of indigenous drugs, its study and systematic cultivation and of course increased use in medical depot. Following this, the government set up the Central Indigenous Drug Committee

(CIDC) rather reluctantly in 1895.[61] The significance of CIDC was that Surgeon Lieutenant Colonel J. Parker McConnell took the advice of the kavirajes and hakims into consideration, rather than Kanai Lal Dey.[62]

CIDC (1896)

The report of CIDC proved far from satisfactory. According to the committee, the raw materials that were so available in India were rather impure and adulterated. Any government initiative of procuring the medicine after removing such impurities would be far more expensive than imported drugs.[63] However, Major J. Parker, the medical storekeeper at Bombay, differed. He submitted to George Watt, the secretary of Drugs Committee, with a list of forty medicines which would act as a proper substitute for imported drugs and were easy to procure.[64] He even provided a list of drugs which could be obtained from Saharanpur and Nilgiris such as *Digitalis, Hyoscyamus, Jalap and Taraxacum.* He even suggested taking assistance from the Forest Department in collection and transfer of the drugs to the medical store. In this regard he even pointed out how previously drugs were supplied to Bombay from the Hewra Garden near Poona and suggested a revival of the garden there.[65] It is no surprise that Parker's idea had no takers. Instead, the view of J. Cleghorn was found more suitable to colonial interest who considered setting up of Indigenous Drug Committee was futile and was in favour of leaving the testing of indigenous drugs to individuals.[66] George Watt, the secretary, proposed formation of provincial committees for collection of information on indigenous drugs, with the head of the Medical Department acting as the president.[67] However, after four years, the committee reported that the functioning of the provincial committees was far from satisfactory and recommended its replacement with 'by one or more selected physicians in important towns who would be required to give the various inquiries entrusted to them their special and personal consideration'.[68]

C. J. Warden, a member of the committee, had doubts about the sincerity of the government from the beginning. In his opinion until the government makes considerable changes in its medical policy, compiling these pharmacopoeias was futile as the previous experiences have led them to believe. Waring's book *The Pharmacopoeia of India* contained substitute for several drugs enlisted in the British pharmacopoeias. But Warden remarks how very few of the indigenous drugs were in government depots.[69]

It is interesting to see that despite much dependence on European and American countries for drugs, the Government of India took monopoly over production of morphine from opium and quinine from cinchona bark. In India, cinchona febrifuge was used by English East India Company apothecaries from eighteenth century. It was first used by James Lind in 1765 in Madras and then by John Clark during Bengal malaria in 1768–1771. In 1839, Dr J. F. Royle first drew the attention of the government officials towards the cultivation of cinchona. After the failure of the first experiment, subsequent experimentation was undertaken simultaneously at Nilgiris, Sylhet, Chittagong, Tenasserim and Darjeeling. Among them only the plantations of Darjeeling and Ootacamund showed positive signs.[70] In 1888, after J. Gemmie was successful in extracting quinine, it annually saved Rs. 3 lakhs for the government. Despite such success, a long-term planning for large-scale investment for quinine production was never entertained.[71] Apart from cinchona, the colonial government exerted monopoly over opium as well. The poppy plant grew profusely in the Himalayas. The first opium factory was set up at Ghazipur in 1820 and by 1872 centres came up at North Western Province and Oudh. Good quality morphine equivalent to that described in British pharmacopoeia was produced in the factories. A circular of 1871 from Bengal General Hospital advises use of locally manufactured morphine in order to reduce the expenditure.[72]

Often the quality of the drugs depended upon the parameters set by the British pharmacopoeia. The British pharmacopoeia became the compendium of the officially recognized drugs along with their weight, measurements and correct method of preparing them. The aim of the first British pharmacopoeia (1864) was modest but later editions of it increasingly became an effective tool of empire.[73] This standardization of Western drugs led the practitioners of Western medicine in India to be conscious of the refinement of Western drugs available in India. They too demanded refined Western drugs but the cost associated with it made government to emphasize on the use of local drugs. As a result, conflict arose between the government and local practitioners on the issue of availability of European drugs at the Medical Store Department in Calcutta.[74] Since it was much cheaper to procure dry, medicinal substances in the bazaars, Medical Department agreed on using indigenous drugs and in regard to those available in crude forms, they were required a prior treatment in the laboratory.[75] Poonam Bala argues that the motive behind this move was that either through medium of medical store or assistance of the Commissariat Office such native drugs were to be made available in the government dispensaries.[76]

A valuable pharmacopoeia of indigenous drugs was composed. The commissary general was even instructed to procure information on indigenous drugs from the best market. Administrative medical officials were directed to use good native medicine instead of European medicines. In this process of compilation of pharmacopoeias, the botanists also provided assistance. Joseph Hooker provided assistance to William Dymock and Warden while preparing *Pharmacographia Indica*. Nathaniel Wallich, the superintendent of botanical gardens, assisted O'Shaughnessy while preparing *Pharmacopoeia of India*.

Despite the search of alternative herbs of Indian origin, the contents of the pharmacopeia lacked an overall consistency.[77] According to the Proceedings of 1866, A. P. Holwell instructed that only supply of such Western medicine be available for which no indigenous drugs could be found.[78] The *Pharmacopoeia of India* was published in 1868 but it lacked the legal status of British pharmacopoeia. David Arnold (1985) and Ram Nath Chopra (1933) both argue that it was only compiled to introduce certain drugs within the British pharmacopeia. The idea of drug substitution too was finally rejected by the government in 1901. Anil Kumar argues that the colonial interest in serving India as an exporter of raw material and importer of finished goods suited perfectly with the colonial agenda. Until the First World War the export ratio of raw material used by the international pharmaceutical firms was quite high. These included plants such as *Nux vomica, Belladonna, Asafoetida, Senna, Camphor, Cinchona bark, tea waste, oil and oil seeds*.[79]

EXPORT OF ESSENTIAL OIL AND OILSEEDS YEAR

55,483 gallons 169,632 cwts 1912–1913

56,170 gallons 155,273 cwts 1915–1918[80]

During the First World War, things started to change for a while as the government accepted that most of the drugs approved by British Pharmacopeia were already available in India. Hence, in order to reduce the expenses, it made more sense to produce them in India. Thus, initiatives were undertaken to meet such wartime requirements. Several drugs were attempted to be grown in the botanical garden at Ootacamund, in Punjab and in Madras Presidency as well. Anil Kumar points out how even private cultivation of such plants was encouraged. But with end of war such efforts of making India self-sufficient in drugs were brought to an end. Sukumar Chattopadhyay too argues that until the First World War, British did not realize the need for a drug industry in India.[81] Raymond Crawford in 1917 began an exploration of resources from Indian herbs. He was in favour of formation of an assorted body of knowledge and was eager to utilize the existent knowledge of Hindu medicine.[82] But he identifies certain basic problems that lay in the compilation of the pharmacopoeia. The foremost being almost no reference to the local names. Second, the study of the medicinal herbs conducted by the colonial officials lacked a proper base.[83]

Stuart Anderson argues that the export of drugs to India was a lucrative trade and could not be given up lightly. In 1866, some £20,000 was spent for importing drugs into India. He states that 50% of the drugs in 1898 and 1914 were indigenous to India. However as regards the traditional drugs, there was no regular cultivation of these. This in turn helped in importing drugs from Britain. Between 1912 and 1937 the total value of import drugs from UK rose from £373,000 to 590,000.[84] There was a continued demand for Indian medicinal herbs as Subrata Pahari has focused upon. He says that a double profitable trade was conducted by the colonial government. For instance, the colonial government procures 50000 maund of Kuchla leaf for 3200 rupees for manufacturing strychchine which was then sold at much higher price in the Indian market.[85] Thus, imperial imperative to reduce expenses steered the need for drug substitution but adequate initiative to ensure its implementation was never undertaken as was proven by the CIDC. Moreover, export of drug was a profitable trade which meant its termination would harm the fiscal interest of the government.

The Drug Enquiry Committee of 1930 and Indigenous Responses

After repeated efforts of George Watts and Kanai Lal Dey, the Indian National Congress included extended investigation and use of indigenous drugs in its demands. In response to their continued demands, the Indigenous Drugs Committee was set up which survived till 1920s. In a report of 1909, it called for establishing a school of tropical medicine, all but in name. Two committees under R. N. Chopra were formed – first in 1930s and the later in 1946.[86] The Drug Enquiry Committee was constituted in 1930 to enquire into the strength of the drugs and medicinal preparations as these drugs were now viewed with suspicion. The objective of the committee was to enquire the extent to which the impure drugs were sold in Indian markets. This of course made the nationalist leaders indignant as the European drugs by this time had already gained a hold over drug market and the government was accused of not providing enough encouragement to the Indigenous Drug Industry.[87] The indigenous response was not uniform either. In 1869, Dr Bholanath Bose, civil surgeon from Bengal, framed a scheme to meet the demands of the ailing population by proposing to establish temporary medical school in each district of Bengal. He even proposed to familiarize the students with a practical knowledge of indigenous drugs, namely, *Bhaunt*, *Indrajb* and others. Bhaunt was used as a general cure for all febrile ailments and latter for diarrhoea, dysentery and cholera. Dr D. B. Smith, the sanitary commissioner of Bengal, showed his unwillingness to implement these reforms. A part of this refusal was based on Bose's overreliance on indigenous medicine.[88] However, Smith agreed that the indigenous products were important and the only way to acquire this knowledge is from the kavirajs. So, the kaviraj/vaidya families continued their hereditary profession in the mofussil. Bramhananda Gupta provides a list of eminent kaviraj families like that of Gangaprasad

Ray, Gangaprasad Sen and Haracharan Chakraborty who lead the school of traditional Ayurveda in nineteenth-century Bengal.[89] Despite much criticism from the practitioners of Western medicine, the practitioners of indigenous medicine established a dispensary at Calcutta to propagate the knowledge of Indian medicine through publication of inexpensive books.[90] They themselves funded pharmaceutical concerns to manufacture and sell indigenous drugs. According to Brahmananda Gupta this made them 'the one time the richest men of the country'.[91] Just as the interest in indigenous medicine among the Western medical professionals weakened and did not completely die down, similarly interest in indigenous drugs such as *Neem*, *Chirata*, and *Anantamul* continued as well.[92] Even the best doctors of Western medicine in Bengal Presidency in the first decade of the century used *Makara dhawaja* for the treatment of cases of typhoid and other ailments.[93] Many committees were even asked to submit local drugs which were used for treatment of malarial fevers and bowel problems. As a consequence, the supply of European medicines was continued.[94] J. C. Ghosh in his *Indigenous Drugs of India: Their Scientific Cultivation and Manufacture* (1918) attributes the increasing utilization of indigenous drugs from abroad as a consequence of the First World War. According to him, acute necessity was then felt for developing and utilizing local resources as far as possible. The Englishman of Calcutta 1917 reported the cutting off of central Europe, following the war, as a source of supply of medicinal plants, which gave impetus to the cultivation of more vegetable drugs in India.[95] Ghosh, who was a graduate from England and a pharmaceutical chemist at the government medical stores dept in Bombay, proposed the attachment of an experimental drug farm to the cultivation of vegetable drugs.[96] Much like their colonial counterpart, confusion regarding identification of plants distressed the indigenous practitioners as can be seen in Horolal Gupta's *Ayurbed Bashabidahn* and Kaviraj Bijoyorotna Sen's *Bonosudhi Darpan*.[97] The growth of nationalist fervour had its impact in the study of medicinal herbs. A strong nationalist argument was gradually gaining ground. One strand of the nationalists centred their argument on the economic drain of the drugs. This line of argument resisted such a drain of the nation and its drugs as they belonged rightfully to her children. Another strand of this argument focused on how Indian herbs are suited for Indian constitution. It was argued in texts such as *Native Constitution and Treatment* by Gourinath Sen and *Arya Griha Chikitsha* by Binodlal Sengupta. K. M. Nadkarni too conducted researches in indigenous drugs. His influential book *Bharat Mata* depicts her holding herbs.[98] In this construction of herbal knowledge, the household remedies prevalent among the women were also appropriated. Works like that of Nobin Chandra Pal's *Indian Herbalist* (1873) and Ramchondro Bidyabinod's *Ayurbed Kusumnajali* (1897) talk about the herbal knowledge that usually preserved by mothers and grandmothers. But in this new project of reasserting the native control, women are completely marginalized. The proliferation of vernacular journals devoted to medicine also allowed insertion of this feminine botanical tradition into professional repertoire through regular columns devoted to *Garhosthya Chikitsa*, *Bonosudhi* and *Totka.*[99] Journals such as *Bamabodhini Patrika* dedicated articles on traditional household remedies.[100]

CONCLUSION

The expansion of trade routes helped in greater spread and accumulation of knowledge on indigenous herbs. As regards the native botanical knowledge, an important question has been raised been by Deepak Kumar regarding the recognition of the native collaborators who were often not acknowledged. Early colonial rulers always took local help while identifying medicinal plants which were regularly published in the *Philosophical Transactions*. Henry Noltie mentions some of the Indian collaborators like Luchman Singh, Rungiah and Govindoo.[101] These works on native medicinal herbs relied heavily on the knowledge of the locals whether it was the Ezhavas, fakirs, *Molues*, *Bediyas* or *Koibortos*.[102] Medicine, thus, became a rhetoric of progress and colonial efficiency. It is needless to say that the British officials classified the natural world on scientific lines. This indeed improved our understanding of the natural world. But such research later contributed to a repertoire of power knowledge. They adopted a negative attitude towards the native knowledge on medicine. In times of crisis, drug substitution was emphasized upon. Also, it is important to remember that prior to the opening of the Suez Canal in 1869, they encouraged the use of bazaar drugs at the medical depots for reducing the expenses. Drug committees were constituted and pharmacopoeias were constituted but to no avail. No fruitful result came out of them.[103]

NOTES

1. V. Sujatha, "Globalisation of South Asian Medicines: Knowledge, Power, Structure and Sustainability," *Society and Culture in South Asia* 6, no. 1 (2020): 7–30; V. Sujatha, "Pluralism in Indian Medicine: Medical Lore as a Genre of Medical Knowledge", *Contributions to Indian Sociology* 41, no. 2 (2007): 169–202.
2. Sujatha, "Globalisation,"7–30; Sujatha, "Pluralism," 169–202.
3. Sujatha, "Globalisation," 7–30.

4. "Introduction," in *Histories of Medicine and Healing in the Indian Ocean World, vol, 1: The Medieval and Early Modern Period,* ed. Anna Winterbottom and Facil Tesfaye (Basingstoke, Palgrave Macmillan, 2016), 2.

5. Haripriya Rangan, Judith Carney, and Denham Tim, "Environmental History of Botanical Exchanges in the Indian Ocean World," *Environment and History* 18, no. 3 (2012): 311–42.

6. Rangan, Carney, and Tim, "Environmental History," 311–42.

7. Michael Pearson, "Concluding Remarks," in *Histories of Medicine and Healing in the Indian Ocean World, vol, 2: The Modern Period*, ed. Anna Winterbottom and Facil Tesfaye (Basingstoke, Palgrave Macmillan, 2016), 245–53.

8. David Arnold, "The Indian Ocean as a disease zone, 1500–1950, South Asia," *Journal of South Asian Studies* 14, no. 2 (1991): 1–21.

9. Michael Pearson, "Concluding Remarks," 245–53,

10. Richard H. Grove, *Green Imperialism: Colonial Expansion, Tropical Island Eden and Origin of Environmentalism, 1600–1860* (New Delhi: Oxford University Press, 1995), 73–94.

11. Grove, *Green Imperialism*, 73–94.

12. Grove, *Green Imperialism*, 73–94.

13. Deepak Kumar, *Science and the Raj: A Study of British in India* (New Delhi, Oxford University Press 2006), 36. Deepak Kumar, "Botanical Exploration and the East India Company," in *East India Company and the Natural world*, ed. Vinita Damodaran, Anna Winterbottom, Alan Lester (London: Palgrave Macmillan, 2015), 16–34.

14. Rangan, Carney, and Tim, "Environmental History," 311–42. Arnold, "The Indian Ocean", 1–21.

15. Londa Schiebinger, "Prospecting for Drugs: European Naturalists in West Indies," in *Colonial Botany: Science, Commerce, Politics in early modern World*, ed. Londa Schiebinger and Claudia Swan (Philadelphia: University of Pennsylvania Press, 2007), 132–47.

16. Schiebinger, "Prospecting," 132–47.

17. Daniela Bleichmar, "Books, Bodies and Fields: Sixteenth Century Transatlantic Encounters with New World Materia Medica," in *Colonial Botany: Science, Commerce, Politics in Early Modern World*, ed. Londa Schiebinger and Claudia Swan (Philadelphia: University of Pennsylvania Press, 2007), 93–110.

18. For details see Bleichmar, "Books, Bodies and Fields," 93–110.

19. Bleichmar, "Books, Bodies and Fields," 93–110.

20. Bleichmar, "Books, Bodies and Fields," 93–110.

21. Bleichmar, "Books, Bodies and Fields," 93–110.

22. H. Pols, "European Physicians and Botanists, Indigenous Herbal Medicine in the Dutch East Indies, and Colonial Networks of Mediation", *East Asian Science* 3 (2009): 173–208.

23. Joanna Bishop, "The First Line of Defence: Domestic Health Care in Colonial New Zealand, 1850s–1920s," *Health and History* 16, no. 2 (2014): 1–23.

24. J. Roberts, "Medical Exchange on the Gold Coast during the Seventeenth and Eighteenth Centuries," *Canadian Journal of African Studies / Revue Canadienne Des Études Africaines* 45, no. 3 (2011): 480–523.

25. Garcia Da Orta (1563) *Colloquies dos simples e drogas he consas medicinas da Indica*, Goa. His works and contributions have been discussed at length in Poonam Bala (ed.), Learning from Empire: Medicine, Knowledge and Transfers under Portuguese Rule, 2018, Newcastle upon Tyne: Cambridge Scholars Publishing.
26. Grove, *Green Imperialism*, 73–94.
27. O.P. Jaggi, *Ayurveda: Indian Systems of Medicine* (New Delhi, 1981).
28. Jaggi, *Ayurveda*.
29. Kapil Raj, "Surgeons, Fakirs, Merchants and Craft People: Making L. Empereurs Jardin in Early Modern South Asia," in *Colonial Botany: Science, Commerce, politics in early modern World*, ed. Londa Schiebinger and Claudia Swan (Philadelphia: University of Pennsylvania Press, 2007), 270–88.
30. Raj, "Surgeons, Fakirs, Merchants," 270–88.
31. Anna Winterbottom, "Medicine and Botany in the Making of Madras," in *East India Company and the Natural world*, ed. Vinita Damodaran, Anna Winterbottom, Alan Lester (London: Palgrave Macmillan, 2015), 35–57.
32. Chittabata Palit, "Ayurveda in Colonial Bengal: Survival and Revival," in *Scientific Bengal: Science, Technology, Medicine and Environment under the Raj*, ed. Chittabrata Palit (Kolkata: Kalpaz Publication, 2006), 15.
33. Deepak Kumar, "Botanical Exploration and the East India Company", in *East India Company and the Natural world*, ed. Vinita Damodaran, Anna Winterbottom, Alan Lester (London: Palgrave Macmillan, 2015), 16–34.
34. Kumar, "Botanical Exploration," 16–34.
35. Mark Harrison, "Medicine and Orientalism: Perspectives on European Encounter with Indian medical system," in *Health, Medicine and Empire: Perspectives on Colonial India*, ed. Biswamoy Pati and Mark Harrison (New Delhi: Orient Longman, 2001), 37–81.
36. Harrison, "Medicine and Orientalism," 37–81.
37. Projit Bihari Mukharji, "Pharmacology, Indigenous Knowledge, Nationalism: A Few Words from the Epitaph of Subaltern Science," in *Social History of Health and Medicine in colonial India* ed. Biswamoy Pati and Mark Harrison (New York: Routledge, 2009), 195–212.
38. Deepak Kumar, "Botanical Exploration and the East India Company," in *East India Company and the Natural World*, ed. Vinita Damodaran, Anna Winterbottom, Alan Lester (London: Palgrave Macmillan, 2015), 16–34.
39. Harrison, "Medicine and Orientalism", 37–81.
40. B.D. Basu, *History of Education under the Rule of the East India Company* (Kolkata, 1867).
41. Projit Bihari Mukharji, "What in a Name? The Crisis of Botanical Identification and Production of Economic Man," *Social Scientist* 33, no. 5/6 (2005): 3–25.
42. Harkishan Singh, "Whitelaw Ainslie: Pioneer in Promoting Indigenous Indian Drugs," *Pharmacy in History* 58, no. 3–4 (2016): 103–106.
43. Singh, "Whitelaw Ainslie," 103–106.
44. Singh, "Whitelaw Ainslie," 103–106.
45. Harrison, "Medicine and Orientalism," 37–81.
46. Harrison, "Medicine and Orientalism," 37–81.

47. Poonam Bala, *Imperialism and Medicine in Bengal* (Kolkata: Sage Publications, 1991), 41–64.

48. Palit, "Ayurveda in Colonial Bengal," 15.

49. Mukharji, "What in a Name?," 3–25.

50. Harrison, "Medicine and Orientalism," 37–81.

51. Deepak Kumar, "Botanical Exploration and the East India Company," in *East India Company and the natural World*, ed. Vinita Damodaran, Anna Winterbottom, and Alan Lester (London: Palgrave Macmillan, 2015), 16–34,

52. W.B. O' Shaughnessy et al. (1838) First Report of the Committee for the Preparation of a Pharmacopoeia for Bengal in *Quarterly Journal of the Medical and Physical Society of Calcutta*, no,6, 153–65.

53. Bala, *Imperialism and Medicine in Bengal*, 41–64.

54. Bala, *Imperialism and Medicine in Bengal.*

55. Eugene Irschik, *Dialogue and History: Constructing South India, 1795–1895* (Berkeley: California University Press, 1994); Projit Bihari Mukharji, "What in a Name? The Crisis of Botanical Identification and Production of Economic Man," *Social Scientist* 33, no. 5/6 (2005): 3–25.

56. Harrison, "Medicine and Orientalism," 37–81.

57. Projit Bihari Mukharji, "What in a Name?: The Crisis of Botanical Identification and Production of Economic Man," *Social Scientist* 33, no. 5/6 (May-June 2005): 3–25.

58. Mukharji, "What in a Name?," 3–25.

59. Bala, *Imperialism and Medicine in Bengal,* 41–64.

60. Anil Kumar, "Indian Drug industry under the Raj, 1860–1920," in *Health, Medicine and Empire: Perspectives on Colonial India,* ed. Biswamoy Pati and Mark Harrison (New Delhi: Orient Longman, 2001), 356–82.

61. Kumar, "Indian Drug Industry under the Raj," 356–82.

62. Projit Bihari Mukherji, "Vishalyakarani as Eupatorium Ayapana: Retro-Botanizing, Embedded Traditions, and Multiple Historicities of Plants in Colonial Bengal, 1890–1940," *The Journal of Asian Studies* 73, no. 1 (2014): 65–87.

63. G. King, *Report of the Central Indigenous Drug Committee*, 1896 (Kolkata: Government of India Press, 1901).

64. Kumar, "Indian Drug Industry under the Raj," 356–82.

65. *Report of the Indigenous Drug Committee*, 1930–31 (Kolkata: Government of India Press, 1931).

66. Anil Kumar, "Indian Drug Industry under the Raj, 1860–1920," in *Health, Medicine and Empire: Perspectives on colonial India*, ed. Biswamoy Pati and Mark Harrison (New Delhi, Orient Longman), 2001, 356–82.

67. Kumar, "Indian Drug Industry under the Raj," 356–82.

68. Home Medical, March 1901, nos, 48–62, National Archives of India.

69. Anil Kumar, "Indian Drug industry under the Raj, 1860–1920," in *Health, Medicine and Empire: Perspectives on Colonial India*, ed. Biswamoy Pati and Mark Harrison (New Delhi, Orient Longman), 2001, 356–382.

70. Kumar, "Indian Drug Industry under the Raj," 356–82.

71. Kumar, "Indian Drug Industry under the Raj," 356–82.

72. Kumar, "Indian Drug Industry under the Raj," 356–82.
73. Stuart Anderson, "Pharmacy and Empire: The "British Pharmacopoeia" as an Instrument of Imperialism 1864 to 1932," *Pharmacy in History,* 52, no. 3/4 (2010): 112–21.
74. Proceedings of the Government of India (1866) Home Department, Medical Branch, July-December.
75. Proceedings of the Government of India (1866) Home Department, Medical Branch, July-December.
76. Poonam Bala, *Imperialism and Medicine in Bengal*, 41–64.
77. Sukumar Chattopadhyay, "The search of last resources of medicinal herbs of India: Role of pharmacopeial literature," in *Science, Technology, Medicine and Environment,* ed. Chittabrata Palit (Kolkata: Kalpaz Publication, 2006), 159–69.
78. Poonam Bala, *Imperialism and Medicine in Bengal,* 41–64.
79. Anil Kumar, "Indian Drug industry under the Raj, 1860–1920," in *Health, Medicine and Empire: Perspectives on Colonial India*, ed. Biswamoy Pati and Mark Harrison (New Delhi: Orient Longman, 2001), 356–82.
80. Source Anuradha Roy, Growth and Development of chemical industry in Bengal 1900–47 PhD dissertation in Anil Kumar, "Indian Drug industry under the Raj," 356–82.
81. Sukumar Chattopadhyay, "The search of last resources of medicinal herbs of India: Role of pharmacopeial literature," in *Scientific Bengal: Science, Technology, Medicine and Environment under the Raj,* ed. Chittabrata Palit (Kolkata: Kalpaz Publication, 2006), 159–69.
82. Chattopadhyay, "The Search of Last Resources of Medicinal Herbs of India," 159–69.
83. Chattopadhyay, "The Search of Last Resources of Medicinal Herbs of India," 159–69.
84. Stuart Anderson, "Pharmacy and Empire: The "British Pharmacopoeia" as an Instrument of Imperialism 1864 to 1932," *Pharmacy in History* 52, no. 3/4 (2010): 112–21,
85. Subrata Pahari, "Sources Relating to the Recent History of Traditional Medicine: Somc Problems and Possibilities," in *Science, technology, Medicine and Environment in India: Historical Perspectives*, ed. Chittabarta Palit and Amit Bhattacharya (Kolkata: Bibhasa, 1988), 128–58. Subrata Pahari, *Drug Imperialism in Modern India* (Corpus Research Institute, Kolkata, 2011).
86. Projit Bihari Mukharji, "Pharmacology, Indigenous Knowledge, Nationalism: A Few Words from the Epitaph of Subaltern Science," in *Social History of Health and Medicine in colonial India*, ed. Biswamoy Pati and Mark Harrison (New York: Routledge, 2009), 195–212.
87. *Report of the Indigenous Drug Committee*, 1930–31 (Kolkata: Government of India Press, 1931).
88. Proceedings of the Government of India,(1866) Home Department, Medical Branch, July-December.
89. Palit, "Ayurveda in Colonial Bengal," 15
90. Poonam Bala, *Imperialism and Medicine in Bengal,* 41–64.

91. Bramhananda Gupta, "Indigenous Medicine in Nineteenth and Twentieth Century Bengal," in *Asian Medical System: A comparative Study*, ed. Charles Leslie (New Delhi: Motilal Banarsidas Publishers, 1998), 368–80.

92. Poonam Bala, *Imperialism and Medicine in Bengal* (Kolkata: Sage Publications, 1991), 41–64.

93. Bala, *Imperialism and Medicine in Bengal,* 41–64.

94. Bala, *Imperialism and Medicine in Bengal,* 41–64.

95. Poonam Bala, *Imperialism and Medicine in Bengal* (Kolkata: Sage Publications, 1991), 41–64.

96. Bala, *Imperialism and Medicine in Bengal,* 41–64.

97. Projit Bihari Mukharji, "Pharmacology, Indigenous knowledge, Nationalism: A Few Words from the Epitaph of Subaltern Science," in *Social History of Health and Medicine in colonial India*, ed. Biswamoy Pati and Mark Harrison (Routledge, New York, 2009), 195–212.

98. Mukharji, "Pharmacology, Indigenous knowledge, Nationalism", 195–212.

99. Mukharji, "Pharmacology, Indigenous knowledge, Nationalism", 195–212.

100. Nupur Dasgupta, "A Bridge for Passing: Journey of Indigenous Medicine in a world of Medical pluralism in Bengal (1870s–1930s)," in *Essays in History of Science, Technology and Medicine,* ed. Nupur Dasgupta and Amit Bhattacharya (Kolkata: Setu Prakshani, 2014), 264–95.

101. Deepak Kumar, "Botanical exploration and the East India Company," in *East India Company and the Natural World,* ed. Vinita Damodaran, Anna Winterbottom, and Alan Lester (London: Palgrave Macmillan, 2015), 16–34.

102. Projit Bihari Mukharji, "Pharmacology, Indigenous Knowledge, Nationalism: A Few Words from the Epitaph of Subaltern Science," in Biswamoy Pati and Mark Harrison ed, *Social History of Health and Medicine in Colonial India* (New York: Routledge, 2009), 195–212.

103. Anil Kumar, "Indian Drug Industry under the Raj, 1860–1920," in *Health, Medicine and Empire: Perspectives on Colonial India,* ed. Biswamoy Pati and Mark Harrison (New Delhi: Orient Longman, 2001), 356–82.

BIBLIOGRAPHY

Anderson, Stuart. "Pharmacy and Empire: The 'British Pharmacopoeia' as an Instrument of Imperialism 1864 to 1932". *Pharmacy in History* 52, no. 3/4 (2010): 112–121.

Arnold, David. "The Indian Ocean as a Disease Zone, 1500–1950". *Journal of South Asian Studies* 14, no. 2 (1991): 1–21.

Bala, Poonam. *Imperialism and Medicine in Bengal.* Kolkata: Sage Publications, 1991.

Bala, Poonam. "Physicians, Knowledge and Curiosities in Colonial Goa". In *Learning from Empire: Medicine, Knowledge and Transfers under Portuguese Rule,* edited by Poonam Bala, 9–17. Newcastle upon Tyne: Cambridge Scholars Publishing, 2018.

Basu, B.D. *History of Education under the Rule of the East India Company*. Kolkata: The Modern Review Office, 1867.

Bishop, Joanna. "The First Line of Defence: Domestic Health Care in Colonial New Zealand 1850s–1920s". *Health and History* 16, no. 2 (2014): 1–23.

Bleichmar, Daniela. "Books, Bodies and Fields: Sixteenth Century Transatlantic Encounters with New World Materia Medica". In *Colonial Botany: Science, Commerce, politics in early modern World*, edited by Londa Schiebinger and Claudia Swan, 93–110. Philadelphia: University of Pennsylvania press, 2007.

Chattopadhyay, Sukumar. "The Search of Last Resources of Medicinal Herbs of India: Role of Pharmacopoeial Literature". In *Science, Technology, Medicine and Environment*, edited by Chittabrata Palit, 159–69. Kolkata: Kalpaz Publication, 2006.

Dasgupta, Nupur. "A Bridge for Passing: Journey of Indigenous Medicine in a world of medical pluralism in Bengal (1870s–1930s)". In *Essays in history of Science, technology and Medicine*, edited by Nupur Dasgupta and Amit Bhattacharya, 264–95. Kolkata: Setu Prakshani, 2014.

Grove, Richard. *Green Imperialism: Colonial Expansion, Tropical Island Eden and Origin of Environmentalism, 1600–1860*. New Delhi: Oxford University Press, 1995.

Gupta, Bramhananda. "Indigenous Medicine in Nineteenth and Twentieth Century Bengal". In *Asian Medical System: A comparative Study*, edited by Charles Leslie, 368–80. New Delhi: Motilal Banarsidas Publishers, 1998.

Harrison, Mark. "Medicine and Orientalism: Perspectives on European Encounter with Indian medical system". In '*Health, Medicine and Empire: Perspectives on colonial India*', edited by Biswamoy Pati and Mark Harrison, 37–81. New Delhi: Orient Longman, 2001.

Home Medical. March 1901, nos. 48–62, National Archives of India.

Irschik, Eugene. '*Dialogue and History: Constructing South India, 1795–1895*', Berkeley: California University Press, 1994.

Jaggi, O.P. *Ayurveda: Indian systems of medicine*. New Delhi: Atma Ram and Sons, 1981.

King, G. '*Report of the Central Indigenous Drug Committee 1896*'. Kolkata: Government of India Press, 1901.

Kumar, Anil. "Indian Drug industry under the Raj, 1860–1920". In *Health, Medicine and Empire: Perspectives on colonial India*, edited by Biswamoy Pati and Mark Harrison, 356–82. New Delhi: Orient Longman, 2001.

Kumar, Deepak. "Botanical exploration and the East India Company". In *East India Company and the natural world*, edited by Vinita Damodaran, Anna Winterbottom, Alan Lester, 16–34. London: Palgrave Macmillan, 2015.

Kumar, Deepak. *Science and the Raj: A Study of British in India*. New Delhi: Oxford University Press, 2006.

Mukherji, Projit Bihari. "Pharmacology, Indigenous Knowledge, Nationalism: A Few Words from the Epitaph of Subaltern Science". In *The Social History of Health and Medicine in Colonial India*, edited by Biswamoy Pati and Mark Harrison, 195–212. London: Routledge, 2009.

Mukharji, Projit Bihari. "What in a Name? The Crisis of Botanical Identification and Production of Economic Man". '*Social Scientist*' 33, no. 5/6 (2005): 3–25.

Pahari Subrata. "Sources Relating to the Recent History of Traditional Medicine: Some Problems and Possibilities". In *Science, technology, Medicine and Environment in India: Historical Perspective,* edited by Chittabarta Palit and Amit Bhattacharya, 128–58. Kolkata: Bibhasa, 1988.

Pahari, Subarta. *Drug imperialism in Modern India.* Kolkata: Corpus Research Institute, 2011.

Palit, Chittabrata. "Ayurveda in Colonial Bengal: Survival and Revival." In *Scientific Bengal: Science, Technology, Medicine and Environment under the Raj,* edited by Chittabrata Palit, 15. Kolkata: Kalpaz Publication, 2006

Pearson, Michael. "Concluding Remarks". In *Histories of Medicine and Healing in the Indian Ocean World, vol. 2: The Modern Period,* edited by Anna Winterbottom and Facil Tesfaye, 245–53. Basingstoke: Palgrave Macmillan. 2016.

Pols, Hans. "European Physicians and Botanists, Indigenous Herbal Medicine in the Dutch East Indies, and Colonial Networks of Mediation". *East Asian Science* 3 (2009): 173–208.

Proceedings of the Government of India, Home Department, Medical Branch, July-December, 1866.

Raj, Kapil. "Surgeons, Fakirs, Merchants and Craft People: Making L'Empereur's Jardin in Early Modern South Asia". In *Colonial Botany: Science, Commerce, Politics in Early Modern World,* edited by Londa Schiebinger and Claudia Swan, 270–88. Philadelphia: University of Pennsylvania press, 2007.

Rangan, Haripriya, Judith Carney, and Tim Denham. "Environmental History of Botanical Exchanges in the Indian Ocean World". *Environment and History* 18, no. 3 (2012): 311–42.

Report of the Indigenous Drug Committee 1930–31. Kolkata: Government of India Press, 1931. Schiebinger, Londa. "Prospecting for Drugs: European Naturalists in West Indies". In *Colonial Botany: Science, Commerce, Politics in Early Modern World,* edited by Londa Schiebinger and Claudia Swan, 132–47. Philadelphia: University of Pennsylvania Press, 2007.

Roberts, Jonathan. "Medical Exchange on the Gold Coast during the Seventeenth and Eighteenth Centuries". *Canadian Journal of African Studies / Revue Canadienne Des Études Africaines* 45, no. 3 (2011): 480–523.

Shaughnessy W. B. O., et al. "First Report of the Committee for the Preparation of a Pharmacopoeia for Bengal". *Quarterly Journal of the Medical and Physical Society of Calcutta* no. 6 (1838): 153–65.

Sujatha, V. "Globalisation of South Asian Medicines: Knowledge, Power, Structure and Sustainability". *Society and Culture in South Asia* 6, no. 1 (2020): 7–30.

Sujatha, V. "Pluralism in Indian Medicine: Medical Lore as a Genre of Medical Knowledge". *Contributions to Indian Sociology* 41, no. 2 (May 2007): 169–202.

Winterbottom, Anna. "Medicine and Botany in the making of Madras". In *East India Company and the natural world* edited by Vinita Damodaran, Anna Winterbottom, Alan Lester, 35–57. London: Palgrave Macmillan, 2015.

Chapter 8

Disease and Dependency in Kweneng, Botswana (ca. 1880–1930)

Jeff Ramsay

At the end of the nineteenth century, indigenous communities in south-east Botswana (then the Bechuanaland Protectorate) were becoming dependent on migrant labour. By the 1920s, working on contract in the South African mines was the shared life experience of most able-bodied adult males, while women and children struggled to sustain domestic production at below subsistence level. Although ultimately reinforced by colonial state impositions, this transformation had been initially driven by the catastrophic appearance of a series of epidemics that, when coupled with other natural disasters, undermined domestic social reproduction. While the significance of labour migration in shaping Botswana society has been a focus of considerable scholarship, the epidemiology associated with its emergence has received little attention.[1] In this respect, recent works on colonial era medical history have focused more on the evolution of health care delivery than the social legacy of major disease outbreaks.[2] More broadly, although there has been regional recognition of the trauma caused by past epidemics, such as smallpox and rinderpest, the significance of disease in the shaping of twentieth-century Southern Africa social order was relatively neglected.[3] As Howard Phillips observed:

> Epidemics – the unusually high prevalence of lethal human disease in a town, country or region – loom small in accounts of South Africa's past, almost in inverse proportion to the anxious attention they attracted while they raged. In part this is because, until quite recently, historians have not known how to incorporate them into their versions of history, dominated as they were by political, economic social and cultural issues. . . . In this short-sightedness, they failed to recognise that, far from existing outside of these frameworks, in some separate medical paradigm, epidemics (and disease generally) are integral to every aspect of life, death and society.[4]

As a contribution to the broader study of disease as a factor in the consolidation of imperialist hegemony, this chapter focuses on the contribution of invasive pathogens, when coupled with colonial state impositions, in the underdevelopment of Kweneng or the Bakwena Tribal Reserve as it was gazetted under colonial rule, where virtually the entire population suffered severe material losses and a consequent decline in livelihoods. The abruptness of this change gave rise to domestic turmoil as people struggled to recover their welfare and sense of social order.

SHAKEN KINGDOM

As a polity Kweneng had grown in wealth and regional influence during the mid-nineteenth century under a king or 'kgosi' (plural 'dikgosi') named Sechele (reign 1833–1892), when it was a nexus for regional commerce, Christian proselytization and armed indigenous resistance to the expansion of white settlers from today's South Africa.[5] Although here collectively referred to as Bakwena, the territory's population is divided between Bakwena proper and other ethnic Batswana clans concentrated in the more arable east, along with smaller numbers of Bakgalagari and Kua (Basarwa, San or 'Bushmen') who are predominant in its sandy west. Historically, members of the latter two groups commonly occupied positions of servitude, being obliged to provide labour and tribute to members of Kweneng's social elite. After the 1885 imposition of British overrule, the indigenous population as a whole remained the subjects of the Bakwena paramount ruler, who was given the colonial title of 'chief'.

By 1890, the kingdom's earlier prosperity as well as political autonomy had waned, but most Bakwena were able to sustain local livelihoods through agropastoral production supplemented by hunting, with some engaged in additional activities such as transport riding and various cottage industries, including the export of local game products. From the 1870s age-regiments had been sent to acquire firearms and other goods by working in the Kimberly Diamond Fields.[6] While this had set a precedent, labour migration was not as yet a path of long-term livelihood.

Sechele's death in 1892 unleashed public expressions of angst. At the royal village of Molepolole, women invaded the central kgotla or meeting place, crying: 'Our king is dead, where shall we flee?' A certain Rangwadi prophesied that his passing marked the beginning of the end of his kingdom. Ominous songs were sung. One, 'Diremogolo', spoke of an angry white man who would steal the land and chieftainship. Another, 'Rasekete', alluded to impending internal divisions, its lyrics telling of a kgosi who dies in possession of fine black and white cattle, which then grew grey and developed dangerous horns.[7] In the face of these outpourings, a meeting was convened where the senior tribesmen were doctored with protective medicines as they gathered to sanction the dynastic succession of Kgosi Sebele I (reign 1892–1911).

Inasmuch as perceptions of foreboding attributed to Sechele's demise may have evolved with hindsight, there were already grounds for unease. An 1891 Order in Council had empowered the British 'to enact laws, to establish a court system, to levy taxes, and to take additional steps to maintain peace, order and good government of all persons' within the protectorate. This development coincided with Botswana's position as the springboard for the 1890–1893 colonial conquest of Zimbabwe. Legal claims by dikgosi to be the 'Sovereigns of the Soil' were summarily dismissed. Even before his father's death, Sebele's own jurisdictional disputes with the British had threatened to escalate into violent confrontation.[8] In October 1892, Batswana were required to register their firearms as a prerequisite for the controlled purchase of ammunition. Resistance to this decree led to a decline in hunting which during 1893 resulted in a two-thirds drop in the until then lucrative export of ostrich feathers from the territory.[9]

There were also environmental indicators of a coming crisis. Poor rains and locust infestation disrupted crop production. Individually neither of these developments was exceptional. Botswana has always been a semi-arid country prone to drought, with seasons of poor rainfall having occurred in each decade of the nineteenth century, though by 1893 the situation was dire enough for Bakwena to seek the services of an external rainmaker.[10] While locust swarms had not been seen for a generation, their reappearance in 1891 was at first an edible nuisance.

What has been regarded as the first worldwide viral pandemic, the 'Russian Influenza' had also appeared.[11] Carried by railways and steam ships, between 1889 and 1890, the pestilence spread rapidly, globally killing about 1 million people. By the end of 1889, it had reached sub-Saharan Africa as well as western Europe and the Americas; being reported in the western Cape in January 1890, from where it spread into Bechuanaland. In March 1892, the district surgeon at Vryburg, then headquarters for both the Bechuanaland Crown Colony and Protectorate, reported the presence of an influenza epidemic accompanied by whooping cough and diphtheria. This development, combined with concern over the spread of syphilis, led him to recommend that the *Contagious Diseases Act* be enforced at native locations, 'owing to the large number of native servants' then in contact with Europeans. In June 1892, Bechuanaland's administrator confirmed 'an epidemic of what is commonly called Russian Influenza in the district of Mafeking'. In 1895, Mahikeng's district surgeon further reported: 'Influenza in the form of infectious feverish catarrhs of the respiratory organs was present in the district from August 1894 to March 1895. The natives suffered considerably from Influenza and several deaths came under my notice'.[12]

But, given the lack of official focus, much less data collection, on the health of the indigenous population, the Russian Influenza's impact within Botswana is uncertain. Although its communicable nature had caused panicked headlines throughout Europe and the Americas, Bechuanaland medical reports suggest greater concern over potential interracial transmission of syphilis and smallpox from blacks to whites, despite the fact that Europeans had been responsible for the introduction of both maladies into the region.

By March 1896, Kweneng's crops had once again failed due to continued drought coupled with locusts. In the same month, another cataclysm arrived in the form of rinderpest, known locally as 'bolwane', a highly infectious viral disease targeting ruminants.[13] Sebele responded to the epizootic by calling on his subjects to follow the colonial regime's instruction to shoot and bury sick livestock. This control effort was undermined from the beginning by the fact that most of the initially afflicted herds belonged to members of the 'BagaMashadi' faction then resisting the kgosi's authority along with Bakwena faith in the inoculations of their traditional doctors and the general practice of salvaging dried meat from the bovine carcasses. By mid-May it was reported that Sebele I's own herd of some 10,000 had been reduced to just seventy-seven beasts.[14] No one was spared. In May 1896, a traveller wrote:

> Hundreds of dead oxen laying in every stage of decomposition, behind the bushes – in places a dozen a batch! The whole air was vitiated by the stench of them, and amidst them we had to camp! I observed that the natives were busily skinning all the dead beasts, and apparently making biltong of the flesh. . . . I don't see how this country can escape a famine now – their crops have all failed from drought, and the remnants are eaten by locusts; their cattle are nearly all dead! I suppose a score of live cattle where there should have been a thousand or two![15]

Throughout the protectorate, both official and unofficial estimates consistently calculated livestock destruction as ranging upwards from 90%, for example, the Bechuanaland Annual Report for 1896–1897: 'The rinderpest travelled through the country from north to south, at one time at the rate of 25 miles a day, and destroyed not less than 90 per cent – at a low estimate – of the enormous herds of cattle within the Protectorate'. The same report further noted that Batswana had suddenly lost their 'staple product, the chief means of livelihood, an important item of the food supply, and the capital and the currency of the country'.[16] Given its general infection of ruminating animals, rinderpest also wiped out much of the small stock while afflicting wild ungulates. Disappearing wildlife frustrated the resort to communal hunting to stave off famine. In October 1896, many Bakwena were reportedly dying of hunger aggravated by dysentery and typhoid, with dying animals having tainted local water supplies.[17]

For some members of the London Missionary Society (LMS), which then exercised a virtual ecclesiastical monopoly over much of Botswana including Kweneng, this 'time of great spiritual testing' was viewed as a long-term blessing. From Kanye the Rev. Edwin Lloyd observed: 'I have long seen that their cattle stood between our people and their progress. While they possessed so many cattle, the young men and boys were obliged to herd them, and were prevented from coming to our schools to learn. In addition, the cattle-posts were the principal schools of heathenism, were untold evil was both taught and practiced'.[18] Lloyd added that men were now leaving in mass to work on the construction of the Mahikeng-Bulawayo railroad or in South African mines. Molepolole's resident missionaries, Mary Partridge and Rev. Howard Williams, were likewise tempted to look upon the calamities then bedevilling their parishioners as a catalyst for progress.

Partridge: The Bakwena need to learn that next to 'love of God' comes the 'dignity of labour'. Bakwena men are frightfully lazy and selfish. They would infinitely rather kopa food from the whites than do a little work to earn it. Some of them have been persuaded to go to work at the mines at Kimberly and some have gone through sheer necessity. No doubt many more will be driven to go. It will do them good.[19]

Williams: The loss of their cattle has driven large numbers to seek work. Certainly, the best thing that could happen as far a teaching them the value of labour. . . . Work was the last thing thought of except among the poorer classes and with these the period rarely exceeds 6 months. All that is altered. A generation will pass before this country will recover its lost wealth in cattle.[20]

Elements of the colonial regime also saw the crisis as an opportunity to encourage wage labour by distributing imported grain through food-for-work schemes.[21] According to Williams, Bakwena were at first reluctant: 'the Government brought immense supplies of food close to them and the Railway afforded the opportunity to work but scarcely any of the would turn out to work and many more would not go out to get food offered to them at a very small rate'.[22] As providers, dikgosi were expected to cater for the most needy from their communal grain stores, resulting in them initially rejecting aid offered through a charitable London Relief Committee. Sebele observed: 'The offer has come through the wrong channels. The very fact that the government officials have written to the missionaries for information has caused my people to look upon the offer with suspicion. The government in some of their dealings with my people have not been true to their word'.[23]

Overwhelmed by desperate circumstance, however, he soon relented, sending wagons to regularly pickup relief supplies. By December 1898, over 1,400 women and children in Molepolole were receiving rations from the committee.[24]

Throughout 1897–1898, reports spoke of horrific mortality rates in south-east Botswana due to famine and disease. When the Rev. Williams visited the Kweneng settlement at Kolobeng in June 1898, where several thousand members of the BagaMashadi faction had relocated three years earlier, he was shocked to find the place nearly deserted. The local kgosi told him that his followers were either 'in graves or scattered in all directions seeking food or work'. Williams supported this observation with statistics for four of the community's kinship wards showing recent death to former population ratios of 57/150, 21/70, 11/14 and 14/40. He further noted that fifteen out of thirty-four church members had died at neighbouring Kumakwane, along with most members of its once predominant Griqua community and one-fifth of the residents at Tlokweng. In Kanye an estimated 1,500 perished in 1898, while over a third of all students at the mission school in Molepolole reportedly died in the same year.[25] Children's health had been especially compromised by the absence of milch cows.

MIGRANT LABOUR

Between March and September 1897 many Bakwena were employed constructing the railway line from Mahikeng to Bulawayo, whose completion had an adverse effect on those who worked as transport riders along the route. A few thereafter made a living harvesting timber for rail shipment, reducing previous forest to bush scrub.[26] For most, the only option then was to seek work in the mines of South Africa or other neighbouring territories. The protectorate's Annual Report for 1897–1898 observed that: 'All of the tribes, except perhaps Linchwe's, are at present very short of food, and many have not the means of purchasing sufficient food for their families. They are, however, making an effort to obtain money for the purpose of buying food by going out to work in Kimberley, Jagersfontein, Johannesburg, and other places'. Affirming that 'so many men have gone that most villages present a quite deserted appearance', the report added that the territory was 'flooded by both white and coloured persons calling themselves Labour Agents'.[27] The licencing of such agents was introduced in 1899. By 1905, the South African Native Affairs Commission calculated that out of 22,206 able-bodied men in the protectorate between fifteen and forty years of age, two-thirds sought labour of which only 9% found work within the territory. An indicator of labour migration's importance among the Bakwena was the practice from

1898 of sending royal representatives to South Africa to look into the welfare of, and later collect taxes and levies from, fellow tribesmen.[28]

Inasmuch as food for work lured Batswana into wage labour, the imposition of Hut Tax served as a stick. Upon its introduction, one official observed: 'it has a twofold advantage, it drives young men to work and it raises revenue'.[29] While in Britain in 1895, Sebele, along with Bathoen and Khama, had accepted the inevitability of taxation during negotiations with the Colonial Office.[30] But, when tax was imposed in April 1899, Bathoen protested: 'Owing to famine not many people were left in his country; that most had gone to work or look for food, that this was the fourth year in succession that their crops had failed; that he was almost alone in the village; that the young men had gone out to the mines and were now living there'.[31]

Thereafter, enforcement of Hut Tax payments became a factor in assuring the continued flow of migrant workers. The link between mining contracts and Hut Tax payments was explicit in 1909 when officials were made responsible for overseeing contracts.[32] Those dikgosi, like Sebele, who were recognized chiefs of 'tribal territories', were allowed to annually pocket up to 10% of the Hut Tax money collected within their reserves. Many also imposed additional levies and expected gifts from returning migrants. By the 1920s, dikgosi were ordering any able-bodied men in tax arrears to sign contracts with local labour recruiters. In 1924, out of the £3,725 in Hut Tax receipts paid in Molepolole, £1,768 was directly remitted by labour recruiters as cash advances on 861 new contracts.[33] Among the Bakwena, Rev. William Clissold observed that 'nearly all the men go to work for periods of 6 to 12 months from time to time as the need for Hut Tax arises'.[34]

Almost all of the Hut Tax revenue was applied to meet recurrent administrative costs. In Kweneng, this meant paying for the local white magistrate and his externally recruited police. Ironically, for many years the major function of this establishment was the prosecution of tax defaulters. Of the 335 criminal cases brought before Molepolole's Resident Magistrate between 1921 and 1925, 262 concerned failures to pay Hut Tax.[35] Other laws, such as those against poaching, cattle smuggling and vagrancy, were also enforced whose effect was to further encourage migration.[36] Indeed, the construction of the Police Camp was the only infrastructure project initiated by the British during their 81-year occupation of Kweneng. Otherwise, the few public works that existed prior to 1966 were the products of local initiative, at times assisted by non-government actors. The Hut Tax thus not only contributed to the local economy's loss of the surplus value of its labour but also deprived it of revenue that could have contributed to internal development. In 1916, Bechuanaland's financial secretary, in a minute on new taxation proposals, commiserated: 'I am not sure that we are not gradually putting the territory into an economically unsound position by seeing interest and I believe capital go out of the country and laying no foundations for new trade nor for the betterment of existing ones'.[37] By 1910, the total value of protectorate exports in non-crisis years, mostly maize, livestock, hides and skins, was less than two-thirds the value of imports.[38]

Notwithstanding the widespread decline in local livelihoods during its early decades, as well as popular resentment of the Hut Tax and other administrative impositions, the Bechuanaland Protectorate stands out as one of the few jurisdictions in Southern Africa that largely avoided violent confrontation by indigenous residents against colonial authority. In this respect, Protectorate Batswana were mindful of the fate of neighbouring communities that had by then been pushed into uprisings, including Batswana in the former British Bechuanaland region of the Cape Colony. In his kgotla, Kgosi Bathoen praised the slain Motlhaping rebel Luka Jantjie as a hero, saying 'they have killed him, but they did so after he had fought'. Then turning to a local policeman, he asked: 'How do the white men fight?' The reply: 'When the government fights no one gets the best against it; the Government always wins'.[39]

War did finally arrive at the end of 1899 when eastern Botswana became a theatre of operations in second Anglo-Boer War (1899–1902). On the eve of hostilities, the chiefs were collectively instructed to assist the British in repelling Boer incursions into their territories. With the south-east protectorate temporarily abandoned by the British, in February 1900, Sebele reached an understanding with the Boer Commandant that they would keep their men on opposite sides of the rail line. But the agreement broke down the following month with the return of reinforced British forces.[40] Beyond its military-related death and destruction, the war caused economic distress through the disruption of farming, mining and other commercial activities. With the restoration of peace, rural-urban migration across the region surged with the long-term effect of lowering wages. In terms of public health, the conflict was associated with a regionwide rise in typhoid and measles.[41] It also coincided with popular alarm over the appearance of bubonic plague in Cape Town, resulting in vigorous containment measures along Bechuanaland's railway.[42]

DRIEDAG

At the end of 1914, the southern protectorate was briefly once again a war zone as Boer rebels passed through areas attempting to reach German South West Africa. Thereafter, up to 4,000 Protectorate Batswana enlisted in the South African auxiliary units were posted elsewhere. They included seventy-four Bakwena, led by the future Sebele II (reign 1918–1931), who served in France as part of South African Native Labour Contingent (SANLC).[43] Yet in local folk memory the 'Kaiser's War' is remembered less for its military tribulations than the die-off that accompanied its ending. By 25 November 1918, when the last German army surrendered at Mbale, Zambia, the whole of Southern Africa was already being convulsed by the twentieth century's most lethal pandemic – the 1918 H1N1 Influenza or 'Spanish Flu'. It is estimated that the influenza infected over a quarter of the world's population, with the figure of 50 million being commonly accepted as an estimate of its death toll.

In 1918, the influenza swept across globe in two waves. While hardly benign, its transmission between March and August 1918 was less lethal than what followed, with many thus believing that it did not pose an exceptional threat. However, in August 1918, a more virulent strain of the virus was detected whose advance was spearheaded by end of war troop movements. Both strains hit Southern Africa at almost the same time, with contrasting impacts. By the first week of September, the milder strain had landed in Durban, from where it expanded across Natal and the eastern Transvaal. For those in its path, this 'Eastern wave' was a relative blessing as the affected population proved to be resistant to the second, more deadly 'Western wave' that proliferated from Cape Town in mid-September, after being introduced by ships bringing home discharged SANLC troops.[44] Advancing along the rail lines in 'Black October' of 1918 the Western wave swept through eastern Botswana, along western South Africa, rapidly killing over 150,000 in the region. To many the influenza came to be known as 'driedag', Afrikaans for 'three days', which was said to be the time it took for the afflicted to either die or recover. In Botswana, stories are still told of passengers boarding trains, only to arrive at their destinations as corpses. With about half of its then approximately 6.7 million people afflicted, as well as a final death total of up to 500,000 by 1919, the Union of South Africa was among the world's most heavily hit jurisdictions.

Union death toll estimates, dovetail with Bechuanaland's 1918–1919 Annual Report, which noted: 'In October 1918, the disease known as Spanish Influenza broke out in the Southern Protectorate, and, spreading rapidly, eventually affected the whole Territory except the western Kalahari and the Ngami littoral; the native population suffered, more or less severely, in proportion as they were concentrated in large communities or scattered. The mortality, all round, amongst them, from the disease and its complications, has been estimated at between 4 and 5 per centum'. The estimate was in line with rough fatality figures totalling over 7,000 out of a population of some 150,000. Elsewhere, in the Cape Colony, the Khoikhoi faced a similar fate when smallpox epidemics and Dutch colonial policies had far-reaching consequences on the lives and overall health of the Khoikhoi, causing fear, resentment and mistrust of the Cape colonists (Viljoen in this volume).

In October 1918, the Protectorate's resident commissioner expressed his conviction that the ongoing tragedy should lead to the long sought-after break-up of the large royal settlements, adding 'this visitation has, however, afforded a painful object lesson which, it is hoped, will not be without its effect on Chiefs and people, and it will be my care to see that they at any rate understand it'.[45] Otherwise, beyond cancelling their war victory celebrations, the colonial regime's response to the pandemic was to let local communities fend for themselves. Batswana across the protectorate tried to stem the virus through movement restrictions and quarantines, while resorting to both indigenous and Western medicine. In the case of Kgatleng, traditional medicines were prepared, with Kgosi Linchwe I ascending Modipe Hill to gather vomit from its 'kgwanyape' (preternatural serpent). Thereafter, boys were dispatched across Kgatleng to 'doctor the boundaries', while movement between villages was temporarily banned.[46]

In April 1919, Kweneng's resident magistrate reported an 80% infection rate and 400 deaths in Molepolole. A sharp decline in agricultural output for the 1919–1920 season was attributed to labour shortages due to influenza. Although it was observed that 'there has been no recurrence of epidemic influenza' during 1920, in 1922 'influenza' was once more included among the prevalent diseases in district. A 1922 LMS report further claimed that the return of influenza had killed four out of five children in the mission school.[47] Annual reports for the period provide further evidence of the sporadic presence of influenza persisting elsewhere in the protectorate culminating in an upsurge in 1929: 'There was an epidemic of influenza throughout the country in October and November, Serowe and Gaberones being the most severely affected. Though 762 sought treatment from Government Medical Officers, this number is only a fraction of the total cases, as the greater proportion occurred in the native villages and were not brought to the notice of the doctors'.[48] Corresponding patterns of spiking influenza recurrence during the decade were also documented in Europe and the United States, as the virus morphed into a strain of seasonal flu.[49]

FAITH AND FITNESS

In the influenza's wake, public health in the protectorate also continued to suffer from additional diseases whose transmission was aggravated by labour migration. In 1920, the principal medical officer observed: 'The Bechuanas are, physically, not probably what they were in the old days. Contact with civilization has not benefitted them in this respect'.[50] Such perceptions fuelled deeper concern about the declining fitness of Batswana labour recruits.[51] While already present in the pre-colonial era, the prevalence of pneumonia, tuberculosis and syphilis as well as smallpox became endemic, with the latter reportedly afflicting 40% of the population by 1920.[52] In addition to venereal syphilis, Bechuanaland, especially in the Kgalagadi including western Kweneng, experienced high instances of non-sexually transmitted syphilis whose aetiology is unclear.[53]

Emerging health challenges coincided with demand for the limited medical services offered by the state and various missions, as well as traditional healers. The link between LMS missionaries and healing among the Bakwena can be traced back to David Livingstone and other pioneer medical missionaries, Batswana's acceptance of inoculation against smallpox being documented in 1862.[54] In Kweneng, the healing role of the church had been revived during the 1901–1914 tenure of Hayden Lewis who had received limited medical training.[55] By 1904, over 400 patients a month were being treated at his small dispensary. But this proved inadequate to meet the post-influenza demand for health services, which ultimately resulted in the LMS giving way to the medical missionaries of the Seventh Day Adventist Church in Kanye as well as the United Free Church of Scotland in Molepolole.[56]

Then as now, Batswana commonly combined indigenous with Western treatment, which the colonial state along with many missionaries perceived as an anathema: 'The Witchcraft and the influence of native medicine-men continue to play a very serious part in the lives of most of the native inhabitants and are responsible for much suffering. It is the aim of the Administration so to develop the Medical Service that these evil factors will be replaced by confidence in qualified medical men'.[57]

'THE WRONG PEOPLE RULE'

By 1920, the spiritual convictions of Kweneng's bible literate population had been shaken by the full gamut of 'God's punishments'. As a result, some were deepened in their Christian commitment, others embraced calls for reform, while others rejected the church and its associated colonial order altogether. In the temporal realm, although old social order seemingly remained intact, its authority was undermined by material losses. Kweneng's cattle population gradually increased after rinderpest, reaching 23,727 in 1921. But the great royal herds never returned, in contrast to those of the Bangwato and Batawana dikgosi to the north.[58] In 1932, Kgosi Sebele II had only 521 cattle, including 253 uninherited 'personal' cattle, which he claimed to have accumulated from his earnings at Johannesburg.[59] Loss of cattle by previously well-to-do Bakwena eroded the quasi-feudal system of patronage that tied junior to senior lineages through the distribution of loan cattle or 'mafisa'. In the upshot, the trend in Kweneng, along with neighbouring Gangwaketse, was towards a more diffuse, though by no means egalitarian, distribution of cattle, as migrants accumulated stock independent of their fathers and elder brothers.[60]

Declining circumstance among the traditional elite also diminished their material hold over former servants among Bakalagari and Kua in western Kweneng and the central Kgalagadi. Indeed, the inclusive nature of migrant labour within Kweneng is reflected in the fact that all levels of society, from former servants to royal family members, ultimately participated in it.[61] Examples of royalty and leading headmen spending much of their youth in outside employment are consistent with a pattern of elite inclusion found elsewhere in the Southern Protectorate.[62] Whereas Bakwena rulers had long drawn upon commoners in their kgotla as a political counterweight to their royal relatives, this balance shifted with the decline in the latter group's wealth. Some became vocal in their indignation over their loss of social and political status, for example, Motswakhumo Kgosidintsi before the resident commissioner in 1921: 'The son of our Chief (i.e. Sebele II ruling on behalf of his late father) respects the common people better than the elders. He is trying to replace them with common people – to drive them away. If the Bakwena meet, the common people alone agree with the Chief – not his relatives. This is a thing that makes me feel like a sick man. . . . We have no position among the Bakwena. The wrong people rule!'[63]

In 1929, one such 'wrong person' observed: 'I greet His Honour the Resident Commissioner and the Magistrate. I am glad today because we dogs now speak before His Honour. I am Sebele's dog. I stand up because of what Motswakhumo said. He speaks of Sechele I. How did he live with Sechele I? He used to make fire for him. No headman lived outside the kgotla then, they were Councillors. We do not know these Councillors of today, they only think of their money and do not make fire for the Chief'.[64]

Noble families in the outlying villages of Kweneng also experienced material decline accompanied by their participation in labour migration and a consequent loss of status. Among the Bahurutshe at Mmankgodi, Kgosi Letlole relinquished control of his village in July 1908 to the self-styled prophet Sentso Legong, who claimed that the overthrow of European oppression would come about if Batswana abandoned the white man's religion and culture. After setting fire to the village's Lutheran chapel, which had lost all but two of its members to his movement, he was apprehended by Sebele I.[65]

In Molepolole, calls for the restoration of pre-Christian practices subsequently found royal support when Sebele's successor, Kgosi Kealeboga Sechele II (reign 1911–1918), broke the LMS monopoly by embracing syncretic elements of the Anglican Church. In 1916, this new 'Chief's Church' gave its blessing to the Kgosi's decision, in face of LMS opposition, to revive traditional initiation school for boys (bogwera). As the sectarian division deepened, the rival denominations were led by two matriarchs, Sechele II's estranged senior wife Mohumagadi Phutego championing the LMS and his Anglican third wife Lena Rauwe. Other women also found a political platform as well as spiritual refuge in the churches. Given its financial obligations and literacy requirements, most female LMS members were originally drawn from the ranks of the relatively privileged, it being at the time observed that: 'all through Bechuanaland, membership in an LMS Church puts a touch of distinction upon even the best born in the community and add much to the strength of a political intriguer'.[66]

Unlike the male-only kgotla, in the congregational assemblies there was no gender barrier to voting status. With woman increasingly being left to manage domestic affairs due to male labour migration, other factors also contributed to the churches' feminine appeal. Their institutional stand in favour of monogamy and the fact that Christian 'white weddings' were legally recognized by the colonial civil courts were attractive. Another lure was the mission schools whose enrolment continued to be predominately female. The LMS headmistress of the Molepolole School from 1895 to 1918, Partridge, was notably committed to female empowerment: 'But Bechuana women, even the wives of Christians, have none of their proper place yet. The men have always been taught that they are far superior to women and they find it hard to part with the notion'.[67] Her feminist vision was shared by some of her male colleagues, including Lloyd:

> The women too are finding their feet, and are not ready to be imposed upon, or disposed of. One feels that the seeds are in the hearts of the women, which, when matured, will bring forth a harvest which will astonish the men. We do not hear yet of the 'Suffragette', but come she will, and the men will find her a very terror when she arrives . . . 'the peculiarities of the feminine mid' are likely, through the slow working of evolution, to cause Bechuana men considerable astonishment, and they will deserve it. I am on the side of the women.[68]

In 1922, the resurgence of influenza along with crop failure, low cattle prices and 'the unfortunate Joburg revolution which threw hundreds of young men out of employment and cut off their only means of earning money for food for their starving people' were together linked to Kgosi Sebele II's decision to finally submit himself for initiation. After several months of seclusion at Botlhapatlou, he re-emerged with a new regiment 'Malatakgosi' ('those who follow the chief') as well as the now initiated members of his own SANLC veteran-led 'Mathubantwa' (those who break up the battle). Thereafter, he became a staunch champion of both male and, unlike his father, female initiation (*bojale*). When Molepolole's Anglican Church, now under the supervision of a white missionary, closed ranks with the LMS to oppose the practice, Sebele announced that in his eyes the white man's church no longer existed since it opposed Bakwena law and custom.[69]

Developments in Kweneng were paralleled elsewhere. Among the Bakgatla-baga-Mmanaana at Moshupa the influenza-related death of Kgosi

Kgabophuti was followed by the revival of the schools under his successor, Kgosi Gobuamang, which also attracted candidates from Kanye. Gobuamang further aligned himself with the previously banned African-led church movement of Mothowagae Mothohelwe, which supplanted the LMS in his village.

In the face of these developments, the LMS lamented that: 'At Kanye as at Molepolole there has been a revival of heathenism." The forward movement chronicled in 1921 report was met by a 'counter move in 1922 from the Powers of Darkness'. Thereafter, the LMS sponsored the formation of Christian Boy's and Girl's Life Brigade Companies, while banning initiates from their congregations.[70] When in 1923, the missionaries further tried to prevent initiates from attending their schools, Sebele II retaliated by taking control of the school board.[71] This 'nationalization' of education was accompanied by further initiatives to increase royal regulatory control over local commerce and natural resources.[72]

Throughout the 1920s, Sebele II clashed with colonial officials as well as missionaries and his disaffected royal relatives, while Molepolole emerged as a place where Gauteng jazz and smuggled booze mixed with pre-Christian customs.[73] In response, malcontents encouraged to draw up petitions for the creation of Tribal Councils that would be more amenable to colonial control. But these efforts failed in the face of the Kgosi's staunch support among male commoners. At the end of the decade, the British authorities were increasingly concerned about Sebele's influence with his peers in other reserves, as well as the increasingly militant majority of his subjects. Using thin allegations of forced recruitment into initiation school as an excuse, in 1931, they detained him without charge and removed him to Ghanzi, where he died as a political prisoner in 1939. His banishment proved to be a political turning point. Today, chieftainship survives among the Bakwena. But as Rangwadi had prophesied after the great Sechele's death within hours of his great-grandson Sebele II's birth, the pre-colonial Bakwena kingdom had been broken, having been brought down by the hidden hand of pathogens, as well as heavy handed imperial overrule.

CONCLUSION

It is likely that even in the absence of the series of diseases and ecological disasters that afflicted Kweneng from 1890, the area would still have been incorporated into Southern Africa's twentieth-century archipelago rural labour reserves, but with less trauma and a different time frame. As it was, the accelerated near collapse of the pre-colonial social order has left an enduring legacy. Kweneng's pathogenic descent into economic underdevelopment and resulting dependency is a case study in how 'acts of God' can facilitate a radical reset in socio-economic and political power.

NOTES

1. While the extent of literature on labour migration in Botswana practically defies citation, the classic study remains. Isaac Schapera's *Migrant Labour and Tribal Life, a Study of Conditions in the Bechuanaland Protectorate* (London: Oxford University Press, 1947). Early labour migration from Kweneng previously explored in J. Ramsay, "The Rise and Fall of the Bakwena Dynasty of South-Central Botswana, 1820-1940" (PhD diss., Boston University, 1991), 250-264. Also W. Duggan, "The Kweneng in the Colonial Era: A Brief Economic History" *Botswana Notes and Records,* Vol. 9 (1977): 41–48 and M. Leepile, "The Impact of Migrant Labour on the Economy of Kweneng 1940-1980" *Botswana Notes and Records*, Vol. 13 (1981): 33–43, which focus on the period from 1940 in the context of Native Recruitment Corporation statistics.

2. R.K.K. Molefi, *A Medical History of Botswana, 1885–1966* (Gaborone: Botswana Society,1996); also "Of rats, fleas, and peoples: towards a history of bubonic plague in southern Africa, 1890–1950" *Pula: Botswana Journal of African Studies* Vol. 15, no. 2 (2001): 259–267 and "Smallpox and History: The Example of Botswana, 1930–1964" *Pula* Vol. 17 (2003): 20–36. S. Khupe, *An Uneasy Walk to Quality: a history of the evolution of Black Nursing education in the Republic of Botswana* (Marceline: Walsworth, 1993). P. Landau, "Explaining Surgical Evangelism in Colonial Southern Africa: Teeth, Pain and Faith", *The Journal of African History,* Vol. 37, no. 2 (1996): 261–281.

3. R.S. Viljoen, "Disease and Society: VOC Cape Town, its people and smallpox epidemics of 1713, 1755 and 1767" *Kleio,* Vol. 27 (1995): 22–45. C. van Onselen, "Reactions to Rinderpest in Southern Africa 1896–97" *The Journal of African History*, Vol. 13, no. 3 (1972), 473–48.

4. H. Phillips, *Epidemics: The Story of South Africa's Five Most Lethal Human Diseases* (Ohio University Press, 2012), 9. Also H. Phillips, *Black October: The Impact of the Spanish Influenza Epidemic of 1918 on South Africa* (PhD diss., University of Cape Town, 1990): https://open.uct.ac.za/handle/11427/7852.

5. Ramsay, "The Rise and Fall of the Bakwena Dynasty," pp. 50–166. J. Ramsay, B. Morton and T. Mgadla, *Building a Nation: A History of Botswana from 1800 to 1910* (Gaborone, Longman, 1996).

6. Public Records Office – Colonial Office (UK) (PRO CO) 879/14/162 Sechele to Lanyon, March 24, 1877. London Missionary Society papers (LMS) in Council of World Mission Archive at School of Oriental and African Studies, London – "Annual report for Molepolole 1872".

7. Willoughby Papers at Shelly Oaks (WCW/SO) File 739 – Kgabo aTebele manuscript. Botswana National Archives (BNA) PP1/1/10 Kwadira Lesele.

8. J. Ramsay, "The Establishment and Consolidation of the Bechuanaland Protectorate" in W. Edge & M. Lekorwe, eds. *Botswana Politics and Society* (Pretoria: Van Schaik, 1998), 62–98.

9. *Annual Report of the Colonies. Bechuanaland 1892–93*: Proclamation of October 4, 1892.

10. P.T. Mgadla & S.C. Volz, eds. *Words of Batswana, Letters to Mahoko a Becwana* (Cape Town: Van Riebeeck, 2006), 249–55.

11. William C. Scholtz, M.D., "The Influenza Epidemic at the Cape" *British Medical Journal* (March 15, 1890). Local Government board Reports – "Report on the Influenza Epidemic of 1889–90" Local Government Board (1891). 33. "Further Report and Papers on Epidemic Influenza, 1889–92" (1893), 38.

12. *British Bechuanaland Annual Reports for 1894–95.* Cited Bechuanaland Annual Reports are available online Digital Content Creation Unit University of Illinois at Urbana-Champaign.

13. LMS H. Williams March 27, 1896.

14. LMS H. Williams May 15, 1896.

15. *Diamond Fields Advertiser* (Kimberly) November 7, 1896. Also, WCW/SO Willoughby to Harry, June 3, 1896. Lugard Papers, Rhodes House, Oxford: Ngamiland Expedition Private Diaries, May-June 1896.

16. *British Bechuanaland, Annual Report 1896–97.* LMS correspondence by Willoughby April 21 and June 29, 1896, Wookey, April 28 and September 18, 1896 and Good September 24,1896.

17. LMS H. Williams October 12, 1896. *Diamond Fields Advertiser*, November 7, 1896, letter by John Brown.

18. LMS E. Lloyd, September 15, 1896; H. Williams May 5, 1896.

19. LMS M. Partridge, November 27, 1896.

20. LMS H. Williams "Annual Report Molepolole, 1896"

21. PRO CO879/46/515 Secretary of State (SS) to High Commissioner (HC), April 16 1896 and HC. SS May 5, 1896. *Bechuanaland Annual Report 1896–97.*

22. LMS H. Williams October 12, 1896.

23. LMS Sebele to H. Williams, July 31, 1896. Also, PRO 879/46/515 Newton to Robinson, October 24, 1896. Annual report of the London Missionary Society (1897) showing £604 raised by Bechuanaland Relief Fund.

24. LMS Wookey December 29, 1898, also September 11, 29 and November 10, 24 1898, Lloyd September 17, 1897, September 22, 1898.

25. LMS H. Williams June 6 and June 27, 1898. Wookey September 11, and 29, 1898, which speak of many deaths in Molepolole. LMS "Annual Report for Kanye, 1898."

26. A. Murray and N. Parsons, "The Modern Economic History of Botswana," in *Studies in the Economic History of Southern Africa*, Vol. 1, The Front-line States, Z.A. Konczacki, J. Parpat and T. M. Shaw eds. (London, Frank Cass, 1990), see also B. N. Ngwenya, "The Development of Transport Infrastructure in the Bechuanaland Protectorate, 1885–1966," *Botswana Notes and Records*, Vol. 16 (January, 1984): 73–84. 58; B. Mocheregwa, *Underdevelopment in Eastern Bechuanaland: The Dynamic Role of The Mafikeng – Bulawayo Railway, from The Late 1800s to 1960s* (MA diss. Trent University, 2016).

27. *British Bechuanaland Annual Report 1896–97.*

28. National Archives of Zimbabwe, Jules Ellenberger Diary, September 15, 1898. BNA SOC Sebele to Poultney, June 30 and September 15, 1908; to the Manger of the Golden Reef Company, July 23, 1908, to Manager of Jumpers Reef Mine, September 15, 1908. BNA DC Molepolole 2/9 Annual report, 1927, which observed the

necessity of the practice given the "comparatively large number of Bakwena residing there in in various employments."

29. D. Massey, "Labour Migration and Rural Development in Botswana" (PhD diss., Boston University, 1981), 70.

30. PRO CO 879/44/498: Khama, Sebele and Bathoen to Colonial Office, September 24, 1895.

31. PRO 879/52/552 Surmon to Goold-Adams, April 21, 1899.

32. Bechuanaland Proclamation No. 7 of 1909: https://botswanalaws.com/Bechuanaland/Subsidiary/1890-1929/PROCLAMATION,%20NO.%207%20OF%201909.pdf.

33. BNA Molepolole annual reports, 1919–29: report for 1923–24, dated March 8, 1925.

34. W.J. Clissold, unpublished 1926 manuscript at St. Paul's Church, Molepolole (Clissold MS), p. 80. The reverend further observed that the Kimberly mines, which did not directly recruit labour, were preferred by Bakwena than those in the Reef.

35. BNA 2DC Mol/13, Criminal Record Book 1918–37.

36. The Cape Vagrancy Acts, which were applied in the protectorate, gave local officials the power to arrest those who were deemed "idle and disorderly persons." BNA BNB 979 M. Williams: "Applicability of the Cape Acts under the Order-in-Council of June 10, 1891," confirmed by the Order-in-council of the General law Proclamation of 1909. BNA S 47/3 "Forced Labour" Resident Commissioner (RC) to HC August 1926 further cites Cape Vagrancy act no. 23 of 1879 and 27 of 1886 to procure labour.

37. BNA S 25/3 "Hut Tax, 1916–28" Financial Secretary to Acting Government Secretary July 17, 1916.

38. "British South Africa, Annual statement of trade and shipping in the Colonies and Territories of the South African Customs Union, 1906–10". Bechuanaland Annual Reports for 1906–07, 1907–08.

39. PRO CO 879/53/552 "Extract from Diary kept in Assistant Commissioners Office Gaberones, August 5, 1897." The colonial authorities were initially suspicious that Bathoen and Sebele had been in friendly contact with the insurrectionist: HC to SS August 10, 1997 w/enclosures. LMS Howard Williams September 2, 1897.

40. LMS Wookey, November 28, 1899 and May 6, 1900; Lloyd December 4, 1899. D. Will & T. Dent "The Boer War as seen from Gaborone" *Botswana Notes and Records*, Vol.4, (1972): 195–209.

41. D. Lowbeer et.al. "Disease and Death in the South African War: Changing Disease Patterns from Soldiers to Refugees" *Social History of Medicine*, Vol. 17, Issue 2, (August 2004): 223–245. For post-war assessment BNA BNB 3240 Donald Mackenzie Macrae "The Bechuanaland Protectorate, Its People and Prevalent Diseases with a Special Consideration of the effects of Tropical Residence and Food in Relation to Health and Disease."

42. R.K.K. Molefi (2001), 260–61.

43. BNA RC 1/29, DCMol 4/11. M.O.M. Seboni *Sebele II* (Pretoria: Van Schaik, 1956).

44. H. Phillips *Epidemics: The Story of South Africa's Five Most Lethal Human Diseases*, 68–93.

45. *Bechuanaland Annual Report for 1918–19*, October 23, 1918 correspondence by James Comyn Macgregor.

46. J. V. Spears "An Epidemic among the Bakgatla: The Influenza of 1918" *Botswana Notes and Records*, Vol. 11, (Botswana Society, 1979): 69–76.

47. BNA DCMol 2/9 Annual Reports 1919–1929. LMS Report for Molepolole 1922, which contrasts with the District Report that "the influenza outbreaks were mild and of the ordinary catarrhal type; most of the cases recovering after a week or ten days."

48. BNA DCMol 2/9 – Annual Report 1929.

49. S. Collins "The Influenza Epidemic of 1928–1929 with Comparative Data for 1918–1919" in *American Journal of Public Health*, Vol XX, no. 2 (1930): 119–29. W. Nicol "Influenza in Relation to the City of Birmingham" *Postgraduate Medical Journal* (1963): 604–10. J. Taubenberger "Influenza: The Once and Future Pandemic" *Public Health Reports*, Supplement 3, Vol. 125, 2010:16–26.

50. BNA BNB 3240 Macrae, 4.

51. J. Livingstone, "Physical Fitness and Economic Opportunity in the Bechuanaland Protectorate in the 1930s and 1940s" *Journal of Southern African Studies*, Vol. 27, no. 4 (2001): 793–811.

52. BNA BNB 3240 Macrae, p. 40. This figure was echoed in the Medical Report for 1930, which observed that "nearly 40 per cent of the work of the Medical Department at the Dispensaries once more being reported as dealing with syphilitics."

53. J.H. Murray et al., "Endemic Syphilis in The Bakwena Reserve of The Bechuanaland Protectorate: A Report on Mass Examination and Treatment" *Bulletin of the World Health Organisation*, no. 15 (1956): 975–1039. Alfred Merriweather *The Desert Doctor Remembers* (Gaborone: Pula Press, 1999), 172–86.

54. J. Mackenzie, *Ten Years North of the Orange River* (Edinburgh: Edmonston and Douglas, 1871), 251–253.

55. A. Digby, *Diversity and Division in Medicine: Health Care in South Africa from the 1800s* (Bern: Peter Lang AG, 2006), 10; P. Landau, "Explaining Surgical Evangelism": 261–281; H. Lewis "Medicine in Molepolole" *Chronical of the London Mission Society* (1906): 183.

56. P.M. Shepard, *Molepolole, A Missionary Record* (Edinburgh: United Free Church of Scotland, 1947).

57. *Annual Report for Bechuanaland Protectorate, 1930*, 23.

58. BNA DCMOL 2/30: According to the 1921 census, Bangwato cattle then numbered 180,608, Batawana 103,989, Bangwaketse 16,866 and Bakgatla-bagakgafela 33,731, the latter can be attributed to their restocking during the 1899–1902 Boer War.

59. BNA S 225/8, Acting Resident Magistrate to Government Secretary May 21, 1932. BNA DCMol 2/31-32 and DCMol 2/2.

60. A. Pim, *Financial and Economic Position of the Bechuanaland Protectorate* (London: HMSO, 1933), 25–27, which found that between 1914 and 1933 the stockholdings of larger owners had declined by some 50% while the total number of cattle had remained the same.

61. Material circumstance of royal lineages in Ramsay, "The Rise and Fall of the Bakwena Dynasty," 264–273.

62. Schapera, *Migrant Labour and Tribal Life*, 42 noted such inclusion among the Bakgatla, Balete and Batlokwa, as well as Bakwena, while stating that in Gangwaketse, along with Gamangwato and Ngamiland "hardly any prominent members of the ruling dynasty have been abroad to work." Sebele II had worked for five years as a clerk at the Rand mines.

63. BNA BNB 233 "Minutes of the Native Advisory Council, March 21–22, 1921".

64. BNA S 23/6/2 "Minutes of meeting held in Chief's kgotla, Molepolole, November 18–19, 1929".

65. H. Lewis, "Sencho, the Mad Prophet" in *Chronicle of the London Missionary Society* (April 1913), 91–92. BNA SOC June-August, 1908. BNA DC Molepolole 5/11. Interview with Kobedi Seribe August 5, 1985. Instability in Mmankgodi persisted under Letlòle's successor Kgosi Maenga II (1922–1928).

66. WCW/SO 382. For broader discussion of role of women missionaries, see T. Mgadla Missionary wives, women and education: the development of literacy among the Batswana 1840–1937 @https://ubrisa.ub. bw/handle/10311/475

67. Mary Partridge, "Bechuana Women" *The Chronicle of the London Missionary Society* (January 1903), 37–38.

68. LMS E. Lloyd, September 21, 1913, 266.

69. Clissold MS, p. 14. LMS Burns, June 8, 1925.

70. *Bechuanaland Report of the London Missionary Society for the year ending March 31, 1923*, p 81. Also, LMS Papers at Moedeng College, Otse: Burns to Hail, November 21, 1924 and Report by Violet Taylor on "Woman's Work" 1929. BNA DCMol 3/2, S 361/1/1.

71. BNA S 598 "Bakwena School Committee."

72. Sebele II's rule and downfall in Ramsay (1991), 318–393. Also F. Morton & J. Ramsay, eds., *Birth of Botswana a History of the Bechuanaland Protectorate 1910–1966* (Gaborone: Longman, 1988), 30–44.

73. Sebele II was, himself, a performer as well as consumer of jazz and marabi. At the time, blacks in Botswana were prohibited from buying imported alcohol, but Sebele worked with local traders to frustrate the ban.

BIBLIOGRAPHY

Primary Sources

Archives

Botswana Laws online digital archive https://botswanalaws.com/

Botswana National Archives (BNA) Gaborone, Botswana. Correspondence Secretary of State for Colonies, (SOC), High Commissioner (HC), Resident Commissioner (RC), Secretariat (S)-1932; District Commissioner Molepolole (DCMOL) 1919-37; Private Papers (PP) Isaac Schapera.

BNB (Library, special holdings).
Bechuanaland Annual Reports 1890–1930 [also available online through University of Illinois Urbana-Champaign Digital Library https://libsysdigi.library.illinois.edu/
London Missionary Society papers (LMS) in Council of World Mission Archive at School of Oriental and African Studies, London: Southern Africa In and Out correspondence, annual reports Southern Africa 1872-30.
LMS Papers at Moedeng College, Otse, Botswana various correspondence.
Lugard Papers, Rhodes House, Oxford: Ngamiland Expedition Private Diaries, May-June 1896.
National Archives of Zimbabwe: Jules Ellenberger Diary.
Papers of Prof. William Charles Willoughby, Shelly Oak Colleges (WCW/SO) Library, Birmingham, UK.
Public Records Office (PRO), Kew Gardens, London, UK: Colonial Office (CO) Confidential Print series 879 1877-97.
St. Paul's Church, Molepolole, Unpublished and incomplete 1926 manuscript by Rev. W.J. Clissold on life among the Bakwena.

BOOKS AND ARTICLES

Lewis, Hayden. "Medicine in Molepolole". *Chronicle of the London Mission Society* (1906): 183.
Lewis, Hayden. "Sencho, the Mad Prophet". *Chronicle of the London Missionary Society* (April 1913): 91–92.
Partridge, Mary. "Bechuana Women". *The Chronicle of the London Missionary Society* (January 1903): 37–38.
Mackenzie, John. *Ten Years North of the Orange River*. Edinburgh: Edmonston and Douglas, 1871.
Pim, Allan. *Financial and Economic Position of the Bechuanaland Protectorate*. London: HMSO, 1933.

Secondary Sources

BOOKS, ARTICLES

Collins, Selwyn. "The Influenza Epidemic of 1928–1929 with Comparative Data for 1918–1919". *American Journal of Public Health*, Vol. 20, no. 2 (1930): 119–29.
Diamond Fields Advertiser (Kimberly) November 7, 1896.
Digby, Ann. *Diversity and Division in Medicine: Health Care in South Africa from the 1800s*. Bern: Peter Lang AG, 2006.
Duggan, William. "The Kweneng in the Colonial Era: A Brief Economic History". *Botswana Notes and Records*, Vol. 9 (1977): 41–48.
Khupe, Serara. *An Uneasy Walk to Quality: A History of the Evolution of Black Nursing Education in the Republic of Botswana*. Marceline: Walsworth, 1993.
Landau, Paul. "Explaining Surgical Evangelism in Colonial Southern Africa: Teeth, Pain and Faith". *The Journal of African History*, Vol. 37, no. 2 (1996): 261–81.
Leepile, Methaetsile. "The Impact of Migrant Labour on the Economy of Kweneng 1940–1980". *Botswana Notes and Records*, Vol. 13 (1981): 33–43.

Livingstone, Julie. "Physical Fitness and Economic Opportunity in the Bechuanaland Protectorate in the 1930s and 1940s". *Journal of Southern African Studies*, Vol. 27, no. 4 (2001): 793–811.

Low-Beer, Daniel, et al. "Disease and Death in the South African War: Changing Disease Patterns from Soldiers to Refugees". *Social History of Medicine*, Vol. 17, no. 2 (August 2004): 223–45.

Macrae, Donald Mackenzie. "The Bechuanaland Protectorate, Its People and Prevalent Diseases with a Special Consideration of the effects of Tropical Residence and Food in Relation to Health and Disease". MD diss., University of Edinburgh 1920.

Massey, David. "Labour Migration and Rural Development in Botswana". PhD diss., Boston University, 1981.

Merriweather, Alfred. *The Desert Doctor Remembers*. Gaborone: Pula Press, 1999.

Mgadla, Themba. "Missionary Wives, Women and Education: The Development of Literacy among the Batswana 1840–1937". https://ubrisa .ub. bw/handle/10311/475.

Mgadla, Themba (P. T.), and Steven Volz, eds. *Words of Batswana, Letters to Mahoko a Becwana*. Cape Town: Van Riebeeck Society, 2006.

Mocheregwa, Bafumiki. "Underdevelopment in Eastern Bechuanaland: The Dynamic Role of the Mafikeng—Bulawayo Railway, from the Late 1800s to 1960s". MA diss., Trent University, 2016.

Molefi, Rodgers (R. K. K.). *A Medical History of Botswana, 1885–1966*. Gaborone: Botswana Society, 1996.

Molefi, R. K. K. "Of Rats, Fleas, and Peoples: Towards a History of Bubonic Plague in Southern Africa, 1890–1950". *Pula: Botswana Journal of African Studies*, Vol. 15, no. 2 (2001): 259–67.

Molefi, R. K. K. "Smallpox and History: The Example of Botswana, 1930–1964". *Pula*, Vol. 17 (2003): 20–36.

Morton, Fred, and Jeff Ramsay, eds. *Birth of Botswana a History of the Bechuanaland Protectorate 1910–1966*. Gaborone: Longman, 1988.

Murray, Andrew, and Neil Parsons. "The Modern Economic History of Botswana". In *Studies in the Economic History of Southern Africa*, Vol. 1, The Front-line States, Z. A. Konczacki, J. Parpat, and T. M. Shaw, eds. London: Frank Cass, 1990.

Murray, John, et al. "Endemic Syphilis in The Bakwena Reserve of The Bechuanaland Protectorate: A Report on Mass Examination and Treatment". *Bulletin of the World Health Organisation*, no. 15 (1956): 975–1039.

Ngwenya, Barbara. "The Development of Transport Infrastructure in the Bechuanaland Protectorate, 1885–1966". *Botswana Notes and Records*, Vol. 16 (January 1984).

Nicol, W. "Influenza in Relation to the City of Birmingham". *Postgraduate Medical Journal* (1963). https://pmj.bmj.com›postgradmedj›605.full.pdf.

Onselen, Charles van. "Reactions to Rinderpest in Southern Africa 1896–97". *The Journal of African History*, Vol. 13, no. 3 (1972): 473–48.

Phillips, Howard. *Epidemics: The Story of South Africa's Five Most Lethal Human Diseases*. Ohio University Press, 2012.

Phillips, Howard. "Black October: The Impact of the Spanish Influenza Epidemic of 1918 on South Africa." PhD diss., University of Cape Town, 1990. https://open.uct.ac.za/handle/11427/7852.

Ramsay, Jeff. "The Establishment and Consolidation of the Bechuanaland Protectorate". In W. Edge and M. Lekorwe, eds., *Botswana Politics and Society*, 62–98. Pretoria: Van Schaik, 1998.

Ramsay, Jeff. "The Rise and Fall of the Bakwena Dynasty of South-Central Botswana, 1820–1940". PhD diss., Boston University, 1991.

Ramsay, Jeff, Barry Morton, and Themba Mgadla. *Building a Nation: A History of Botswana from 1800 to 1910*. Gaborone: Longman, 1996.

Schapera, Isaac. *Migrant Labour and Tribal Life, a Study of Conditions in the Bechuanaland Protectorate*. London: Oxford University Press, 1947.

Scholtz, William C. "The Influenza Epidemic at the Cape". *British Medical Journal* (March 15, 1890).

Seboni, Michael (M. O. M.). *Sebele II*. Pretoria: Van Schaik, 1956.

Spears, John. "An Epidemic among the Bakgatla: The Influenza of 1918". *Botswana Notes and Records*, Vol. 11, Botswana Society (1979): 69–76.

Shepard, Peter. *Molepolole, a Missionary Record*. Edinburgh: United Free Church of Scotland, 1947.

Taubenberger, Jeffery. "Influenza: The Once and Future Pandemic". *Public Health Reports*, Supplement 3, Vol. 125 (2010): 16–26.

Viljoen, Russel. "Disease and Society: VOC Cape Town, Its People and Smallpox Epidemics of 1713, 1755 and 1767". *Kleio*, Vol. 27 (1995): 22–45.

Will, Denzil, and Tommy Dent. "The Boer War as Seen from Gaborone". *Botswana Notes and Records*, Vol. 4 (1972): 195–209.

Chapter 9

Colonialism, Epidemics and the Indian Experience (ca. 1817–1920)

Saurav Kumar Rai

Colonialism and spread of diseases shared an integral link. Out of various other things that were exchanged between the metropole and the colonies, exchange of diseases was the most devastating one.[1] Not only new diseases were introduced in the lands which were hitherto unexposed to them, the scale of spread of a particular disease was heightened in an unprecedented manner in the era of colonialism. It would not be an exaggeration to say that colonialism provided wings to the spread of diseases. Firstly, the colonial mobility imparted swiftness to the spread of many epidemic diseases thereby turning them into pandemics.[2] Secondly, owing to the colonial interconnectedness of different regions and continents of the world, diseases which were hitherto endemic to a particular region started finding new terrains for their spread.[3] Thus, colonialism not only raised the status of erstwhile endemic diseases to the level of epidemics, but it also broadened the horizon of epidemics transforming them into pandemics. It is in this context that a medical historian goes on to characterize colonialism as 'literally a health hazard'.[4] Commenting further on this linkage between colonialism and spread of diseases, Ira Klein argues, 'western intrusion unleashed a disease holocaust on other peoples, which probably reduced their numbers by half'.[5]

The aforesaid transforming capacity of colonialism was best epitomized through outbreak of various epidemics in colonial India between 1817 and 1920. The present chapter would analyse various dimensions of this interconnectedness of colonialism and epidemics in India by looking into cholera outbreaks of first half of nineteenth century, bubonic plague outbreak of 1890s and Spanish influenza epidemic of 1918–1920 in India. One interesting aspect which emerges out of this analysis is that the Indian experience of epidemic diseases had far-reaching impact on formulation of public health policies of not only British India but also that of the metropole.

Further, a cursory glance through the literary works revolving around the aforesaid epidemics as discussed in this chapter brings out the socio-emotional quotient of these historical experiences. Although here there are chances of anachronistic trap as most of these literary pieces were written not during the epidemic but in its aftermath, in some cases even a few decades after the actual epidemic moment. However, this temporal distance between the events under analysis and their much later revisiting in literature does not make these literary pieces historiographically less significant. This is largely because epidemics often create rolling stones of memories passed from one generation to other in the form of lived realities. Also, in many cases, the litterateurs such as Master Bhagwan Das and Suryakant Tripathi 'Nirala' had personally experienced in their lifetime the moments of described epidemics. It makes their literary representation of epidemics more authentic and significant.

CHOLERA PANDEMIC AND THE EMERGENCE OF 'SANITARY REGIMES'

The havoc created by the cholera pandemic in nineteenth century earned much notoriety for the tropics. It played an important role in conceptualization of the tropics as the 'diseased other'.[6] However, research shows that earlier cholera was by and large endemic to the lower Ganga valley.[7] It was through networks of colonial mobility that the outbreak of cholera was raised to epidemic proportion. In fact, there were occasional outbreaks of cholera from 1761 to 1781 through pilgrims who carried it to different places. Nevertheless, it remained confined to eastern India only. In the nineteenth century for the first time it was under the aegis of the British colonialism that cholera not only stepped out of the lower Ganga valley, but also crossed the geographical boundaries of the Indian subcontinent.[8] Here, as David Arnold remarks, the spread of cholera was widely identified with the British occupation of India and was absorbed within a broader 'trauma of conquest'.[9]

Beginning from 1817, the whole world witnessed several waves of cholera pandemic, all of them invariably starting from India, in quick succession. The first wave began from Jessore where it broke out in August 1817. It soon spread to major cities of the Bengal Presidency sparing only the elevated regions of Oudh and Rohilkhand.[10] In the coming few years through colonial trade routes it dispersed from the Indian subcontinent to Southeast Asia, West Asia, Europe and East Africa. This first wave of cholera pandemic is believed to have lingered till 1824 providing only a brief intermittent relief before the beginning of the second wave in 1826. The second wave of cholera pandemic which lasted from 1826 to 1837 moved further to take even the North

American continent within its sphere of influence. After almost a decade, the third wave started in 1846 which persisted even longer till around 1860. The third wave of cholera pandemic engulfed North Africa and the South American continent as well.[11] This was followed by a few other waves of cholera pandemic in the second half of nineteenth and early twentieth century. In fact, as Ira Klein shows that with the introduction of modern transport and railways the instances of cholera outbreak went on increasing in the Indian subcontinent in the second half of the nineteenth century. Explaining this crucial linkage between modern means of transport and spread of cholera, Klein states:

> Modern transport multiplied domestic commerce and labour mobility and even social or religious travel, and people often staggered down dusty roads when rains failed, to seek succour from starvation in towns or on relief works. India's vast human mobility and commerce brought the disease bacillus in profusion to new locales, where it often found circumstances propitious for its acculturation.[12]

Nevertheless, the third wave of cholera pandemic (1846–1860) in England eventually prompted the passage of the landmark Nuisances Removal and Diseases Prevention Act by the British parliament in 1846. This Act was designed as a temporary legislation to restrict the spread of cholera. It increased the powers of the Privy Council to make regulations to prevent the spread of infectious disease. Simultaneously, the Sewerage and Drainage of Liverpool Act was also passed in 1846 which provisioned for the appointment of a medical officer of health to inspect and report on the sanitary state of the area and point out 'nuisances' that might contribute to disease. These Acts were updated alongside the introduction of Public Health Act in 1848. These Acts led to the creation of a General Board of Health with powers to initiate and assist local sanitary reform projects. It consisted of Lord Morpeth, Lord Ashley and Edwin Chadwick. It was Ashley and Chadwick who together with the medical inspectors Grainger and Sutherland did most of the works to restrict the spread of cholera in England.[13]

Actually, the frequent outbreak of cholera pandemic wreaked havoc in the industrial cities of England, such as Liverpool, especially in the areas inhabited by the mill workers.[14] This was largely due to poor sanitary conditions of the working-class quarters. This, in turn, affected production thereby posing serious economic challenges in front of the English state. The matter soon caught attention of the legislators. Speaking on the epidemiology of sanitation, Lord Morpeth, quoting Dr Thomas Southwood Smith, in the British parliament on 30 March 1847, stated that 'if you trace down the fever districts on a map, and then compare that map with the map of the commissioners of sewers, you will find that wherever the commissioners of sewers have not been, there fever is prevalent; and, on the contrary, wherever they have been, there fever is comparatively absent'.[15]

This concern regarding the linkage between the spread of disease and poor sanitary condition overlapped with the growing consciousness in England regarding the relation between economy of the country and health of its citizens. The central figure in promoting the latter consciousness was Edwin Chadwick who also happened to be one of the chief architects of 1834 Poor Laws. Chadwick made an economic argument in his 1842 text *The Sanitary Condition of the Labouring Population of Great Britain* that much poor relief was given to the families of men who had died from infectious diseases due to poor sanitary conditions. Hence, he claimed that money spent on improving public health was therefore cost effective, as it would save money in the long term. Proper sanitary measures could also be the key to 'a contented, healthy and docile working class' – something which the state was looking for in the era studded with frequent revolutions.[16] In such an atmosphere, the outbreak of third wave of cholera pandemic provided opportune moment for passage of the above acts which, in turn, precipitated a new era of 'sanitary regime' in England where the state became extra sensitive and interventionist in matters related to health and sanitation.

The aforesaid 'sanitary regime' was introduced in India as well following the transfer of powers from the East India Company to the British crown in the aftermath of the 1857 uprisings.[17] The colonial sanitary regime in India introduced far-reaching changes in the city landscape having lasting impact on the Indian populace, on their lifestyle and on their dwelling places.[18] However, one significant question to ask here is 'What was colonial about colonial sanitary regime?' The answer lies in the tremendous stereotyping which was carried out regarding the sanitary habits, cleanliness and dwelling places of the Indians in the post-1857 period which, in turn, paved the way for racial division of space as well. It was most visible in the case of transformation of cities like Lucknow (the capital of Oudh province) and the colonial arguments accompanying this transformation.[19]

Incidentally, knowledge about exact reason and cure for cholera was still primitive in nineteenth century. However, the disciples of miasmatic theory firmly argued in favour of relationship between poor sanitary conditions and outbreak of cholera. Once this relationship was established, habitual disregard for sanitation by the 'native' population appeared as the most potent colonial explanation behind frequent outbreak of cholera in the Indian subcontinent.

Noticeable in this regard are the remarks and comments made by the colonial officials and reports. As for instance, the *Report of the Royal Commission on the Health of the Anglo India Army* in 1863 stated that 'habits of the natives are such that, unless they are very closely watched, they cover the whole neighbouring surface with filth'. It further argued that 'there is no such thing as subsoil drainage. . . . Neither latrines nor urinals are drained. For all purposes to which drainage is applied in this country, as a means of preserving health, *it is unknown in India*'.[20] In this connection, Dr Bonavia, the civil surgeon at Lucknow, identified numerous 'filthy depots' that dotted the cityscape and were referred to as 'a disgrace to civilization'.[21] These 'filthy depots' were seen as perfect breeding ground for diseases like cholera and were to be removed at the earliest. Bonavia also envisioned a citywide revolution in the Lucknow latrine system as the old ones were seen as 'stinking filthy holes'. These efforts completely transformed the city landscape as old structures were demolished in the name of decongesting the lungs of the city, building of new drainage system and public utilities.

At the same time the aforesaid notions regarding the sanitary habits of the Indians promoted the post-1857 phenomenon of racial division of space in order to provide a 'healthier' and 'safer' living place for the Europeans. In fact, it provided a kind of pseudoscientific sanctity for strategically planned racial division of space. The carving out of civil lines in most of the old cities manifested this twin ambition of providing 'safe' and 'clean' dwelling space to the Europeans. There were stances of forcible removal of 'native' villages and hamlets from within and around civil lines and cantonments 'to preserve the health and life of the remaining and more important section of the community'.[22] The uprooting of the 'native' village of Nimi Bagh in 1901, as an insanitary eyesore, which was viewed as located too close to Government House in the city of Allahabad, is a prominent example of the mentality that prevailed in colonial sanitary regime. Related to this was the unequal focus of the municipal committees of the respective cities on the sanitary conditions of the 'old' and 'new' part of the town. Reporting this imbalanced approach the *Oudh Akhbar* of Lucknow reported that the places inhabited by the Europeans received far greater consideration with one or two other places emerging as 'favoured places'.[23] Elsewhere the project to elevate the sanitary condition remained more haphazard, chaotic and occasionally punitive to the 'native' inhabitants.

The aforesaid colonial negligence and lack of will to restrict the spread of cholera among the 'native' inhabitants overlapped with the societal prejudices of the Indians regarding this disease. The fear of cholera and resultant sufferings led to its ritualization in deltaic Bengal. In order to escape from the wrath of cholera, the inhabitants of the region worshipped a specific cholera deity known as Ola Bibi among the Muslims, and Olai-Chandi among the Hindus. Olai-Chandi (literally 'the goddess of the flux') was usually worshipped on Tuesdays and Saturdays throughout the cholera season. Although propitiation of cholera deity was not new to Bengal, it reached new heights in the nineteenth century in the wake of frequent outbreaks of cholera pandemics. As David Arnold argues, 'before 1817 the Goddess (of cholera) enjoyed far less popular devotion than Sitala (the smallpox goddess), but she was thereafter extensively propitiated during the season when cholera was most prevalent'.[24] Not only instances of fictive appearance of the cholera deity in popular countryside imagination multiplied in nineteenth century, Olai-Chandi was now accommodated in a regular temple structure as well. In fact, in 1818, the Christian missionary Rev. J. Keith reported the appearance of an incarnation of Ola Bibi at Salkia in Howrah district of Bengal. According to Keith, so much was the popularity of this incarnation of Ola Bibi that she even competed with the goddess Kali (one of the most popular deities of Bengal) for the attention and offerings.[25] Such instances of incarnation of cholera deity made its appearance in Bombay Presidency and in Konkan area as well.[26] These engagements of epidemics with religious associations were important aspects of public health policies in India (Bala in this volume).

Further, as Arabinda Samanta argues, cholera sharpened caste animosities, raked up interpersonal rivalry and broke down traditional social relation beyond repair.[27] It can be best understood by resorting to some of the literary works revolving around the episodes of outbreak of cholera. As for instance, Fakir Mohan Senapati, often described as the 'father of Odia literature', writes about deepening of social prejudice associated with women education during the outbreak of an extremely virulent cholera epidemic. In the first-ever short story published in Odia titled 'Rebati' (1898), he writes about Rebati, a young girl from a backward village hit by cholera, who is determined to get an education. However, her conservative grandmother attributes the girl's desire for an education and the steps taken by her father to fulfil his daughter's wish as the reasons behind the cholera outbreak.[28]

In a similar vein, the noted Bengali novelist Sarat Chandra Chattopadhyay in his novel *Pandit Moshay* (1914) portrays the deepening of social tensions between the orthodoxy and the progressive people of the locality in the wake of outbreak of *bishuchika* or cholera. It depicts how cholera in due course of time became a part of 'divine curse' which could be inflicted upon a person or village for not succumbing to or disbelieve in *shastric* authority. The way protagonist of the novel Brindaban, a rational man, was cursed by the Brahmin that his whole family would be wiped out by cholera for going against the *shastric* beliefs reflects this spectacular juxtaposition of age-old superstitions and outbreak of cholera. The fact that Brindaban's mother died of cholera and his son also got infected with this deadly disease following the aforesaid curse by the Brahmin must have confirmed this divinity of cholera in the eyes of the common people of the countryside.[29]

Similarly, *Arogya Niketan* (1953), a novel belonging to a relatively later date, written by Tarashankar Bandyopadhyay exquisitely portrays the panic and rumours associated with cholera epidemic in the Bengali countryside. Interestingly, the imagery of cholera deity which appears in *Arogya Niketan* overlaps more with the popular imagery of a 'witch' than a goddess – lean and thin body with raised bones, fiery eyes, rough disheveled hairs, long teeth, wearing ragged cloth, carrying tattered mat to carry the corpse and treading on the way to cremation ground. The street dogs start wailing out of fear at the very sight of her.[30] Here, it would not be an exaggeration to assume if during cholera epidemic a few women were put to death under false premises for spreading cholera.

BUBONIC PLAGUE AND THE EPIDEMIC DISEASES ACT

The colonial sanitary regime reached new heights during the bubonic plague epidemic of 1890s in India. Incidentally, the outbreak of bubonic plague in the subcontinent during the closing years of the nineteenth century was yet another glaring example of integral linkage between colonialism and spread of diseases. The plague which was brought from Hong Kong to Colombo to Bombay via the colonial trading route created havoc in British India.[31] The catastrophic memories of the British pertaining to Black Death (1348) and 'the great plague' of London (1665) compelled the colonial sanitary regime to respond quickly. It resulted into introduction of severe measures in order to restrict the spread of bubonic plague.

However, as Anil Kumar remarks, the colonial anti-plague campaign of the time 'was directed more against the natives than the plague bacillus'.[32] The Epidemic Diseases Act, which was passed in February 1897 in the wake of outbreak of bubonic plague in the Indian subcontinent, gave draconian powers to the colonial government. While introducing the Epidemic Diseases Bill in the Council of the Governor-General of India in Calcutta for 'better prevention of the spread of dangerous epidemic diseases', John Woodburn, the council member who introduced it, himself considered the powers mentioned in it as 'extraordinary' but 'necessary'. Woodburn emphasized that people must 'trust the discretion of the executive in grave and critical circumstances'.[33]

This Act empowered the colonial authorities to detain the plague suspects, destroy or demolish infected property and dwellings, prohibit fairs and pilgrimages and examine the passengers at will. Simultaneously, it made disobedience of any regulation or order made under this Act a punishable offence. It also carried provisions for protection of persons/officials acting under this Act as no suit or other legal proceeding could be initiated against any person for anything done or in good faith intended to be done under this Act.[34] Thus, it gave unbridled power even to those working at the lower rung of colonial officialdom. It soon precipitated into numerous instances of executive excesses whereby dignity of people was often encroached upon and occasionally tarnished as well. A natural outcome of this was widespread anti-plague riots that took place around this time against the obtrusive nature of state intervention.[35] Occasionally mob attacks on search parties and even the assassination of British officials took place.

Commenting on such instances of fierce resistance Raj Chandavarkar argues that the widespread hostility which can be seen during the outbreak of plague epidemic in India had little to do with the fear associated with the epidemic itself and was primarily due to the most coercive manifestation of a brutally intrusive state.[36]

In the aforesaid context, particularly emotive was the issue of the 'check-up' or medical examination of Indian women at railway stations and public places especially by *firangi* (viz. foreign) male doctors. It was soon translated by the Hindu and the Muslim elites alike as colonial interference in the 'private sphere' and an attempt to 'dishonour' Indian women. As a corollary, opposition started brewing among Indians against colonial anti-plague interventions in order to restrict the colonial encroachment in the private sphere. An integral part of this opposition was the rhetoric around 'safeguarding' the 'honour' of Indian women which brought various sections of Hindu society as well as Muslims together. As Charu Gupta puts it, 'interference with women's bodies was effectively used to give an emotive appeal to anger against plague orders, linked as it was to honour, *purdah*, domestic privacy, public examination, and forcible removal to segregation camps and hospitals'.[37] That is why nearly a thousand of millhands attacked Bombay's Arthur Road hospital on 29 October 1896 after a woman worker was reported to be taken there as a suspected plague sufferer. In a similar vein, the Plague Riot of Kanpur in April 1900 was fuelled largely by the rhetoric around the issue of women's 'honour' whereby a mob comprising both the Hindus and the Muslims along with the untouchables attacked the local plague segregation camp partly inspired by reports of women being detained there against their will.[38]

Actually, if we look at the entire modus operandi of the plague check-ups then it was primarily based upon the identification of swollen lymph nodes which generally appeared in the underarms or groin area of the infected person. Hence, the person had to be stripped during the plague examination which was disrespectful, particularly in the case of women. Added to this were instances of misbehaviour on the part of colonial authorities during inspections. Depicting a scene of plague check-up by the colonial authorities and humiliation involved in it, Sarat Chandra Chattopadhyay in his novel *Srikanta* writes:

> Eventually the time to commence the medical examination for plague arrived. There appeared on the scene a white doctor along with compounder, peon, and other staffs. . . . The grossly insensitive and ruthless manner in which the

doctor was pressing and examining the private parts of each person was enough to enrage even the clay effigy, however, people were helpless. . . . In different circumstances people would have burnt the doctor alive.[39]

Likewise gender, caste and class issues also put the colonial authorities in difficult situations while carrying out the provisions of the Epidemic Diseases Act. In this context, a report published in *The British Medical Journal* on 28 November 1896, while discussing the riots caused in Bombay because of government policies of quarantine, noted that many people belonging to upper caste and class requested evasion from being quarantined with low caste or class people. In other words, upper caste or class people demanded special considerations under the Epidemic Diseases Act in accordance with their 'caste' prejudices. The report suggested that a sensible way out of this difficulty was to throw the responsibility on the particular caste or class demanding special consideration to carry out their own expense for such modifications (such as a separate isolation cell or quarantine at home) as they wish.[40]

In fact, as Arnold argues, while the British saw the hospital as a sanitized and healing site, it was to many Indians (not least to the higher castes) a place of pollution, contaminated by blood and faeces, inimical to caste, religion and *purdah* or veil.[41] Actually, in a general hospital it was very difficult to segregate the patients belonging to different castes. At the same time it was equally difficult to maintain the prescribed taboos pertaining to food, cooking and touch, and so on in hospitals. Hence, British-style colonial hospitals posed serious challenge to a caste-based social structure obsessed with concerns of 'purity' and 'pollution'. That is why we see various caste hospitals being set up during the plague epidemic in India through communitarian efforts in order to ensure the caste norms of the patients belonging to respective castes. Bhatia Plague Hospital, Memon Plague Hospital, Parel Road Jain Hospital, Telugu Hospital, Parsi Fever Hospital, and so on were few examples of this network of caste-based hospitals that emerged during this period in India. Incidentally, by April 1898, in Bombay Presidency alone there were as many as thirty such private caste-based hospitals which came into existence.[42]

Likewise hospital, quarantine shelter was yet another site to which Indians were sceptical. As Rajinder Singh Bedi in his Urdu short story 'Kwaranteen' (1940) points out that people feared being sent to these quarantine shelters more than they feared the plague itself. In popular perception, these shelters were hellish and were seen no less than a morgue. To them it was also a place where hardly any ritual was followed before disposing the dead body. Echoing the aforesaid popular perception, Bedi in his story writes:

Keeping in mind the large number of deaths inside the quarantine shelters, a unique way had been adopted to dispose the dead bodies infected with plague.

> Hundreds of dead bodies were used to be dragged like dogs and piled up in the form of a big mound. Subsequently, they used to sprinkle petrol on them and burn without performing any last rite. The very sight of rising flames out of this mound used to send chills down the spines of rest of the inmates.[43]

It naturally resulted into cases where the family members of the infected person deliberately tucked him away from the eyes of the authority so as to safeguard him from the hellish quarantine shelters. This, in turn, often necessitated forceful inspection of dwelling places and forcible removal of the infected person to quarantine shelters by the authorities which bred further discontent.

Nevertheless, the issues of gender and caste during the bubonic plague outbreak became so significant that even someone as progressive as Vivekananda had to take them into account while drafting his 'Plague Manifesto'. In May 1898, the bubonic plague started spreading in the city of Calcutta. At this crucial juncture Vivekananda-led Ramakrishna Mission played a commendable role in running special hospitals and other relief operations for plague-infected people of the city. When the terror-stricken residents of the city started fleeing the city, Vivekananda also issued a 'Plague Manifesto' which was originally written in Bengali and was printed and freely distributed among the people. Out of several other points, the manifesto stated categorically: 'There will be no lack of effort in treating the afflicted patients in our hospital under our special care and supervision, paying full respect to religion, caste and the modesty (*purdah*) of women'.[44] Noticeable here is the utmost attention which was paid on 'religion, caste and the modesty of women'.

The entire situation got further aggravated owing to various rumours that were generated during the plague epidemic. According to Arnold, these rumours flourished in the atmosphere of fear and uncertainty generated by the plague and the colonial medical intervention against it.[45] These rumours ranged from deliberate poisoning of Indians by Western doctors to cutting up of the bodies of the natives in order to extract *momiai*[46] in the hospitals and at quarantine shelters. At the same time, hospitalization was also seen as the tactics to corrupt the caste status of upper caste Hindus so that they could be converted to Christianity. Again, in Bengal Presidency it was rumoured that the then viceroy of India, Lord Elgin, had promised a yogi to sacrifice two lakhs of human lives to the Goddess Kali in order to save the British Empire in India.[47] Such rumours obviously gave rise to disturbances and riots.

The traditional beliefs of Indians regarding plague also posed a serious challenge in front of the government. Likewise cholera, plague was also ritualized and feared. Any interference in the natural course of its spread was seen as messing with the divine intervention. The Bengali novelist Premankur Atarthi recounts an interesting anecdote in this regard:

> One day the news spread that one woman arrived at Howrah station by Bombay Mail and then moved forward to Calcutta after hiring a carriage. When she

> reached Harrison Road in central Calcutta the carriage driver asked her, 'Which place do you wish to go?' The woman replied, 'Don't you know who I am? I am the goddess of plague'. Then all on a sudden she disappeared.

The story spread like a wildfire and people started shouting, 'Plague, plague, plague everywhere. Better flee the city'.[48]

Thus, fleeing was seen as the only option to save life from the 'Plague Goddess'. Any attempt to restrict her advance was tantamount to sacrilege. In a different context, Master Bhagwan Das in his story 'Plague ki Chudail' (1902) explores the fear psychosis in Allahabad during the plague epidemic.[49] In the story, the fear of infection from plague leads to the hasty disposal of the body of an unconscious woman, who happens to still be alive. When she regains consciousness, people believe that she is 'plague ki chudail' or 'the plague witch'. In a similar vein, the eminent Hindi poet, Kedarnath Singh, in one of his reminiscences recounts that how plague in his village was deemed by many as a man-eating demon.[50] Thus, plague was one disease which was deified as well as demonized both at the same time depending upon the context. However, what was common in both the phenomena was that it always invoked some sense of fear.

Irrespective of riots and disturbances against the anti-plague measures of the government, the colonial sanitary regime kept its wheels moving thereby introducing far-reaching changes in the topography of the Indian cities. In February 1898, the colonial government set up the Bombay Improvement Trust (BIT) with the proposed aim of redressing the problem of 'sanitary disorder' of the city. Dwelling upon its role on the occasion of laying of foundation stone of the Improvement Trust Scheme at Nagpada (Bombay), on 9 November 1899, the then viceroy Lord Curzon remarked that it was to bring 'the fresh breezes of the sea into the congested lungs of Bombay'.[51] Guided by miasmatic theory, just like cholera, plague was also seen as a disease of filth and overcrowding. Consequently, BIT cleared large-scale commercial and residential areas to make way for relatively open boulevards such as Princess Street at Marine Lines and Sandhurst Road. Simultaneously, poor quarters of Nagpada, Agripada and Pydhonie were uprooted and planned to be rehabilitated to the newly developed areas of Dadar, Matunga, Wadala and Sion of south Bombay. However, as Prashant Kidambi argues, the poorly conceived rehabilitation programmes of BIT rendered a large number of people either homeless or trapped in single rooms. According to Kidambi, in July 1919, it was reported that nearly 892,000 inhabitants out of a total urban population of 1,200,000 resided in single rooms and there was an overall shortfall of 64,000 tenements in the city.[52] Thus, epidemic was once again used by the colonial regime as a handy pretext to introduce far-reaching changes in the urban landscape.

Nevertheless, as argued before, the anti-plague measures adopted by the colonial sanitary regime bred severe discontent. Bal Gangadhar Tilak wrote a series of articles against such measures in his newspapers *Mahratta* and *Kesari*. An anonymous letter published in *Mahratta* on 25 April 1897 went on to designate the whole scenario as a 'reign of terror'. Even Tilak, in the context of Poona, claimed that the Plague Committee and its officers ran riot in the city as if the city was a silent cemetery inhabited by dead bodies.[53] In fact, Tilak was quite critical of the ways adopted by W. C. Rand, plague commissioner of Poona, especially his mechanism of unique search parties assisted by armed soldiers. He claimed that 'Mr. Rand is perhaps too callous and heartless to realize that a night surprise by the dreaded soldiers strikes fearful panic in the already panic stricken people'.[54] Even in the issue of *Mahratta* published immediately after the assassination of Rand by Chapekar brothers, Tilak deemed it a natural outcome as he believed that 'ever since the establishment of the British rule in India no measure was undertaken by Government which interfered so largely and in such a systematic way with the domestic, social and religious habits of the people'.[55] Incidentally, following the assassination of Rand, Tilak was charged with sedition by the colonial government for his aforesaid writings against colonial anti-plague measures.

SPANISH INFLUENZA AND THE UNFATHOMABLE TRAGEDY

The deadliest of epidemics which ravaged India under the colonial rule was the Spanish flu/influenza of 1918–1920. Starting from Camp Funston in Kansas (United States of America) in early 1918, it soon spread throughout the world. The mobility of soldiers engaged in the First World War facilitated its spread. However, owing to the war time censorship, the governments of most of the belligerent countries suppressed any news associated with its spread. Nevertheless, as Spain was not involved in the First World War, the Spanish media reported it extensively thereby sending a wrong impression to the common people across the globe that it was started from Spain and hence termed as 'Spanish flu/influenza'.[56] In fact, many rumours got circulated regarding the origin of this disease linking it to Spain during this period. According to one such rumour, the Spanish flu virus was developed by the Germans in a laboratory located in the city of Madrid (Spain) as a biological weapon intended to infect the American soldiers, so that the United States could not help the Allies. However, due to the negligence and some mutual discord among scientists, this virus broke out in the city of Madrid and slowly spread throughout the world. The effect of this rumour was such that even the noted Indian woman social activist, Rameshwari Nehru, in her editorial of the much acclaimed Hindi journal *Stree Darpan* (1919) presented the same version of the origin of Spanish influenza epidemic.[57]

In India, likewise many other countries of the world, the Spanish flu disease came through the soldiers returning from the First World War. The first case was reported in June 1918 in Bombay. Subsequently, within a few months it acquired the epidemic proportion spreading throughout the Indian subcontinent. The death toll from Spanish influenza reached its peak in the Bombay Presidency in September 1918, in the Madras Presidency in October 1918 and in the Calcutta Presidency in November 1918. The worst affected age group from this epidemic was of 20–40 years. Also, women were disproportionately affected by this disease.[58] It led to serious problems related to livelihood and raising of children in front of most families. It is noticeable that ever since the census began in India in 1872, the decade from 1911 to 1921 is the only decade when the population decline between the two censuses was observed.[59] One of the major reasons for this was the Spanish flu pandemic of 1918–1920. India, in fact, reported the highest number of deaths from Spanish influenza disease.

Mortality estimates for India due to Spanish influenza outbreak are wide ranging, from 12 to 20 million.[60] Families of many well-known Indians were also among those infected with this disease. Gulab Gandhi, the eldest daughter-in-law of Mahatma Gandhi, died untimely in this epidemic. The wife of Khan Abdul Ghaffar Khan also passed away during the same time after being infected with Spanish flu. Suryakant Tripathi 'Nirala', one of the leading Hindi poets, lost nearly half the family, including his wife and daughter during this epidemic.

The main reason for this unexpected havoc of the Spanish flu pandemic in India was the lax attitude adopted by the colonial regime for its prevention. It was probably the natural outcome of the severe discontentment, as discussed before, which the colonial government had to face for its measures taken during the bubonic plague epidemic. It is quite possible that the colonial government did not want to conflagrate through its interventionist medical approach the same kind of discontentment which it had to face at the end of the nineteenth century, especially keeping in mind the context of world war as well as rising nationalist movement in India. At the same time, the massive deaths during Spanish influenza epidemic also exposed the dilapidated condition of colonial health infrastructure in India. In fact, the colonial government always refrained from the massive 'non-colonial' public investments. There was a belief that such investments were 'unfruitful' and 'undesirable' as it could demoralize private initiatives besides adding to the budgetary deficits and national debt. In the specific context of the colonial health expenditure, Mark Harrison argues that the colonial state's investment in expanding medical infrastructure in India was severely restricted by this sort of fiscal conservatism.[61]

However, despite *en masse* deaths in India during Spanish influenza pandemic, we hardly have enough archival sources as well as historiographical works which may capture this unforeseen tragedy. What is more ironic in this regard is that the British Indian government, known for its high-level inquiry commissions even on minor incidents, did not set up a single high-level inquiry commission to investigate and study the spread of Spanish influenza and the number of deaths it caused. For this very reason, we do not have enough archival records to reconstruct the history of Spanish influenza in India.

In fact, scholars have deemed Spanish influenza a kind of 'forgotten pandemic'.[62] Forgetting this pandemic in the Indian context is even more surprising because, as argued before, India experienced the highest number of deaths across the globe from Spanish influenza. One can only guess the factors responsible behind obliteration of this pandemic from popular memories. Actually, the second half of the 1910s was a period of 'great tragedies'. In the First World War, numerous soldiers and ordinary people lost their lives. In addition to it, in the particular context of India, the drought and famine of 1918 made the condition even more serious. There was an orgy of death everywhere. In such a situation, probably deaths due to pandemic started appearing as a 'normal' phenomenon.

One of the reasons behind its obliviscence in the Indian context may also be the political instability of the time. It is worth mentioning that the years 1918–1920 was a period of Rowlatt satyagraha, Khilafat movement, Jallianwala Bagh massacre and non-cooperation movement in Indian politics. The entire country was engaged in these burning political issues. In such a situation, the issue of pandemic might have been left behind. The intensity of the Spanish flu might also be a reason behind its obliteration from popular memory. Earlier timeline of an epidemic spanned for many years. Epidemic like cholera created havoc throughout the nineteenth century. Similarly, bubonic plague epidemic remained more or less widespread in India from 1896 to 1910. On the other hand, the 'reign of terror' of Spanish influenza did not go beyond two years, that is, 1918–1920. Also, prior to Spanish influenza, Indian public had already been battling various epidemics for the past several decades. The Spanish influenza was just a part of this long series of epidemics. All these factors probably contributed in its erasure from historical consciousness of the public.

Nevertheless, some of the Hindi writers do inscribe extremely moving portrayal of this period. A cursory glance through them helps us to comprehend the gory times of Spanish influenza epidemic. The famous Hindi poet Suryakant Tripathi 'Nirala' describing the indiscriminate deaths of this period writes in his memoir *Kulli Bhat* (translated into English as *A Life Misspent*, 2016) that the Ganga river was laden with human corpses during the Spanish flu epidemic.[63] He further recalls:

> This was the strangest time in my life. . . . My family disappeared in the blink of an eye. All our sharecroppers and labourers died, the four who worked for

> my cousin, as well as the two who worked for me. My cousin's eldest son was fifteen years old, my young daughter a year old. In whichever direction I turned, I saw darkness.[64]

In a similar vein, capturing the gruesome situation during the Spanish influenza epidemic in India, Pandey Bechan Sharma 'Ugra' in his short story 'Vibhatsa' writes: 'In most parts of the country, there was a deadly panic of war-fever or influenza. Everyday hundreds of people were dying in each city and many more in each village. . . . Nobody used to go to the market because of fear as they had heard that this disease spreads by contagion'.[65] In such a situation, there was no one left even to shoulder the corpse of a person died of this disease. Whoever shouldered the corpse of the person died of Spanish flu, he himself would soon be suffering from fever as soon as he returned from cremation ground. It was in this context that spotting an opportunity to make a small fortune, the central character of the story, Sumera, starts carrying dead bodies to cremation sites. Indeed, he earns a handsome sum for this service but gets infected and pays with his own life.

In his novel *Meri Teri Uski Baat* (1974), the famous Hindi novelist Yashpal mentions the origin of the Spanish influenza in popular parlance and how people in India dealt with it in the following words:

> Owing to non-disposal of corpses in a terrible massacre for nearly four years during the First World War and as a consequence of other lethal effects of the War, the dreadful storm of a new epidemic started from Europe which soon engulfed the whole world. This storm of epidemic also reached this country. The name, diagnosis and treatment of this disease were completely unknown to doctors, vaids and hakims. With the new disease came a new name: *Falanja* (influenza). Coughing and fever with nasal congestion were its foremost symptoms. No one remained untouched by this disease. Two to three persons out of every ten people infected from this disease died. One could see biers round the clock in the streets and markets. As soon as people used to return from cremation sites, two or three more corpses would be ready for disposal. The biggest cause of terror was that even doctors failed to suggest any remedy to prevent this disease. Many neighbourhoods, streets, and villages were uprooted due to fear of this disease. It was said that the disease was everywhere in the air. People continuously applied decoction of Eucalyptus oil in front of the nose and drank concoction of cinnamon and large cardamom to safeguard themselves from such contagious air.[66]

Besides Hindi literature, we have references of Spanish flu in other languages as well.[67] Also, more recently Madhu Singh has used the 'native' press reports, monitored and collected by the colonial rule as part of colonial supervisory mechanisms, to reconstruct the history of Spanish influenza in India. Based on the reports, Singh argues that 'with no effective cure in sight and an understaffed bureaucracy, not to speak of the state of the public health system, the colonial government was largely ineffective in this crisis, which affected the Bombay presidency and many other parts of India'.[68] Thus, literature as well as newspaper reports may be the potential sources to reconstruct the history of Spanish influenza in the absence of official archives.

CONCLUSION

The aforesaid discussion on the three major epidemics faced by India under the colonial rule attempts to bring out the complex relationship between colonialism, spread of diseases and subsequent response of the masses. It aims to provide a better understanding of the way people, society and regimes react towards such outbreaks. Incidentally, one cannot make sense of an epidemic merely as spread of a disease caused by certain microorganism and consequent deaths; rather, one has to essentially look at it from political, social and economic angle as well. In this context, one may categorically suggest that any epidemic begins as a biological phenomenon, but it soon turns into political, social and economic phenomena. In fact, any epidemic outbreak churns the established settlements thereby fast-forwarding historical processes. Here Yuval Noah Harari, commenting on a more recent outbreak, rightly argues that epidemics set in motion many short-term emergency measures thereby making them a fixture of life. This is the nature of emergencies. Decisions that in normal times could take years of deliberation are passed in a matter of hours. Immature and even dangerous technologies are pressed into service, because the risks of doing nothing are bigger.[69]

Ironically, there persists a historiographical amnesia about the 'age of pandemics'[70] that devastated India for a century, wiping out its significant population. Pandemics, except for bubonic plague outbreak, could hardly manage to come out of the footnotes of Indian history. This amnesia itself may be a subject of analysis, which is outside the scope of this chapter. One thing is clear, frequent outbreaks severely undermined the 'civilizing' presence of the British in India. That is why the colonial masters always blamed the 'dirty' and 'unhygienic' living habits of Indians as the primary reason behind spread of epidemics. Later on, the 'enlightened' Indian middle class and intelligentsia tried to shift this blame to their fellow countrymen belonging to lower castes and class. The poor quarters of a locality were particularly looked as the storehouse of diseases. In fact, in the middle class/upper caste imagination, out of several other essentialized characterization of a particular caste, sanitary sense became one of the characters on the basis of which a particular caste could be identified. Incidentally, lower castes and classes were indifferently seen as having unclean, insanitary, infectious and dirty habits providing the perfect breeding ground for epidemics to spread.

NOTES

1. For specimens of this devastating impact of colonialism in terms of exchange of diseases, see Tzvetan Todorov, *The Conquest of America: The Question of Other* (New York: Harper Perennial, 1992), 136. It is noticeable that along with the Spanish and Portuguese conquistadors several diseases like plague, smallpox and measles also reached the American continents. Having no clue of these diseases, the natives of America died in large numbers in sixteenth and seventeenth century due to frequently occurring plague and smallpox epidemics in these newly found continents. In a similar vein, syphilis, the sexually transmitted disease, supposedly entered Europe from the American continents and then passed on to Asia and Africa.

2. Complex web of trade and frequent movement of armed forces coupled with modern means of communications such as railways and steam ships contributed significantly in rapid spread of diseases under the aegis of colonialism. For role of railways in spreading contagious diseases such as cholera and plague in colonial India, see Ritika Prasad, *Tracks of Change: Railways and Everyday Life in Colonial India* (Cambridge: Cambridge University Press, 2015), 165–99.

3. The classic example of this phenomenon is metamorphosis of cholera from a disease endemic to parts of eastern India into a global pandemic in nineteenth century.

4. Donald Denoon, *Public Health in Papua New Guinea: Medical Possibility and Social Constraint, 1884–1984* (Cambridge: Cambridge University Press, 1989), 52.

5. Ira Klein, "Imperialism, Ecology and Disease: Cholera in India, 1850–1950", *Indian Economic and Social History Review*, vol. 31, no. 4 (1994): 493.

6. Burton Cleetus, "Tropics of Disease: Epidemics in Colonial India", *Economic and Political Weekly Engage*, vol. 55, no. 21 (May 23, 2020).

7. It was known locally by various names such as *sitanga*, *bishuchika* and *murree*. See J.N. Hayes, *Epidemics and Pandemics: Their Impacts on Human History* (Santa Barbara: ABC-CLIO, 2005), 193.

8. It does not mean that cholera as a disease was unknown to the West. There is ample evidence which shows that the Europeans were already aware of this disease and also there are stances of its occurrence in Europe prior to 1817 (see Srabani Sen, "Indian Cholera: A Myth", *Indian Journal of History of Science*, vol. 47, no. 3 (2012): 345–74). However, what was unique about the nineteenth-century outbreaks of cholera was its simultaneous spread across regions and continents. Incidentally, the epicentre of this spread was always located in the Indian subcontinent which earned for the region the reputation of being the 'homeland of cholera'.

9. David Arnold, *Colonizing the Body: State Medicine and Epidemic Disease in Nineteenth-Century India* (Berkeley: University of California Press, 1993), 150.

10. Arabinda Samanta, *Living with Pandemics in Colonial Bengal, 1818–1945* (New Delhi: Manohar, 2017), 56.

11. These initial waves of cholera pandemics that broke out in the nineteenth century have been studied extensively by a range of scholars for different regions. Rosenberg has worked upon cholera epidemic in the United States of America, McGrew on Russia, Delaporte on France, Durey on Britain, and many others on various other countries have undertaken similar studies. See C.E. Rosenberg, *The Cholera Years: The United States in 1832, 1849 and 1866* (Chicago: Chicago University Press,

1962); R.E. McGrew, *Russia and the Cholera, 1823–32* (Madison: University of Wisconsin Press, 1965); Francois Delaporte, *Disease and Civilization: The Cholera in Paris, 1832* (London: MIT Press, 1986); Michael Durey, *The Return of the Plague: British Society and the Cholera, 1831–32* (Dublin: Gill and Macmillan, 1979). In fact, many cartoons and caricatures were produced during nineteenth century denoting the extensiveness of cholera pandemic. Notable is the 1832 French allegory of cholera pandemic 'Le cholera morbus' where cholera has been personified hugging the fellow human beings.

12. Klein, "Imperialism, Ecology and Disease", 499. However, this whole argument regarding connection between modern means of communication, such as railways, and spread of epidemic diseases was not something infallible. Ritika Prasad, in her study of railways and everyday life in colonial India, has shown that the official opinion in this regard was quite variegated. According to Prasad, while in the 1860s, India's expanding railway map was used as proof that cholera was indeed disseminated through contact; in the next two decades, the same railway map was used to support anti-contagionist views, putting India considerably at odds with international medical consensus (see Prasad, *Tracks of Change*, 171).

13. Edwin Hodder, *The Life and Work of the Seventh Earl of Shaftesbury* (London: Cassell and Company, 1887), 417.

14. Durey, *The Return of the Plague.*

15. *Hansard's Parliamentary Debates 3rd Series*, 91 (March 30, 1847): 621.

16. Here it should be kept in mind that this was the period roughly coinciding with what Eric Hobsbawm has deemed as the 'age of revolution'. See Eric Hobsbawm, *The Age of Revolution, 1789–1848* (London: Weidenfeld & Nicolson, 1962).

17. The uprisings of 1857 ended the rule of the English East India Company (also referred to as the 'Company Raj') in the subcontinent and marked the beginning of direct rule of Britain over India (known as the 'British Raj'). This shift in power apparently linked India more organically to the political developments of Great Britain.

18. It was coupled with the racial restructuring of the British Raj in India as well. The threatening disorder and 'putrid air' were understood to characterize the old cities. In contrast, the British created separately demarcated spaces for themselves. In cities these areas were labelled 'civil lines', with associated 'cantonments' for the military. In mountainous regions they established 'hill stations' that served as summer refuges not only for individuals but for the colonial governments. See Barbara D. Metcalf and Thomas R. Metcalf, *A Concise History of Modern India* (Cambridge: Cambridge University Press, 2006), 108–11.

19. Veena Oldenburg, *The Making of Colonial Lucknow, 1856–1877* (Princeton: Princeton University Press, 1984), 96–144.

20. J.B. Harrison, "Allahabad: A Sanitary History", in *The City in South Asia: Pre-modern and Modern*, eds. K. Ballhatchet and J. Harrison (London: Curzon Press, 1980), 173 (emphasis mine).

21. Oldenburg, *The Making of Colonial Lucknow*, 102.

22. Harrison, "Allahabad: A Sanitary History", 178.

23. *Oudh Akhbar*, December 5, 1865.

24. David Arnold, "Cholera and Colonialism in British India", *Past and Present*, vol. 113, no. 1 (1986): 130.

25. Interestingly, the woman who claimed to be an incarnation of Ola Bibi at Salkia was later on arrested by the colonial authorities for imposture and sentenced by the magistrate for six months in the House of Correction where, ironically, she contracted cholera but survived (see Arnold, "Cholera and Colonialism", 132).

26. Arnold, *Colonizing the Body*, 173–74.

27. Samanta, *Living with Pandemics*, 70.

28. Fakir Mohan Senapati, "Rebati", trans. Leelawati Mohapatra, Paul St. Pierre and K.K. Mohapatra, in *Outbreaks: An Indian Pandemic Reader*, ed. Madhu Singh (Delhi: Pencraft International, 2022), 316–25.

29. Sarat Chandra Chattopadhyay, *Pandit Moshay* (New Delhi: Subodh Publication, 1985).

30. Tarashankar Bandyopadhyay, *Arogya Niketan*, trans. H. Tiwari (Delhi: Rajpal & Sons, 1957), 188–89.

31. According to an estimate, plague-related death rates in Bombay between 1897 and 1900 was 2 per 1,000 among Europeans; around 10 per 1,000 among Parsis, Jews and Eurasians; 15 per 1,000 among Hindu 'Brahmnas'; and 20 per 1,000 for all other Hindu castes. See Chinmay Tumbe, *The Age of Pandemics, 1817–1920: How They Shaped India and the World* (Noida: HarperCollins, 2020), 84.

32. Anil Kumar, *Medicine and the Raj: British Medical Policy, 1835–1911* (New Delhi: Sage Publications, 1998), 197.

33. "Legislative Note: The Epidemic Diseases (Amendment) Ordinance, 2020", Library and Reference Research Documentation & Information Service (LARRDIS), http://164.100.47.193/Refinput/New_Reference Notes/English/10092020_114427_1021205239.pdf, Accessed November 15, 2021.

34. "Epidemic Diseases Act, 1897", https://main.mohfw.gov.in/sites/default/files/1625462448.pdf. Accessed February 25, 2022.

35. For a comprehensive account on anti-plague riots, especially in western India, see Arnold, *Colonizing the Body*, 200–39.

36. Raj Chandavarkar, "Plague Panic and Epidemic Politics in India, 1896–1914", in T. Ranger and P. Slack (eds.) *Epidemics and Ideas: Essays on the Historical Perception of Pestilence* (Cambridge: Cambridge University Press, 1992), 203–40.

37. Charu Gupta, *Sexuality, Obscenity, Community: Women, Muslims, and the Hindu Public in Colonial India* (Delhi: Permanent Black, 2001), 191–92.

38. David Arnold, "Touching the Body: Perspectives on the Indian Plague, 1896–1900", in *Subaltern Studies V: Writings on South Asian History and Society*, ed. Ranajit Guha (New Delhi: Oxford University Press, 1987), 63.

39. Sarat Chandra Chattopadhyay, *Srikanta*, ed. O.P. Sharma (New Delhi: Kitabghar Prakashan, 2008), 173–74 (translation mine).

40. "The Plague in Bombay: Riots and Blackmail", *The British Medical Journal*, vol. 2, issue 1874 (November 28, 1896): 1606.

41. Arnold, "Touching the Body", 62.

42. Arnold, "Touching the Body", 62.

43. Rajinder Singh Bedi, "Kwaranteen", in *Dana-o-Daam* (Delhi: Maktaba Jamia, 1963), 121 (translation mine).

44. Vivekananda, "The Plague Manifesto", in *The Complete Works of Swami Vivekananda*, vol. 9, 3rd revised edition (Kolkata: Advaita Ashram, 2016).

45. Arnold, "Touching the Body", 68.

46. Denoted a magical balm which was believed to cure wounds and make the user invulnerable. As per the popular belief, it was usually extracted by making a hole at the top of the head and hanging the person upside down over a slow fire.

47. *Amrita Bazar Patrika*, May 4, 1898.

48. Cited in Samanta, *Living with Pandemics,* 130.

49. *Saraswati*, 1902 (reprinted in *Hirak Jayanti Granth of Saraswati*, 1950), 162–69.

50. Kedarnath Singh, "Chakia ke Kedar", *Sankalp Srijan*, vol 1, no. 1 (January–March 2022): 11.

51. S.C. Sinha, *Indian Speeches of Lord Curzon, Vol. I* (Calcutta: Sanyal & Co., 1900), 201.

52. Prashant Kidambi, *The Making of an Indian Metropolis: Colonial Governance and Public Culture in Bombay, 1890–1920* (Hampshire: Ashgate, 2007), 112.

53. *Mahratta*, May 30, 1897, Roll No. MFR 213 (New Delhi: Nehru Memorial Museum and Library).

54. *Mahratta*, May 09, 1897, Roll No. MFR 213 (New Delhi: Nehru Memorial Museum and Library).

55. *Mahratta*, June 27, 1897, Roll No. MFR 213 (New Delhi: Nehru Memorial Museum and Library).

56. Howard Phillips and David Killingray (eds.), *The Spanish Influenza Pandemic of 1918–19: New Perspectives* (London and New York: Routledge, 2003), 7.

57. Rameshwari Nehru, "Shleshmajwar, Samarjwar, Influenza", *Stree Darpan* (January 1919).

58. I.D. Mills, "The 1918–1919 Influenza Pandemic: The Indian Experience", *Indian Economic and Social History Review*, vol. 23, no. 1 (1986): 36.

59. See "Variation in population since 1901", Office of the Registrar General and Census Commissioner, India, https://censusindia.gov.in/census_data_2001/india_at_glance/variation.aspx. Accessed March 09, 2022.

60. J.T. Marten, *Census of India, 1921*, Vol. I, Part I (Calcutta: Superintendent of Government Printing, 1923); K. Davis, *The Population of India and Pakistan* (Princeton, NJ: Princeton University Press, 1951); Mills, "The 1918–1919 Influenza Pandemic"; K.D. Patterson and G. Pyle, "The geography and mortality of the 1918 influenza pandemic", *Bulletin of the History of Medicine*, vol. 65, no. 4 (1991): 4–21.

61. Mark Harrison, *Public Health in British India: Anglo-Indian Preventive Medicine 1859–1914* (Cambridge: Cambridge University Press, 1994), 166–67.

62. A.W. Crosby, *America's Forgotten Pandemic: The Influenza of 1918* (Cambridge: Cambridge University Press, 1989).

63. Testifying this, contemporaneous Proceedings of Sanitary Department actually show that rivers became clogged with corpses because firewood available was

insufficient for the cremation of Hindus (Mills, "The 1918–1919 Influenza Pandemic", 35–36).

64. Suryakant Tripathi Nirala, *A Life Misspent*, trans. Satti Khanna (New York: Harper Perennial, 2016).

65. Pandey Bechan Sharma, "Vibhatsa", *Matwala* (September 7–22, 1929) (translation mine).

66. Yashpal, *Meri Teri Uski Baat* (Allahabad: Lokbharti Paperbacks, 2009) (translation mine).

67. As for instance, Sarat Chandra Chattopadhyay in his Bengali novel *Shesh Prashna* (1931) provides a moving description of deserted condition of the city during Spanish influenza pandemic.

68. Madhu Singh, "Bombay Fever/Spanish Flu: Public health and native press in Colonial Bombay, 1918–19", *South Asia Research*, vol. 41, no. 1 (2021): 36.

69. Yuval Noah Harari, "The World After Coronavirus", *Financial Times*, March 20, 2020, https://www.ft.com/content/19d90308-6858-11ea-a3c9-1fe6fedcca75. Accessed March 04, 2022.

70. This phrase has been borrowed from Chinmay Tumbe's recent work on pandemics. According to Tumbe, between 1817 and 1920, more than 5% of the global population died of various pandemic outbreaks thereby making this period an 'age of pandemics'. See Tumbe, *The Age of Pandemics*, 20–21.

BIBLIOGRAPHY

Arnold, David. "Cholera and Colonialism in British India." *Past and Present*, vol. 113, no. 1 (1986): 118–51.

Arnold, David. "Touching the Body: Perspectives on the Indian Plague, 1896–1900." In *Subaltern Studies V: Writings on South Asian History and Society*, edited by Ranajit Guha, 55–90. New Delhi: Oxford University Press, 1987.

Arnold, David. *Colonizing the Body: State Medicine and Epidemic Disease in Nineteenth-Century India*. Berkeley: University of California Press, 1993.

Bandyopadhyay, Tarashankar. *Arogya Niketan*. Translated by H. Tiwari. Delhi: Rajpal & Sons, 1957. Bedi, Rajinder Singh. *Dana-o-Daam*. Delhi: Maktaba Jamia, 1963.

Chandavarkar, Raj. "Plague Panic and Epidemic Politics in India, 1896–1914." In *Epidemics and Ideas: Essays on the Historical Perception of Pestilence*, edited by T. Ranger and P. Slack, 203–40. Cambridge: Cambridge University Press, 1992.

Chattopadhyay, Sarat Chandra. *Pandit Moshay*. New Delhi: Subodh Publication, 1985.

Chattopadhyay, Sarat Chandra. *Srikanta*. Edited by O.P. Sharma. New Delhi: Kitabghar Prakashan, 2008.

Cleetus, Burton. "Tropics of Disease: Epidemics in Colonial India." *Economic and Political Weekly Engage*, vol. 55, no. 21 (May 23, 2020).

Crosby, A.W. *America's Forgotten Pandemic: The Influenza of 1918.* Cambridge: Cambridge University Press, 1989.

Davis, K. *The Population of India and Pakistan.* Princeton, NJ: Princeton University Press, 1951. Delaporte, Francois. *Disease and Civilization: The Cholera in Paris, 1832.* London: MIT Press, 1986.

Denoon, Donald. *Public Health in Papua New Guinea: Medical Possibility and Social Constraint, 1884–1984.* Cambridge: Cambridge University Press, 1989.

Durey, Michael. *The Return of the Plague: British Society and the Cholera, 1831–32.* Dublin: Gill and Macmillan, 1979.

Gupta, Charu. *Sexuality, Obscenity, Community: Women, Muslims, and the Hindu Public in Colonial India.* Delhi: Permanent Black, 2001.

Hansard's Parliamentary Debates 3rd Series, 91 (March 30, 1847).

Harari, Yuval Noah. "The World After Coronavirus." *Financial Times*, March 20, 2020, https://www.ft.com/content/19d90308-6858-11ea-a3c9-1fe6fedcca75.

Harrison, J.B. "Allahabad: A Sanitary History." In *The City in South Asia: Premodern and Modern*, edited by K. Ballhatchet and J. Harrison, 167–196. London: Curzon Press, 1980.

Harrison, Mark. *Public Health in British India: Anglo-Indian Preventive Medicine 1859–1914.* Cambridge: Cambridge University Press, 1994.

Hayes, J.N. *Epidemics and Pandemics: Their Impacts on Human History.* Santa Barbara: ABC-CLIO, 2005.

Hobsbawm, Eric. *The Age of Revolution, 1789–1848.* London: Weidenfeld & Nicolson, 1962.

Hodder, Edwin. *The life and work of the Seventh Earl of Shaftesbury*, London: Cassell and Company, 1887.

Kidambi, Prashant. *The Making of an Indian Metropolis: Colonial Governance and Public Culture in Bombay, 1890–1920.* Hampshire: Ashgate, 2007.

Klein, Ira. "Imperialism, Ecology and Disease: Cholera in India, 1850–1950." *Indian Economic and Social History Review*, vol. 31, no. 4 (1994): 491–518.

Kumar, Anil. *Medicine and the Raj: British Medical Policy, 1835–1911.* New Delhi: Sage Publications, 1998.

Marten, J.T. *Census of India, 1921*, Vol. I, Part I. Calcutta: Superintendent of Government Printing, 1923.

McGrew, R.E. *Russia and the Cholera, 1823–32.* Madison: University of Wisconsin Press, 1965. Metcalf, Barbara D. and Thomas R. Metcalf. *A Concise History of Modern India.* Cambridge: Cambridge University Press, 2006.

Mills, I.D. "The 1918–1919 Influenza Pandemic: The Indian Experience." *Indian Economic and Social History Review*, vol. 23, no. 1 (1986): 1–40.

Nehru, Rameshwari. "Shleshmajwar, Samarjwar, Influenza." *Stree Darpan* (January 1919).

Nirala, Suryakant Tripathi. *A Life Misspent.* Translated by Satti Khanna. New York: Harper Perennial, 2016.

Oldenburg, Veena. *The Making of Colonial Lucknow, 1856–1877.* Princeton: Princeton University Press, 1984.

Patterson, K.D., and G. Pyle. "The Geography and Mortality of the 1918 Influenza Pandemic." *Bulletin of the History of Medicine*, vol. 65, no. 4 (1991): 4–21.

Phillips, Howard, and David Killingray, eds. *The Spanish Influenza Pandemic of 1918–19: New Perspectives*. London and New York: Routledge, 2003.

Prasad, Ritika. *Tracks of Change: Railways and Everyday Life in Colonial India*. Cambridge: Cambridge University Press, 2015.

Rosenberg, C.E. *The Cholera Years: The United States in 1832, 1849 and 1866*. Chicago: Chicago University Press, 1962.

Samanta, Arabinda. *Living with Pandemics in Colonial Bengal, 1818–1945*. New Delhi: Manohar, 2017.

Sen, Srabani. "Indian Cholera: A Myth." *Indian Journal of History of Science*, vol. 47, no. 3 (2012): 345–74.

Senapati, Fakir Mohan. "Rebati". Translated by Leelawati Mohapatra, Paul St. Pierre and K.K. Mohapatra. In *Outbreaks: An Indian Pandemic Reader*, edited by Madhu Singh, 316–25. New Delhi: Pencraft International, 2022.

Sharma, Pandey Bechan. "Vibhatsa." *Matwala* (September 7–22, 1929).

Singh, Kedarnath. "Chakia ke Kedar." *Sankalp Srijan*, vol 1, no. 1 (January–March 2022): 10–12.

Singh, Madhu. "Bombay Fever/Spanish Flu: Public health and native press in Colonial Bombay, 1918–19." *South Asia Research*, vol. 41, no. 1 (2021): 35–52.

Sinha, S.C. *Indian Speeches of Lord Curzon, Vol. I*. Kolkata: Sanyal & Co., 1900.

Todorov, Tzvetan. *The Conquest of America: The Question of Other*. New York: Harper Perennial, 1992.

Tumbe, Chinmay. *The Age of Pandemics, 1817–1920: How They Shaped India and the World*. Noida: HarperCollins, 2020.

Vivekananda. "The Plague Manifesto." In *The Complete Works of Swami Vivekananda*, Vol. 9, 3rd Revised Edition. Kolkata: Advaita Ashram, 2016.

Yashpal. *Meri Teri Uski Baat*. Allahabad: Lokbharti Paperbacks, 2009.

Chapter 10

Colonization, Disease and Displacement in Australia in the Eighteenth and Nineteenth Centuries

Mark F. Briskey

This chapter explores the myriad manifestations of how disease introduced by the colonizers of Australia decimated the indigenous population. Coupled with and amplifying the destruction of indigenous Australia was the concurrent disenfranchisement of rights and forced separation of indigenous Australian peoples to their traditional lands and the destruction of culture. The impact of disease has been a constant from the eighteenth to the twenty-first century that has and continues to destroy indigenous communities around the globe. In exploring how these indigenous littoral communities have been and remain prey to introduced diseases, the chapter also examines the links between the agencies of the state and their historic interactions with indigenous Australians to identify other co-morbid factors in the grievous impact of colonization upon indigenous Australians. The chapter draws upon evidence from historical as well as contemporary sources to illustrate the devastating impact of introduced diseases upon indigenous Australians.

INTRODUCTION

The caves in Juukan Gorge in the remote Pilbara region of the Australian State of Western Australia have been inhabited at various times by Australia's indigenous peoples for the last 45,000 years. Other sites around Australia prove the incredible antiquity of the indigenous Australian presence in this country over the course of recorded human and geomorphic history. Juukan Gorge, similar to other sites of great antiquity in Australia, indicates the enduring presence of indigenous peoples and their culture in Australia. The remains of indigenous peoples located near Lake Mungo, for example in the current-day Australian state of New South Wales, show them to have been ceremonially anointed with red ochre in a funeral rite dated to around 30,000 years ago. The Lake Mungo human remains and Juukan Gorge are evidence of the continuity of human inhabitation and culture in Australia of up to 60,000 years.[1]

The Juukan Gorge caves with a cultural, spiritual and archaeological significance were destroyed in May 2020 by the Rio Tinto mining company in order to mine the mineral resources there valued in the vicinity of $75 million Australian dollars.[2] The act was catastrophic in terms of its physical destruction as well as the grief it caused to indigenous Australians. This act of desecration and destruction was not unusual. A British solar power company allegedly destroying hundreds of indigenous artefacts sometime after the Juukan Gorge incident when they bulldozed a sacred indigenous site near the New South Wales town of Wagga Wagga was fined a paltry $1,500.00. Indigenous people noted the fine hardly acted as an impediment or as a credible deterrent to future acts of cultural vandalism.[3] Perhaps most egregiously in the Juukan Gorge incident were the unconscionable and unscrupulous actions in that the company was alleged to have hired lawyers to prevent any injunctions against their mining activity in the cave area and so allow their destruction of the site to go on unhindered by protest from the indigenous community and other concerned Australians.[4]

With the advent of the COVID-19 pandemic from 2020 onwards, indigenous Australians are among the most at-risk populations in Australia from yet another introduced disease with the capacity to devastate their communities as much as disease introduced by colonization. While this chapter's focus is upon the calamitous tragedies that befell indigenous Australians because of introduced biological diseases, the ongoing psychological trauma since the first European occupation cannot be understated in their collective impact upon the continuing individual and community health of indigenous Australians.

It is important to note the exponential spread of these diseases from the indigenous inhabitants from the littoral areas that had first contact with the invaders and colonizers. Sexually transmitted venereal diseases discussed shortly perhaps illustrate this most starkly, though smallpox was the single most lethal impact upon indigenous Australians. Diseases encompass a diverse and large group of afflictions impacting specific and overall health outcomes.

The chapter, in considering the impact of disease, provides initially some context in which to situate the varied ways that colonization has impacted the indigenous people and their stewardship of the pre-colonial ecology. After providing some idea of the myriad impacts of colonization and its continuing impact upon indigenous Australians, the chapter considers the almost immediate and catastrophic impact of the first smallpox epidemic introduced by the colonizers. The first smallpox epidemic that flourished only one year after European colonization is examined together with contentious arguments that the loss of life from disease has been overstated in order to blur the stark impact of Aboriginal deaths from direct violence inflicted upon them by Europeans. Such arguments fall within those debates upon violence termed as being the 'hidden factor' as opposed to arguments upon the lethality of disease.

The chapter then moves on to briefly address the impact of the British doctrine of *Terra Nullius* as well as the 'White Australia Policy' operating between 1901 and 1975. This is important as the manner in which the British ruled, as much as the diseases they brought with them, had tremendous impact on the health of the indigenous population. The impact of biological disease, as well as the various doctrines and practices of colonization, is considered by this chapter as essentially co-morbid elements of a pathology in which colonization is an active determinant of indigenous health.

Significant attention is then devoted to colonization and sexually transmitted venereal diseases as well as the close connection between this factor and a history of sexual abuse and violence directed against indigenous Australian women. Lastly, the conclusion notes that the impact of colonization continues to cast its impact upon indigenous Australians whether that be in the poor biological health outcomes they continue to suffer or in the continued scourge of poor mental health. The conclusion also notes a cautious optimism borne out of greater representation of indigenous Australians across both services and government in Australia.

COLONIZATION AND INDIGENOUS HEALTH

The impact of colonization has been described by Evans-Campbell as having diverse manifestations and nuances that encompass a litany of negative consequences, including displacement, forced labour, slavery, removal of children from their families, relocation to areas less desired by the colonists, ecological destruction, war, massacres, genocide, spread of noxious and fatal diseases, the destruction of cultures and the forcible replacement of religions, languages, myths and historical heritages.[5]

This is the case with Australia. In contemporary Australia, as with earlier times, the impact of European colonization is vigorously debated with the annual Australian National Day, 'Australia Day' incurring competing arguments as to what there is to celebrate. Conservative government figures and others defend the celebration of Australia Day on 26 January to commemorate the landing of the First Fleet at present-day Sydney Harbour and establishing the first colony are one side of the divide. Indigenous Australians from Australia, Tasmania, the Torres Strait and other islands with indigenous inhabitants and their supporters equally argue and demonstrate that 26 January is no day to celebrate. Placards stating 'Don't celebrate Genocide' and protesters wearing t-shirts printed with slogans stating 'You are standing on stolen land' as well the day being renamed 'Invasion Day' and calls for indigenous mourning are explicitly made, are highly visible and involve both civil and uncivil responses.[6] Counter-protesters as well as those with more sinister platforms rejecting the indigenous perspective of Australia Day are also present. Approaching Australia day in 2021 media reported a group of Australian neo-Nazis hiking in the hills of the Australian state of Victoria brandishing Nazi tattoos, wearing military fatigues, singing nationalistic songs, raising their hands in 'Sieg Heil' salutes and shouting epithets about 'White Power'.[7]

The debate about the impact of colonization also occurs within popular media and within learned journals and books with Kociumbas encapsulating this debate,

> writers are taken to task either for overemphasizing the cruelty and greed of Western colonizers, or for conveniently omitting documentary evidence that does not fit their damning hypotheses.[8]

as well as,

> lofty and often legalistic debates about assimilation, protection, unfree labor, population, Christianization, health, and most recently, historiography, have combined to obscure mass death and trauma, while also helping to silence or erase indigenous perspectives on these issues. . . . The obfuscation of genocide . . .[9]

In his paper on 'Colonisation, racism and indigenous health', Paradies in drawing from a number of authorities notes the ongoing ever-present nature of domination that is an inherent part of colonialism that contains a duality that oscillates between elimination and coercive exploitation.[10] This is an enduring element of the indigenous experience in Australia where indigenous populations have not only been reduced by disease and lethal violence by Europeans, but where Europeans have sought to introduce or consider insidious strategies to manage the indigenous population. These strategies have encompassed at various times eugenicist ideas to dissolve not only the familial bonds of indigenous Australians by taking children from their families, but also in advocating theories of racial dilution that would eventually eliminate an allegedly dying race. A similar situation was seen in case of indigenous communities in the Cape Colony, south-east Botswana and India (Viljoen, Ramsay and Ahmed in this volume). For the indigenous

Australians who lived a satisfying life materially and spiritually before the European invasion and in which it has been argued that excepting for that small element of Europeans who in 1800 were wealthy, Aboriginal Australian life was superior.[11] Aboriginal life was remarkable in regard to nutrition, health and freedom in comparison to the typical European peasant. The British arrival in 1788 ushered in a catastrophic epoch of misfortune, death and disease.

SMALLPOX

Judy Campbell, the noted Australian historian of the impact of disease upon Aboriginal Australia, wrote:

> Smallpox was the worst disease ever seen among indigenous Australians, and was the first and major single cause of the decline of Aboriginal populations on the mainland between 1780 and 1880. Ancient chains of social connections became chains of infection that caused the strange and terrifying disease, which undermined customary life before Europeans did.[12]

'"All dead, all dead!" and then hung his head in mournful silence' (Judge Advocate of the Colony), David Collins, relating in 1789 the impact of the smallpox epidemic upon an indigenous man known to him in present-day Sydney.[13] Smallpox would decimate the Aboriginal population of Australia as it had other indigenous populations once introduced by the colonizer. In a comment lacking empathy made in 1541, a Spaniard writer wrote of the indigenous Indian population of Mexico that 'they died in heaps, like bedbugs' and compared their catastrophe with the biblical plagues of Egypt.[14] Similar devastation was to occur soon after the establishment of the British penal colony in Australia.

A stark illustration of this epoch of misfortune is how in 1789, one year after the arrival of the First Fleet in what is now Sydney Harbour by the British soldiers, sailors and convicts, it was estimated by a number of observers that half of the original indigenous population of current-day Sydney and its environs had perished because of smallpox. John Maynard, Emeritus professor of Aboriginal History at the University of Newcastle and a Worimi man, notes,

> We've got several different accounts that said Aboriginal bodies were littering every crevice and cove of the harbour.[15]

Smallpox and its impact was written on by other colonial figures who wrote that it had in fact killed 80 per cent of the local Cadigal people in their heart-wrenching descriptions of bodies lying in heaps around Sydney.[16] In what was called the smallpox epidemic of 1789, Governor Phillip, the first European governor of the fledgling British convict colony, wrote to London.

> Not possible to determine the number of natives who were carried off by this fatal disorder. It must be great and judging from the information of the native now living with us, and who had recovered from the disorder before he was taken off, one half of those who inhabit this part of the country died . . . it must have spread to a considerable distance, as well inland as along the coast. We have seen the traces of it wherever we have been.[17]

Vice Admiral John Hunter, who would become the colony's second governor, also recorded the unprecedented loss in life of the indigenous population around Port Jackson, current-day Sydney.

> It was truly shocking to go round the coves of this harbour, which were formerly so much frequented by the natives, where in the caves of the rocks which used to shelter whole families in bad weather, were now to be seen, men, women and children laying dead.[18]

Reynolds, the respected Australian historian, devotes one full chapter to explore the contentious possibility and vigorously debated hypothesis that this calamitous smallpox outbreak, so soon after initial European settlement, could have been deliberate. Reynolds's argument draws upon comparative evidence of its use as a biological weapon in North America through the provision of blankets infected with smallpox being passed to Native Americans.[19] The impact of Smallpox on indigenous Australians was catastrophic. In the book American Holocaust it was argued that smallpox was the primary suspect in having reduced the indigenous American population by 90% after the arrival of Columbus. Smallpox's impact on Australia was to be similarly catastrophic.

Compelling arguments debating the possibility of this first outbreak being deliberately inflicted on indigenous Australians appear on both sides. That such an act could have occurred is still being argued while others argue that smallpox pre-existed the calamitous outbreaks brought upon by European settlement.

Broome argues that the disease had made an impact earlier with its arrival with Macassan traders early in the eighteenth century when trading with indigenous Australians in northern Australia and that the indicative pock marks of smallpox were noted on the faces when Europeans first arrived in Port Phillip Bay in 1804.[20] Campbell also argues that smallpox was introduced by visiting trepang fishermen from Macassar who traded with Aborigines in coastal northern Australia and spread inland.[21]

Support for this argument is made in noting that between 1780 and 1783 there was a smallpox epidemic in Sumatra causing death to about one-third of the population[22] and that this could have spread southwards through the archipelago. Campbell argues this was eventually transmitted by Macassans to the Cobourg Peninsula in northern Australia after presumably their annual fishing and trading visit.[23]

Another smallpox epidemic laid waste to great numbers of the indigenous population around Sydney and its environs in 1829–1831. Indigenous accounts of these epidemics noted that there were so many dead from the disease that they were left where they died and could not be properly disposed of in accordance with indigenous customs.[24]

The epidemic of 1829–1831 was possibly even more catastrophic with the *Journal of the Royal Society of NSW* reporting,

> All the very old men . . . say that . . . it followed down the rivers . . . laying its death clutches on every tribe . . . until the whole country became perfectly decimated . . . at last the death rate became so heavy . . . buying their bodies was no longer attempted . . . the whole atmosphere became tainted . . . from decomposing bodies.[25]

There was direct medical reporting of the 1829 epidemic of the significant death rates from Port Macquarie on the central north coast, north to Brisbane in current-day Queensland and spreading out from Bathurst in the NSW central west along the rivers leading to the Darling. Reports at the time noted up to 30% death rates around Bathurst while in the Western District of Victoria there were in some cases total depopulation of tribes and sub-tribes in which survivors coalesced into smaller bands.[26] Smallpox followed the epidemic patterns of the disease in Australia as it had with other exposed Aboriginal populations around the globe. As with other hunter gatherer societies, the impact of smallpox is particularly destructive on hands and feet with pustules cracking and destroying the limbs required for the population to secure food and water. The impact of smallpox on aboriginal peoples of North America corroborates the decimation of exposed Aboriginal populations around the globe including Australia. Between 1837 and 1839, for example, smallpox displayed a regional variance on the West Coast of the United States of mortality ranging from 25% to near total annihilation, ending in an entire death rate in excess of 50%.[27]

In killing large numbers of the indigenous population locally and at more distant locations, smallpox in effect aided the British colonization as it had, as Bennett argued, 'a catastrophic impact on their capacity to resist British expansion'.[28]

SEXUALLY TRANSMITTED VENEREAL DISEASES AND A CONTINUING HISTORY OF VIOLENCE AGAINST INDIGENOUS WOMEN

> What is clear is the presence particularly of gonorrhoea amongst convicts of the First and subsequent Fleets and amongst whalers and sealers off the south-eastern coasts . . . the introduction in the First Fleet, of considerable numbers discharged from British hospitals as suffering from incurable venereal diseases provided a certain infection.[29]

Before effective treatment was available it has been estimated that at least 10% of the adult population of England was infected with syphilis.[30] The spread of white settlement, in which sometimes small numbers of males who would seek sexual relationships with indigenous women by consent or rape, meant that considerable numbers of women could be exposed to the disease by relatively few white men.[31]

Sexually transmitted diseases were among the first of the European diseases introduced into Australia, with this arguably occurring with the arrival of the First Fleet at Sydney Cove in 1788. Within four years of the commencement of the new Colony by the British, both venereal syphilis (hereafter referred to as syphilis) and gonorrhoea were firmly established as an infectious health problem among the indigenous groups inhabiting the environs of the new colony.

Colonization introduced virulent sexual diseases among the indigenous population which was accompanied by an absence of respect for indigenous women that culminated in their abuse as sexual chattels or what we might even describe today as 'sex slaves'. The appalling sexual exploitation of Aboriginal women began from the earliest European colonization as well as the earliest trading settlements with women being bartered for food stuffs and alcohol. In Tasmania then Van Diemen's Land, women were bought for the carcass of a seal or kangaroo and kept in brutal inhumane circumstances.[32] Roberts-Thomson in his examination of the diaries of George Robinson notes the brutality and utter hopelessness for the indigenous women consigned to this life. Robinson wrote on Christmas Eve, 1829, the woman whom I sent to the hospital yesterday bore marks of the lash on her back and had contracted a loathsome disease.[33]

In another instance in a diary full of these tragic observations and writing some years later in 1843, Robinson wrote of a young female named Queen Clara who at twenty-four years of age had succumbed to 'sequelae of syphilis'.[34] Aboriginal women who had outlived their roles as concubines/sex slaves were on some occasion summarily killed and their bodies disposed of, while other young women would be separated from their people and be forced into prostitution.

Venereal disease was referred to obliquely and as noted before as that 'loathsome disease', with Robinson's diary noting how numbers of women were 'afflicted with a loathsome disorder' attributed to their cohabitation with European whalers at Adventure Bay.[35]

All too often these women were punished by their ostracization from their own people when they contracted syphilis.[36] Sexual crimes and abuse of women were widespread wherever the Europeans met with the indigenous inhabitants and especially so where European women were not present or only present in small numbers. Mulvaney notes the tremendous demographic discrepancies, for example in Central Australia, during the 1880s where even in 1901 there were only nine European women in Alice Springs.[37]

Aboriginal women met the sexual appetites, willingly or unwillingly, of the colonizers in these locations with one European police officer William Henry Willshire subsequently charged with murder, drew on divine justification for the seizure and sexual abuse of these indigenous women, stated;[38] 'Men would not remain so many years in a country like this if there were no women . . . and perhaps the Almighty meant them for use as He has placed them wherever the pioneers go . . . what I am speaking about is only natural . . . especially for men who are isolated . . . where women of all ages and sizes are running at large'.[39]

As in other locations where Europeans had conquered, colonized or coerced less powerful or organized states and indigenous populations, venereal disease was rapidly established. This was also the case when the British invaded Australia. Dowling argues that syphilis was prevalent in indigenous populations inland from littoral regions that had either been colonized or regularly visited by Europeans.[40] Dowling analysing the record of the Australian explorer Charles Sturt, and the pathological reactions he recorded when exploring Southeast Australia, argues there was clear evidence of an epidemic of sexually transmitted syphilis with no previous immunological exposure to the syphilis pathogen. Sturt on one occasion, after going beyond the limits of European settlement at that time and travelling via the Murrumbidgee and then Murray river system and exploring its tributaries, observed,

> Syphilis raged amongst them with fearful violence; many had lost their noses, and all glandular parts were considerably affected. I distributed some Turner's cerate to the women, but left Fraser to superintend its application. It could do no good, of course.[41]

Sturt argues in his record and Dowling concurs on the probability of the epidemiological spread of the syphilis was introduced by sealing and whaling ships on the southern coast of Australia. But if we look more closely at his comments in an aetiological and epidemiological context, several points emerge which support an epidemic disease, most likely syphilis. . . . The areas of the body involved according to Sturt's observations included integument tissue over much of the torso, as well as soft tissue and bone destruction of the nasal region. Sturt commented on blindness and lameness . . . destruction of the peri-nasal soft tissue and bone would indicate that the disease was in its tertiary stage. . . . The blindness . . . may have been the result of tertiary syphilis of the central nervous system (neurosyphilis) or interstitial keratitis, a condition of late congenital infection affecting mainly the 4 to 30 years age group. The dissemination of skin lesions is consistent with the primary and secondary stages of untreated syphilis. Foetal involvement also seems to be represented with infants displaying lesions to the surface of the body similar to adults.[42]

Dowling also offers bioarchaeological evidence to support his argument that Sturt was correct in his assessment of the prevalence of syphilis among the indigenous population of the inland waterway areas he was exploring. Furthermore, after Sturt's return to Sydney the superintendent of the Point McLeay mission settlement between 1859 and 1879 noted the testimony of the local indigenous people informing him that they had not known of the disease before advent of Europeans.[43] Extrapolating from Sturt's evidence would suggest that syphilis was introduced in the first decades of the 1800s from the coast of present-day South Australia where the whaling industry operated around the South Australian coast and the islands of Bass Strait and from there it spread upstream along the river systems.

Dowling notes that small base settlements were established on Kangaroo Island around this time and that sealers often landed on the mainland coast to kidnap indigenous women and girls euphemistically as 'wives' and slaves. This is supported by evidence from a number of sources including Captain Sutherland of the brig *Governor Macquarie* who in 1819 recorded in his diary at Kangaroo Island the depredations of the crews of the whaling ships after their mainland raids.

> They have carried their daring acts to extremes . . . seizing on the natives, particularly the women, and keeping them in a state of slavery, cruelly beating them on every trifling occasion, and when at last some of the marauders were taken off the island by an expedition from New South Wales, these women were landed on the main with their children and dogs, to procure a subsistence, not knowing how their own people would treat them after a long absence.[44]

It wasn't only brigands and whalers mistreating the women with the police provided extraordinary powers to seize individuals they suspected of having sexually transmitted venereal diseases. The police undertaking these seizures searched male and female Aboriginals alike with their unqualified diagnoses. Those seized and removed from their communities in remote Western Australia in 1911, for example, were led away shackled by neck chains which could only have the added effect of cross-infecting others if they did indeed have venereal disease and the oft mistaken condition of yaws. Prisoners often shackled to horses suffered horrendous injuries should the horse bolt or if they fell while crossing a water course, as well as instances of women being sexually abused while chained.[45] A West Australian police commissioner as recently as 1958 defended the use of neck shackles as something preferred by Aborigines.[46] In a number of Australian jurisdictions, including the state of Queensland, indigenous Australians suspected of having venereal disease could be detained on in a 'lock' hospital that quarantined them from both their local communities as well as the larger Australian community. Indigenous Queenslanders were between 1928 and 1945 confined on remote Fantome Island off the Queensland coast.[47]

VIOLENCE, DISEASE, *TERRA NULLIUS*, THE WHITE AUSTRALIA POLICY AND COLONIZATION

What is not in doubt though is that there existed a simmering propensity for lethality in early and later colonial European dealings with indigenous Australians. The introduction of diseases and its effect on the depopulation of indigenous Australia has been argued as seeking to distract and conceal the overarching impact of murder, massacre and sexual violence perpetrated against the indigenous population via what has been referred to as the 'Exotic disease theory' of population reduction.

Arguments upon the overstatement of disease as a factor in depopulation though are not as abundant as arguments maintaining the pivotal role of disease as the major factor in the death of indigenous Australians occasioned by the European invasion. The disease and epidemic arguments maintain that the number of indigenous Australians killed as a result of violence is likely 'to have been dwarfed by the spread of introduced diseases such as smallpox and respiratory diseases'.[48] Arguments concerning the role of disease usually maintain the probability of interactions between viral diseases such as smallpox and the bacterial infections brought by Europeans as being pivotal and

> that will increase mortality among immuno-compromised populations like the Aboriginal population exposed to exotic diseases for the first time.[49]

It is therefore important to note that there is not complete agreement on the severity of disease as being a major factor in indigenous population reduction. Some indigenous academics have argued that 'exotic disease theory may be considered as a Eurocentric ideological construct that preaches a cognitive imperialistic sermon of racial superiority' while obfuscating the impact of direct violence applied to the Aboriginal population.[50]

Indigenous Australian authorities challenging the extent of disease mortality explain this theory as follows:

> Exotic disease theory is the belief that Europeans and others unintentionally introduced diseases such as smallpox, measles, influenza, and syphilis with a result that large numbers of Indigenous people died because they had no immunity. Europeans did not succumb at the same rates because they had prior exposure which resulted in acquired immunity. The theory is used within the colonial narrative, as it is in other colonised states, to explain the rapid depopulation of Indigenous peoples in the face of European incursions into their country.[51]

What then of violence as a factor to explain indigenous depopulation? It is for this reason that it is important for this chapter to also address the violence Europeans applied against the indigenous population.

Disturbing reports on the quality of those sent by Britain to establish and maintain the colony can sometimes make for disturbing reading, especially so when considered against the backdrop that these colonizers and invaders from a vastly different society would soon be the interface with a culture largely isolated for upwards of 60,000 years. Military personnel were notorious according to the colony's second governor where he wrote in a dispatch to England in 1796, 'They are sent to guard and to keep in obedience . . . and yet we find among those safeguards men capable of corrupting the heart of the best disposed, and often superior in every species of infamy to the most expert in wickedness among the convicts'.[52]

The collision of the European settlers with indigenous Australians resulted in violent confrontations with a substantial and tragic record of massacres, murders, rape and other brutalities visited upon the original inhabitants by settlers, convicts, whalers, pastoralists, police, military as well as the use of indigenous levies against people from different tribal groups. Owen's 2016 work titled *Every mother's son is guilty* is a particularly searing account of the subjection of West Australia's indigenous population by colonial and early federation authorities and how relatively recent a great deal of this violence occurred with, for example, up to 300 indigenous West Australians killed during the 1926 Forrest River massacre.[53]

Europeans from the beginning believed themselves to be a civilizing influence upon the indigenous population. Governor Hunter being instructed to 'conciliate the affections of the Aborigines, to live in amity and kindness with them, and to prepare them for civilization'.[54] Despite some admonitions it became apparent from the very beginning that the closer the Aboriginal got to the 'civilizing European' the more degraded they became and how rapidly their population decreased. Catching a disease was not the only hazard in the early indigenous collision with the European invaders. One early instance of this civilizing influence involved Europeans murdering the family of a young Aboriginal girl so they could 'adopt' the girl.[55] The Europeans responded violently with countless atrocities should the Aboriginals dare to contest the European affronts against their way of life. Near the end of 1821, Rev. Mr Mansfield was told by one Aboriginal man, 'Black man die fast since white man came, old black man nigh all gone', with Rev. Mansfield ruminating on whether his religious society in London should rather be sending missionaries for the Europeans.[56]

The impunity with which the Europeans dealt violence to the Aborigines was noted in an early history of the Australian colonies:

> Governors had tempered, if they could not quell, the cruel blasts of persecution which raged over the land. But on disappearance of the Governor's active control, there arose a confidence that the Executive Government, dependent on the people's voice, would not dare, if even it should desire, to mete out equal justice to the two races. Dwellers in the outlying Districts denounced as impertinent any questionings as to the number, or the manner of the violent deaths of natives on their cattle stations.[57]

The indigenous population was not protected or policed effectively, with police either delivering this violence themselves or being complicit with other parties.[58] At a select committee of the Queensland Legislative Assembly querying what had occurred to the Aboriginal community, Captain John Coley informed:

Chairman: On the Kilcoy Station owned by Mr. Evan Mackenzie, there were two white men killed . . . and their retaliation was very severe on the blacks – they destroyed hundreds of them. In what way?
Coley: By shooting and poisoning them.
Chairman: What with?
Coley: With strychnine and arsenic, in flour.[59]

Except for some significant matters, such as the Myall Creek massacre of twenty-eight Aborigines where two white settlers were convicted and hanged for their crimes, there was a remarkable indifference to the plight of the Aborigines or the crimes against them.[60]

Similar to other colonialist settler societies, such as the United States, and conducive with the doctrine of *Terra Nullius*, the British did not recognize the indigenous inhabitants who had been in Australia for 60,000 years and viewed them as primitive and without legal rights. The British concept of *Terra Nullius* effectively rendered the Australian landmass as vacant of humanity prior to European arrival. Furthermore, there was a belief from the colonists that these feckless, immature and vulnerable indigenous people in

Australia and elsewhere were dying out 'requiring only some perfunctory palliation of their passing'.[61]

Similarly, influential was the racism explicitly evident in both the colonial period and after Australian Federation, when a 'White Australia' Policy was the officially sanctioned position of the government from 1901 to 1975.[62] Aboriginal Australians were not allowed to vote until the 1960s with the Australian state of Queensland being the last state to grant this right in 1965[63] while the first ever federal minister for Indigenous Affairs who was an indigenous Australian did not occur until 2019.[64] *Terra Nullius* was not fully rejected until a High Court decision in 1992. British attitudes contained admixtures of Social Darwinism, with a belief that because the Aborigines were hunter-gatherers, they did not produce any profit from the land through agriculture or pastoralism and, therefore, the seizure of the lands could be justified.[65] One newspaper referred to the indigenous inhabitants as 'dogs and horses . . . irreclaimable brute[s] . . . the one argument a blackfellow understands is that delivered from a rifle or six shooter'.[66]

INDIGENOUS MENTAL HEALTH, SUICIDE, CHRONIC DISEASE AND COLONIZATION

Mental health issues remain a major health problem with indigenous Australians. Aboriginal youth suicide has been and remains a significant problem into the second decade of the new millennium. Sherwood, an indigenous health professional, argues that Aboriginal Australians have not been the recipients of a balanced and accurate account of the history of colonization in Australia.[67] Sherwood, citing Czyzewski, notes that 'colonization is a determinant of health and requires appreciation that it is not a finished project'.[68]

Colonization is a determinant of indigenous health in Australia and the continuing marginalization and discrimination of Aboriginal Australians following the British invasion and colonization in 1788 have resulted in their socioeconomic disadvantage. This disadvantage is in turn linked to their historically dismal health outcomes and an intergenerational impact should be no surprise.[69] Indigenous Australians have heightened prevalence of risk factors for chronic diseases that do not present among non-Aboriginal Australians at younger ages and with greater frequency.[70] Similarly, poorer mental health outcomes also exist.

In 2019, a coronial inquiry into the deaths of thirteen young indigenous people in the remote Kimberley region involved an enquiry that drew evidence from several remote indigenous communities investigating the suicide of indigenous persons as young as ten years of age. This tragedy, stated the coroner, had been shaped by 'the crushing effects of intergenerational trauma'.[71] The 2019 coronial investigation into these continuing mental health problems significantly found many of the same unsolved problems identified in the previous 2008 coronial investigation into the deaths of twenty-two indigenous Australians in much of the same remote Kimberley region of Western Australia.[72]

CONCLUSION

This chapter has cast a broad view over the history of the colonization of the Australian continent by Europeans from 1788 onwards and the dire impact of this colonization in terms of the destruction of the indigenous societies that had lasted for the previous 60,000 years or so as a result of introduced European diseases and European policy that amplified this impact. What has become apparent is that arguments that conflate disease and European colonization seem to be arguably correct in their premise that 'colonization is a determinant of Indigenous Health'.

Furthermore, the chapter has shown how the belief in *Terra Nullius* the White Australia Policy and related government policies and actions out of either omission or active intrusion and violence have served to demoralize the indigenous population of Australia and contribute to historic and contemporary poor health outcomes. Historically, the evidence strongly indicates the catastrophic nature of introduced diseases while other records noted throughout the chapter have identified the concurrent lethality of violence directed towards indigenous Australians by the colonizers. Indigenous Australians have been subjected to numerous enquiries and interventions since 1788 most lacking any of their real involvement. While some have been overtly paternalistic and others less so there is some cause for cautious optimism. Recent debate on the Australian Constitutional recognition of indigenous Australians as well as activism to improve indigenous health, education and employment is contemporaneous and ongoing. The recent appointment of the first Federal Indigenous Affairs Minister who is indigenous himself is significant.

NOTES

1. Blainey, *The Story of Australia's People – The Rise and Fall of Ancient Australia,* 3–18.
2. British Broadcasting Corporation (BBC), *Rio Tinto Chief Jean-Sebastien Jacques to Quit Over Aboriginal Cave Destruction,* https://www.bbc.com/news/world australia-54112991, 11 September, 2020.
3. Australian Broadcasting Corporation (ABC), *Solar Farm Developer METKA EGN Fined $1,500.00 for Destroying Hundreds of Indigenous Artefacts.* https://www.abc.net.au/news/2021-01-29/indigenous-artefacts-destroyed-in-solar-farm-development/13103390, January 2021.

4. British Broadcasting Corporation (BBC), *Rio Tinto Chief Jean-Sebastien Jacques to Quit Over Aboriginal Cave Destruction.* https://www.bbc.com/news/world-australia-54112991, 11 September, 2020.

5. Evans-Campbell, T., 'Historical Trauma in American Indian/Native Alaska communities: A Multilevel Framework for Exploring Impacts on Individuals, Families, and Communities', *Journal of Interpersonal Violence,* 23(3), 2008, 316–338.

6. Australian Financial Review (AFR), *Communications Minister urges ABC to drop Invasion Day References,* https://www.afr.com/politics/federal/government-urges-abc-to-drop-invasion-day-references-20210125-p56wjx, 25 January 2021.

7. McKenzie, N. & Tozer, J. 'Neo-Nazis Go Bush: Grampians Gathering Highlights Rise of Australia's Far Right', *Sydney Morning Herald,* https://www.smh.com.au/politics/federal/neo-nazis-go-bush-grampians-gathering-highlights-rise-of-australia-s-far-right-20210127-p56xbf.html, 27 January 2021.

8. Kociumbas, J. 'Genocide and Modernity in Colonial Australia, 1788–1850', in Moses, A.D. (ed.), *Genocide and Settler Society – Frontier Violence and Stolen Indigenous Children in Australian History* (New York: Berghahn Books, 2012), 98.

9. Kociumbas, 'Genocide and Modernity in Colonial Australia, 1788–1850', in Moses (ed.), *Genocide and Settler Society – Frontier Violence and Stolen Indigenous Children in Australian History,* 78.

10. Paradies, Y. 'Colonisation, Racism and Indigenous Health', *Journal of Popular Research,* Springer Science Online, no. 33 (2016): 83–96.

11. Blainey *The Story of Australia's People – The Rise and Fall of Ancient Australia,* 213.

12. Campbell, J. *Invisible Invaders: Smallpox and Other Diseases in Aboriginal Australia, 1780–1880* (Melbourne University Press, 2002), 25.

13. National Museum of Australia (NMA), *Smallpox Epidemic–1789: Smallpox Breaks Out in Sydney,* https://www.nma.gov.au/defining-moments/resources/smallpox-epidemic, 12 November 2020.

14. *Plague, Pestilence and Pandemic – Voices from History,* Furtado, P. (ed.) (Thames & Hudson, 2021), 105.

15. Thorpe, N., Willis, O., & Smith, C., 'Dear Devil: The sickness that changed Australia', Australian Broadcasting Corporation (ABC, 2022) https://www.abc.net.au/news/health/2021-06-07/patient-zero-smallpox-outbreak-of-1789/100174988

16. Clark, A., *Making Australian History* (Australia: Vintage Books, 2022), 45–46.

17. New South Wales Government, 'Historical Records New South Wales, Vol. 1, 1783–92', Government Printer, 308.

18. Thorpe, N., Willis, O., & Smith, C., 'Dear Devil: The Sickness that Changed Australia', Australian Broadcasting Corporation (ABC, 2022) https://www.abc.net.au/news/health/2021-06-07/patient-zero-smallpox-outbreak-of-1789/100174988

19. Reynolds, H., *An Indelible Stain – The Question of Genocide in Australia's History* (Melbourne: Viking Books, 2001), 35–48.

20. Broome, R., *Aboriginal Australians* (Allen and Unwin, Sydney, 2019, Fifth Edition), 13.

21. Campbell, J., *Invisible Invaders: Smallpox and Other Diseases in Aboriginal Australia, 1780–1880,* (Melbourne University Press, 2002).

22. Hopkins, D.R., *Princes and Peasants: Smallpox in History* (University of Chicago Press, Chicago, 1983).

23. Campbell, J. *Invisible Invaders: Smallpox and Other Diseases in Aboriginal Australia 1780–1880* (Melbourne: Melbourne University Press), 2002.

24. Broome, *Aboriginal Australians,* 64.

25. Beveridge, P, 'On the Aborigines', *Journal of the Royal Society of NSW,* 1883, 35.

26. Butlin, N. *Our Original Aggression* (George, Allen & Unwin, 1983), 64.

27. Butlin, N. *Our Original Aggression* (George, Allen & Unwin, 1983), 64–65.

28. Bennett, M.J. 'Smallpox and Cowpox under the Southern Cross: the smallpox epidemic of 1789 and the advent of vaccination in colonial Australia', *Bulletin of the History of Medicine*, Vol. 83, no. 1 (2009): 39.

29. Butlin, N. *Our Original Aggression* (George, Allen & Unwin, 1983), 77.

30. Campbell, J. *Invisible Invaders: Smallpox and Other Diseases in Aboriginal Australia 1780–1880* (Melbourne University Press, 2002), 17.

31. Butlin, N. *Our Original Aggression,* (George, Allen & Unwin, 1983), 78.

32. Manning Clark, *Manning Clark's History of Australia – Abridged by Michael Cathcart,* 121.

33. Roberts-Thomson, P.J. 'Impact of Introduced Disease into Tasmanian Aboriginal Populations and its Role in Depopulation', Papers and Proceedings: *Tasmanian Historical Research Association,* Vol.61, Issue 2/3, December 2014, 124, 125, 119–137.

34. Roberts-Thomson, 'Impact of Introduced Disease into Tasmanian Aboriginal Populations and its Role in Depopulation', Papers and Proceedings: *Tasmanian Historical Research Association,* Vol.61, Issue 2/3, December 2014, 124,125, 119–137.

35. Roberts-Thomson, 'Impact of Introduced Disease into Tasmanian Aboriginal Populations and its Role in Depopulation', Papers and Proceedings: *Tasmanian Historical Research Association,* Vol.61, Issue 2/3, December 2014, 124, 125, 119–137.

36. Manning Clark, *Manning Clark's History of Australia – Abridged by Michael Cathcart,* 309.

37. Mulvaney, D.J. *Encounters in Place: Outsiders and Aboriginal Australians 1606–1985* (University of Queensland Press, 1989), 126.

38. Mulvaney, *Encounters in Place: Outsiders and Aboriginal Australians 1606–1985*, 124.

39. Mulvaney, *Encounters in Place: Outsiders and Aboriginal Australians 1606–1985,* 126–127.

40. Dowling, P., 'What Charles Sturt Saw in 1830 – Syphilis Beyond the Colonial Boundaries?' *Health and History,* Vol. 19, no. 1 (2017): 44–59.

41. Sturt, C., *Two Expeditions into the Interior of Southern Australia,* Vol. 2 (London: Smith, Elder and Co, 1830, [facsimile copy] Sydney: Doubleday, 1982).

42. Dowling, 'What Charles Sturt Saw in 1830 – Syphilis Beyond the Colonial Boundaries?' *Health and History,* Vol. 19, no. 1 (2017): 47–48.

43. Dowling, 'What Charles Sturt Saw in 1830 – Syphilis Beyond the Colonial Boundaries?' *Health and History,* Vol. 19, no. 1 (2017): 53.

44. Summers, J. "Colonial Race Relations", in E. Richards (ed.), *Flinders History of South Australia. Social History* (Adelaide: Wakefield Press, 1986), 285.

45. Mulvaney, *Encounters in Place: Outsiders and Aboriginal Australians 1606 –1985,* 185–189.

46. Mulvaney, *Encounters in Place: Outsiders and Aboriginal Australians 1606 –1985,* 188.

47. Parsons, M., 'Fantome Island Lock Hospital and Aboriginal Venereal Disease Sufferers 1928–1945', *Health and History,* Vol. 10, no. 1 (2008), Australia and New Zealand Society of the History of Medicine, Inc.

48. Hunter, B.H and Carmody, J. 'Estimating the Aboriginal Population in Early Colonial Australia: The Role of Chickenpox Reconsidered', *Australian Economic History Review,* Vol. 55, no. 2 (July 2015): 122.

49. Hunter and Carmody, 'Estimating the Aboriginal Population in Early Colonial Australia: The Role of Chickenpox Reconsidered', *Australian Economic History Review,* Vol. 55, no. 2 (July 2015): 112.

50. Blyton, G. 'Seeds of Myth: Exotic Disease Theory and Deconstructing the Australian Narratives of Indigenous Depopulation', *Australian Journal of Indigenous Education*, Vol. 38, Supplement (2009): 17.

51. Blyton, 'Seeds of Myth: Exotic Disease Theory and Deconstructing the Australian Narratives of Indigenous Depopulation', *Australian Journal of Indigenous Education*, Vol. 38, Supplement (2009): 17–18.

52. 'Historical Records of Australia, Series 1', Watson, F. (ed.), Government Printer, Sydney, New South Wales, 1915, 574.

53. Owen, C. *'Every Mother's Son is Guilty': Policing the Kimberley Frontier of Western Australia 1882–1905* (Apollo Books, 2016).

54. Manning Clark, C.H. *Manning Clark's History of Australia – Abridged by Michael Cathcart* (Melbourne University Press, Melbourne, 1993), 23.

55. Manning Clark, *Manning Clark's History of Australia – Abridged by Michael Cathcart,* 23.

56. Manning Clark, *Manning Clark's History of Australia – Abridged by Michael Cathcart,* 96.

57. Rusden G.W., *History of Australia* (Chapman and Hall, 1883), 235.

58. Richards, J, *The Secret War: A True History of Queensland's Native Police* (University of Queensland Press, 2008).

59. Queensland Legislative Assembly, *Report from the Select Committee on the Native Police Force and the Condition of the Aborigines Generally: Together with the Proceedings of the Committee and Minutes of Evidence* (Brisbane: Fairfax and Belbridge Printers, 1861), 19. National Library of Australia, https://nla.gov.au/nla.obj-52862431/view?partId=nla.obj-103371174#page/n19/mode/1up (image 37).

60. National Museum of Australia (NMA), *Smallpox Epidemic–1789: Smallpox Breaks Out in* Sydney. https://www.nma.gov.au/defining-moments/resources/smallpox-epidemic, 12 November 2020.

61. Anderson, W. 'The Colonial Medicine of Settler States: Comparing Histories of Indigenous Health', *Aboriginal Health and History,* Vol. 9, no. 2 (2007); Bates, D. *The Passing of the Aborigines: A Lifetimes Spent Among the Natives of Australia* (London: John Murray, 1947); Hoffman, F.L. 'Are the Indians Dying Out?', *American Journal of Public Health,* Vol. 20, no. 6 (1930); McGregor, R. *Imagined Destinies: Aboriginal Australians and the Doomed Race Theory, 1880–1939* (Melbourne: Melbourne University Press, 1997).

62. National Archives of Australia. *The Immigration Restriction Act, 1901.* https://www.naa.gov.au/explore-collection/immigration-and-citizenship/immigration-restriction-act-1901. 2020.

63. Australian Electoral Commission (AEC), *Electoral Milestones for Indigenous Australians,* https://www.aec.gov.au/indigenous/milestones.htm, 12 November 2020 (accessed 12 January 2021).

64. Australian Electoral Commission (AEC), *Electoral Milestones for Indigenous Australians,* https://www.aec.gov.au/indigenous/milestones.htm, 12 November 2020 (accessed 12 January 2021).

65. Bryett K, Harrison A & Shaw J, *The Role and Functions of the Police in Australia* (New South Wales: Butterworths, 1994).

66. Grassby A & Hill M, *Six Australian Battlefields: The Black Resistance to Invasion and the White Struggle against Colonial Oppression* (Sydney: Angus & Robertson, 1988), 35.

67. Sherwood J, 'Colonisation – It's Bad for Your Health: The Context of Aboriginal Health', *Contemporary Nurse,* Vol. 46, no. 1 (2013): 28–40.

68. Sherwood, 'Colonisation – It's Bad for Your Health: The Context of Aboriginal Health', *Contemporary Nurse,* Vol. 46, no. 1 (2013): 28–40.

69. Dudgeon, P., Wright, M., Paradies, Y., Garvey, D. & Walker, I.. 'The Social, Cultural and Historical Context of Aboriginal and Torres Strait Islander Australians'. in Purdie, N, Dudgeon & P, Walker R (eds.), *Working Together: Aboriginal and Torres Strait Islander Mental Health and Wellbeing Principles and Practice* (Canberra: Australian Department of Health and Ageing, 2010).

70. Gubhaju L, McNamara BJ, Banks E, 'The Overall Health and Risk Factor Profile of Australian Aboriginal and Torres Strait Islander Participants from the 45 and Up Study', *BMC Public Health,* Vol. 13, no. 1 (2013): 661.

71. Australian Broadcasting Corporation (ABC), *Cluster of Kimberley Child Suicides Blamed by Coroner on 'Tragic Intergenerational Trauma'*, https://www.abc.net.au/news/2019-02-*07/kimberley-child-suicides-blamed-on-inter-generational-trauma/10783016*, 7 February, 2019.

72. Australian Broadcasting Corporation (ABC), *Cluster of Kimberley Child Suicides Blamed by Coroner on 'Tragic Intergenerational Trauma'*, https://www.abc.net.au/news/2019-02-07/kimberley-child-suicides-blamed-on-inter-generational-trauma/10783016, 7 February, 2019.

BIBLIOGRAPHY

Anderson, Warwick. 'The Colonial Medicine of Settler States: Comparing Histories of Indigenous Health', *Aboriginal Health and History,* Vol. 9 (2), 2007.

Australian Broadcasting Corporation (ABC). *Cluster of Kimberley Child Suicides Blamed by Coroner on 'Tragic Intergenerational Trauma',* https://www.abc.net.au/news/2019-02-07/kimberley-child-suicides-blamed-on-inter-generational-trauma/10783016, February, 2019.

Australian Broadcasting Corporation (ABC). *Solar Farm Developer METKA EGN Fined $1,500.00 for Destroying Hundreds of Indigenous Artefacts,* https://www.abc.net.au/news/2021-01-29/indigenous-artefacts-destroyed-in-solar-farm-development/13103390, January 2021.

Australian Electoral Commission (AEC). '*Electoral Milestones for Indigenous Australians*', https://www.aec.gov.au/indigenous/milestones.htm, November 2020.

Australian Financial Review (AFR). *Communications Minister Urges ABC to Drop Invasion Day References,* https://www.afr.com/politics/federal/government-urges-abc-to-drop-invasion-day-references-20210125-p56wjx, 25 January 2021.

Bates, Daisy. *The Passing of the Aborigines: A Lifetimes Spent Among the Natives of Australia,* John Murray, London, 1947.

Bennett, Michael J. 'Smallpox and Cowpox under the Southern Cross: The Smallpox Epidemic of 1789 and the Advent of Vaccination in Colonial Australia', *Bulletin of the History of Medicine,* Vol. 83, no. 1 (2009).

Beveridge, Peter. 'On the Aborigines', *Journal of the Royal Society of NSW* (1883): 35.

Blainey Geoffrey. *The Story of Australia's People—The Rise and Fall of Ancient Australia.* Viking, Australia, 2020.

Blyton, Greg. 'Seeds of Myth: Exotic Disease Theory and Deconstructing the Australian Narratives of Indigenous Depopulation', *Australian Journal of Indigenous Education,* Vol. 38, Supplement (2009): 17–18.

British Broadcasting Corporation (BBC). *Rio Tinto chief Jean-Sebastien Jacques to quit over Aboriginal Cave Destruction,* https://www.bbc.com/news/world-australia-54112991, 11 September 2020.

Broome Richard. *Aboriginal Australians 5th Edition.* Allen and Unwin, Sydney, 2019.

Bryett Keith, Arch Harrison, and John Shaw. *The Role and Functions of the Police in Australia.* Butterworths, New South Wales, 1994.

Butlin, Noel. *Our Original Aggression,* George, Allen & Unwin, Australia, 1983.

Campbell, Judith. *Invisible Invaders: Smallpox and Other Diseases in Aboriginal Australia, 1780–1880.* Melbourne University Press, 2002.

Clark, Anna. *Making Australian History,* Vintage Books, Australia, 2022.

Dowling Peter. 'What Charles Sturt Saw in 1830 – Syphilis Beyond the Colonial Boundaries?' *Health and History,* Vol. 19, No. 1 (2017), pp. 44–59.

Dudgeon, Pat, Michael Wright, Yin Paradies, Darren Garvey, and Iain Walker. 'The Social, Cultural and Historical Context of Aboriginal and Torres Strait Islander

Australians'. In N. Purdie, P. Dudgeon, and R. Walker (eds.), *Working Together: Aboriginal and Torres Strait Islander Mental Health and Wellbeing Principles and Practice*. Australian Department of Health and Ageing, Canberra, 2010.

Evans-Campbell, Teresa. 'Historical Trauma in American Indian/Native Alaska communities: A Multilevel Framework for Exploring Impacts on Individuals, Families, and Communities', *Journal of Interpersonal Violence,* 23(3), 2008, 316–338.

Furtado, Peter, ed. *Plague, Pestilence and Pandemic—Voices from History,* Thames & Hudson, UK, 2021.

Grassby Al, and Marji Hill. *Six Australian Battlefields: The Black Resistance to Invasion and the White Struggle Against Colonial Oppression*. Angus & Robertson, Sydney, 1988, 35.

Gubhaju Lina, Bridgett J. McNamara, and Emily Banks. 'The Overall Health and Risk Factor Profile of Australian Aboriginal and Torres Strait Islander Participants from the 45 and Up Study', *BMC Public Health,* Vol. 13, no. 1 (2013): 661.

Hoffman, Frederick L. 'Are the Indians Dying Out?', *American Journal of Public Health,* Vol. 20, no. 6 (1930).

Hopkins, Donald R. *Princes and Peasants: Smallpox in History*. University of Chicago Press, Chicago, 1983.

Hunter, Boyd, and John Carmody. 'Estimating the Aboriginal Population in Early Colonial Australia: The Role of Chickenpox Reconsidered', *Australian Economic History Review,* Vol. 55, no. 2 (July 2015).

Kociumbas, Jan. 'Genocide and Modernity in Colonial Australia, 1788–1850', in Moses, A.D (ed.), *Genocide and Settler Society – Frontier Violence and Stolen Indigenous Children in Australian History*, Berghahn Books, New York, 2012.

Manning Clark, and Charles Hope. *Manning Clark's History of Australia – abridged by Michael Cathcart.* Melbourne University Press, Australia, 1997.

McGregor, Russell. *Imagined Destinies: Aboriginal Australians and the Doomed Race Theory, 1880–1939*. Melbourne University Press, Melbourne, 1997.

McKenzie Nick and Joel Tozer. 'Neo-Nazis Go Bush: Grampians Gathering Highlights Rise of Australia's Far Right', *Sydney Morning Herald,* https://www.smh.com.au/politics/federal/neo-nazis-go-bush-grampians-gathering-highlights-rise-of-australia-s-far-right-20210127-p56xbf.html, 27 January 2021.

Mulvaney, Derek John. *Encounters in Place: Outsiders and Aboriginal Australians 1606–1985*. University of Queensland Press, 1989, 126.

National Archives of Australia. *The Immigration Restriction Act, 1901*. https://www.naa.gov.au/explore-collection/immigration-and-citizenship/immigration-restriction-act-1901. 2020.

National Museum of Australia (NMA). *Smallpox Epidemic–1789: Smallpox Breaks Out in Sydney,* https://www.nma.gov.au/defining-moments/resources/smallpox-epidemic, 12 November 2020.

New South Wales Government. 'Historical Records New South Wales, Vol. 1, 1783–92', Government Printer.

Owen, Chris. *'Every Mother's Son is Guilty': Policing the Kimberley Frontier of Western Australia 1882–1905*. Apollo Books, Australia, 2016.

Parsons, Meg. 'Fantome Island Lock Hospital and Aboriginal Venereal Disease Sufferers 1928–1945', *Health and History,* Vol. 10, no. 1 (2008), Australia and New Zealand Society of the History of Medicine, Inc.

Paradies, Yin. 'Colonisation, racism and indigenous health', *Journal of Popular Research*, Springer Science Online (33), 2016, 83–96.

Queensland Legislative Assembly. '*Report from the Select Committee on the Native Police Force and the Condition of the Aborigines Generally: Together with the Proceedings of the Committee and Minutes of Evidence*' 1861. Fairfax and Belbridge Printers, Brisbane, 19, National Library of Australia, https://nla.gov.au/nla.obj-52862431/view?partId=nla.obj-103371174#page/n19/mode/1up (image 37).

Reynolds, Henry. *An Indelible Stain – The Question of Genocide in Australia's History.* Viking Books, Melbourne, 2001.

Richards, Jonathan. *The Secret War: A True History of Queensland's Native Police,* University of Queensland Press, Australia, 2008.

Roberts-Thomson, Peter J. 'Impact of Introduced Disease into Tasmanian Aboriginal Populations and its Role in Depopulation', Papers and Proceedings: *Tasmanian Historical Research Association,* Vol.61, no. 2/3 (December 2014).

Rusden George William. *History of Australia.* Chapman and Hall, Melbourne, Australia, 1883.

Sherwood Juanita, 'Colonisation – It's Bad for Your Health: The Context of Aboriginal Health', *Contemporary Nurse,* Vol. 46, no. 1 (2013).

Sturt, Charles. *Two Expeditions into the Interior of Southern Australia,* Vol. 2. Smith, Elder and Co, London, 1830, [facsimile copy] Sydney: Doubleday, 1982.

Summers, John. "Colonial Race Relations", in E. Richards (ed.), *Flinders History of South Australia. Social History.* Wakefield Press, Adelaide, 1986.

Thorpe, Nakari, Olivia Willis, and Carl Smith. 'Dear Devil: The Sickness that Changed Australia', Australian Broadcasting Corporation (ABC, 2022), https://www.abc.net.au/news/health/2021-06-07/patient-zero-smallpox-outbreak-of-1789/100174988

Watson, Frederick, ed. 'Historical Records of Australia, Series 1'. Government Printer, Sydney, New South Wales, 1915,

Chapter 11

Epidemic and the Raj

Locating Malarial Fever in Colonial Bengal

Arabinda Samanta

Scholars have emphasized a close correlation between cholera and military conquest in early colonial India.[1] Cholera epidemic of nineteenth-century India, it has been argued, came close on the heels of the most decisive phase of British imperial expansion. The arrival of the epidemic in western India in 1818 coincided in point of time with the decisive defeat of the Marathas and the extinction of sustained military opposition to British power. Thus, linkage between the cholera epidemic and the political conquest, it is argued, was not fortuitous. Was there any such correlation between epidemic malaria and the British conquest of Bengal? To put it more directly, who was responsible for the outbreak of epidemic fever in Bengal? Admittedly, the etiological intelligence is divided. The predisposing causes, it has been argued, were already there in the Bengali countryside, especially in the appalling insanitary condition of the villages and in the poor sense of health and hygiene of the villagers. Still, one has to look for the proximate causes that aggravated the situation and rendered the possibility of the disease into an absolute certainty. And this inevitably calls into question the role of the Raj.

In this chapter, I shall argue that the nineteenth-century British commercial and political intervention in Bengal and the subsequent creation of colonial infrastructures annihilated the geographical barriers. Roads, railways, ports, mine compounds, plantations – all the new colonial spaces, a concomitant result of colonial economic penetration – as also the system of labour migration, military recruitment and civilian administration enhanced, as it did, internal mobility of people. It stirred up the hitherto endemic property of a disease and disseminated it in such a scale that its endemic property turned out to be an epidemic reality. Colonial labour recruitment policies tended to impinge on the health of workers and the communities from which they were drawn. Insanitary conditions emanating from stagnant rivers around homestead, in mine compounds and on plantations created a microenvironment, immensely favourable for mosquito breeding and spreading malaria in the locality. The expansion of irrigation canals and the construction of railway embankment – all corollaries to colonialism – created habitats, favourable for malaria-carrying mosquitoes. Poor management of natural calamities like flood and drought and substitution of food crops by commercial crops were much enmeshed in the very nature of the colonial conquest of Bengal and the ecological changes brought under the colonial rule. Introduction of new infrastructural changes and alterations in the geographical landscape led to the emergence of 'breeding grounds' for existing diseases to re-emerge, aggravating public health and sanitation concerns within British-controlled territories in South Africa and India (Steere-Williams, Dey, Ahmed and Samanta in this volume).

RAILROADS AND EMBANKMENTS

When the outbreak of epidemic malaria first drew interested attention in the early 1860s, the disease was ascribed to the construction of railway embankment. The principal protagonist of this theory was Raja Digambar Mitra, the Indian member of the first committee appointed by the government in 1863 to enquire into the causes of the epidemic.

Mitra referred to cases of continuous line of villages where severe type of fever broke out as and when the railway embankment had progressed along their borders.[2] Mitra asserted that the construction of roads and railway embankments obstructed drainage, and as a result, certain type of waterlogging followed. Stagnant pools were particularly conducive to the multipled breeding of anopheles mosquitoes, the carrier of malaria. The result was a proleferation of devastating fever.[3]

Mitra's embankment theory of malaria found ready acceptance among the indigenous community, for, under it, the colonial government could be blamed for causing the mischief. The *Hindoo Patriot* published a series of articles defending the arguments of Raja Digambar Mitra.[4] Contrary to Mitra's position, a sizeable section of British administrators took pain to shift the emphasis elsewhere. The British administrators, decidedly supported by a section of medical officers, sanitation inspectors and public health engineers, sought to shout down through medical jargon the most powerful arguments in the embankment theory. The commissioner of Burdwan Division, for instance, reported in 1869 that in the Burdwan district, the railways and the roads were not believed by the local officers to have had any interference with the general health of the people.[5] Professional examination of each of the roads, supposedly obstructed drainage, was undertaken by government engineers, and they reported that 'roads and railroads have not obstructed the drainage of the country and thereby contributed to the epidemic fever'.[6]

Nevertheless, received wisdom tells us that pools and swamps were closely associated with railway construction and embankment along the river lines of Bengal. It is difficult to deny that the proliferation of malarial fever in Burdwan and the adjacent districts was largely owing to deficient sanitary arrangement during the aggregation of labour for embankment work. W. W. Clemesha, sanitary commissioner with the Government of India, admitted in 1917 two important things. First, railways authorities often incurred unnecessary expenditure by not taking into consideration expert advice and making adequate sanitary arrangements for the protection of their working staff in unhealthy districts. Consequently, large cases of sickness, death or desertion of the labour did occur. Second, alterations in the natural conditions of a locality caused by the construction of borrow pits, and the blocking of drainage with embankments, sometimes occasioned ill health of the rural population.[7] There could be no doubt, Clemesha argued, that in certain cases, the advent of a railway had resulted in a marked deterioration in the health of the community, which it served. It was fairly certain, he concluded, that the extraordinary epidemic of malaria, which occurred in the Lower Bengal, was 'due to the construction and opening of the railway between Calcutta and Burdwan'.[8]

Dr Christopher and Dr Bentley, two noted British malariologists, had argued in 1909 almost in the same vein.[9] According to them, labour aggregation with all its attendant conditions appeared to provide 'the key to the riddle of epidemic malaria in Bengal'. In fact, whenever the undertaking of large projects in a malarious district involved the employment of huge labourers and the establishment of labour camps, one could find the malarial incidence very high and the virulence of the infection unusually great. This was because when the victims returned to their homes sick, deserting or dismissed, they were replaced by other in whom the process was repeated and virulent malaria was, thus, disseminated in all directions.[10]

While opinions differed among the doctors, sanitation inspectors and civilians on the extent and nature of harm the embankments caused to the civil population, the indigenous people themselves were unequivocal in pointing their accusing fingers to the Raj. Volumes of vernacular literary tracts throughout the second half of the nineteenth and first half of the twentieth centuries poured forth anguished venom against the embankment. In 1917, one Karali Charan Ray, for instance, published a book of poem, *Bange Malaria*, which highlighted the pitiable plight of villagers afflicted by epidemic malaria.[11] Ray contended that expansion of railways had spread malaria in Bengal. In 1924, Haridhan Bandyopadhyay published a Bengali drama, *Banglar Shatru*, in which he argued that embankments were responsible for spreading malaria in the country.[12] Such examples proliferate.

INDIGENOUS WATER MANAGEMENT PRACTICES

It is, however, pertinent at this juncture to look at the traditional irrigation system in Bengal to comprehend the colonial renderings of causation of the disease. In fact, the most debated agenda of the past decade of the Raj in Bengal had been the 'decadence', 'decay' and 'death' of the Bengal delta followed by the degradation of its river system. The writings of Sir William Willcocks, C. A. Bentley, C. Adams Williams, Radha Kamal Mukherji, S. C. Majumdar, M. N. Saha and many others point to a period of ecological disaster.[13] In 1930, Sir William Willcocks, one of the empire's most celebrated hydraulic engineers, delivered a series of lectures on the rivers of Bengal at Calcutta University. He questioned the familiar colonial route for hydraulic manipulation through canal irrigation in the region and advocated for the traditional practice of 'overflow irrigation'.[14] It referred to a system by which the nutrient-rich, silt-laden monsoon floodwaters from the upper regions of various rivers flowing into Bengal were distributed evenly over the delta watering, and more importantly fertilizing fields, spreading fish over the countryside and sweeping away the mosquito population that used to spread malaria. Willcocks argued that one of the major features of flood irrigation practiced by the 'ancient kings' in Bengal delta was its importance as a fertilizing agent and not just a source of water. Moreover, the silt-laden waters combated malaria as they carried the fish eggs which entered the canals; floated into the subsidiary channels, tanks and rice fields and then soon became young fish who instantly fell upon the larvae of the mosquitoes and lived on them.[15] The colonial engineers blundered by mistakenly considering silted up canals to be 'dead rivers'. Moreover, they had built up a railway embankment along the left bank of the Damodar River in the 1850s, which effectively cut off the area north of the river from the flow of silt and floodwater so necessary for the health and prosperity of the region.[16]

The most nuanced ecological analysis of the problems of deltaic Bengal seems to be Radha Kamal Mukherji's *The Changing Face of Bengal*, published in 1938. Mukherji argued inter alia that the rivers were choked with weeds, the *khals*, pools and depressions, no longer served as natural drainage reservoirs and channels, but were converted into breeding grounds of mosquitoes.[17]

Contrary to what had long been debated upon, the colonial rulers viewed the delta's rivers as essentially poised against the surrounding alluvial plains. The rivers, according to them, appeared in two opposing functions: they either burst their banks and injured cultivation or so weakened their flows that crops withered from lack of water. A conception of river hydrology was thus premised as the unstable fluid opposite to settled agriculture. For the colonial rulers therefore the delta's rivers had to be conceived only through the language of control.[18] They shut out the flood with embankments, which led to appalling malaria epidemics, for it allowed mosquito population to multiply alarmingly. Bentley estimated that out of a population of 45 million people in Bengal in 1911, 30 million people were afflicted by malaria, more than 10 million severely so.[19]

DRAINAGE OBSTRUCTION

As early as the 1840s, the British medical officers and engineers had an impression that malaria diffused with works of economic development. The first systematic enquiry in this regard appears to have been conducted by a Canal Committee appointed in the mid-1840s to explore the causes of unhealthy conditions around the Delhi and Jumna canal works.[20] T. E. Dempster, a member of the Canal Committee, noticed the 'astonishing difference' between the numbers of fever cases belonging to the 'irrigated and unirrigated parts' of the region of the West Jumna Canal.[21] The Canal Committee found that the spread of malaria was intimately connected with 'this canal construction in a remarkable degree'. They discovered two remarkable local conditions common to all tracts irrigated from the existing canals where spleen disease was alarming, namely, obstructed drainage and a stiff retentive soil. They observed that where soil condition and drainage were favourable, malaria had not taken hold. In fact, the East Jumna Canal illustrated the best and the worst results of canal irrigation. In the northern and southern sectors of the East Jumna Canal where the soil was light and the drainage perfect, the committee found 'all the blessing of a canal'.[22] But in the central division where drainage had been greatly obstructed and the soil was stiff and clayey, the effect on health was exactly the opposite.

Similar phenomenon was noticeable in Bengal. In January 1863, Dr J. Elliot, civil assistant surgeon of Hooghly, who was placed on a special duty to enquire into the epidemic fever prevailing in the Nadia and Burdwan divisions, reported on a complete absence of drainage in the affected villages. 'The greatest sufferers', he noticed, 'have been the villages on the banks of stagnant rivers filled with vegetation and weeds'.[23] Again in March 1869, Jaykrishna Mukherjee of Uttarpara submitted to the government a memorial from the zamindars, talukdars and traders of Hooghly and Burdwan districts.[24] Mukherjee emphasized, among other things, the case of obstructed drainage, arguing that the gradual deposit of mud and silt had greatly raised the beds of almost all rivers, canals, channels and other streams, which formerly served to drain the country efficiently of its surplus water. He made a special mention of the Damodar River, which was beheaded by embankments for the railway construction.[25]

R. V. Cockerell, the magistrate of Hooghly, corroborated Jaykrishna Mukherjee's observations. Cockerell wrote on 29 January 1868: 'It is very common to hear the remark made in any village in this part of the district that since the Railway has been made, the water in all the khals and rivers has diminished; that the khals and drains have become obstructed; that there have been no inundations etc.'[26] The consequence of the cessation of these periodic floods was that the part of the land ceased to get refreshed by the purer Damodar waters. Worse still, the beds of these canals, being no longer kept clear of the accumulated vegetation by the periodic flush of the flood waters, 'had gradually become obstructed'.[27] Cockerell noticed that in most of them, there was no stream at all, and bunds had been thrown across them in many places to secure water for irrigation purposes.[28] In May 1870, Dr D. B. Smith, sanitary commissioner of Bengal, observed that 'the most important of all the causes of malarious fever was insufficient drainage by the partial or complete obliteration of rivers'.[29] The channels of the rivers Kana and Kunti were deteriorated into miles of damp ground, interspersed with a series of shallow pools with terribly impure water. They were merely broad ditches, and their sides were greatly polluted with vegetable and animal decomposition. It could not be reasonably disputed, Dr Smith argued, that there did in many instances exist a general relation between the extreme unhealthiness of the place and the proximity of old river channels in a half-dry filthy state.

Dr C. J. J. Jackson, the sanitary commissioner of Bengal, however, refused to believe that obstructed drainage had in any way caused malaria in Bengal.[30] Dr Jackson argued that 'there has never been any such connection between the direction of its propagation and that of the lines of drainages'.[31] He noticed that the fever prevailed in both ill- and well-drained village, remained longer in the former, but 'was more intense in the latter. It was more intense in dry than in moist areas'.[32] Dr Jackson's observation deserves careful scrutiny not only because he had contradicted the views of his contemporaries, but also because his arguments had been shared by a good number of health officers and engineers of the government. In fact, when the embanking of the delta tracts began first as a measure of flood prevention and afterwards for railway construction, few realized that the entire exercise was fraught with danger. Even when attention had been drawn to the outbreak of fever that followed the construction of embankments, the term 'water-logging', which was frequently employed by medical officers and engineers without carefully defining it, appeared to have led to a misunderstanding of the situation. In those days, the cause of malaria was not known, but medical authorities were wont to ascribe it generally to 'water-logging' by which they meant a supersaturation of the soil with water. Digambar Mitra, when seeking to explain the epidemic malaria that occurred in association with the construction of embankment, suggested that they were due to 'water-logging' produced by these embankments.[33] By 'water-logging' he, however, appears to have meant 'obstructed flow' rather than supersaturating of the soil.

We intend to engage in the issue of 'obstructed drainage' in more details arguably because it would help one understand the operation of drainage system as it prevailed in Bengal countryside, and help one understand if the British were responsible for any disturbance in the system. The Epidemic Commission observed that the drainage of all villages in the epidemic districts was affected by the water first running into the nearest paddy fields lying in the directions of their slope; thence it collected in the beels from which it rushed through canals into larger streams, which again communicated with navigable rivers. 'An obstruction occurring in any of these conduits', it was argued, 'must interfere with the drainage, and its effects are felt more or less according to the proximity or remoteness of the obstruction from the scene of its influence'. Accordingly, the commission found that 'the stoppage of the mouths of the different streams has not been productive of such serious consequences to the village lying within their influence, as when the same occurred more in the vicinity of those villages'.[34]

No one contradicts that silting up of the rivers was calculated to interfere with the drainage of a village nearly as much as obstruction offered to it at any one of the intermediate conduits. But it was foolish to lay the blame entirely at the door of the river itself. 'Do the engineers pretend to say', the *Hindoo Patriot* rightly questioned, 'that a sufficiently high road or embankment crossing any one of these conduits, will not quite effectually shut out the drainage of a number of villages lying on the upper side of the road or embankment even if the outfall, the river, were perfectly open?'[35] And if so, one may recall the number of roads, which had been constructed in both the affected districts either as railway feeders or as ordinary highways during the last fifteen years.[36] Therefore, it was the waterlogged subsoil of villages, consequent upon impeded drainage, that had mainly contributed to the generation of condition, resulting in the outbreak of the epidemic fever of Bengal. The mischief had been committed chiefly by roads, railroads and embankments, not because as such, but because they had happened to cross the drainage level of villages. In many instances, the mischief had been similarly done by the canals or other natural channels of drainage, having been dammed up by zamindars or their raiyats for purposes of fishery or for retaining monsoon water on their comparatively elevated rice fields.

Viewed in retrospect, it appears that a trend of misunderstanding seems to inform some of the recent writings on the subject. Ira Klein, for instance, remarked that 'the building of river embankment did not originate with the British raj' and by way of exoneration he seems to argue that the British government was not responsible for the consequent mischief.[37] It is true that river walls were used to be constructed locally by individual zamindars in Bengal to protect their holdings from flood. Truer still, the phenomenon of bunding operation is as old as the human civilization. But Ira Klein never took to ask, why did the malarial epidemic in Bengal occur at a time when it did? Instead, he argued that where riverbanks rose more and more above the cultivated plain, embankments become within the tidal area, an absolute necessity.[38] It is difficult to buy this argument. In the tidal zone of Bengal, the large tracts of the country were situated in depressions or hollows. The drainage channels being tidal, drainage in the hollows was only possible at ebb tide. People used to live in these areas by excluding, on the one hand, sweet water from the rivers above by embankment, and by excluding the saline water on the other hand, of the creeks coming from below by a system of sluices with automatic doors closing at flow tide and opening out at ebb tide along with embankments. Here, one can see, it was not possible to prevent malaria by ordinary anti-mosquito measure on account of excessive waterlogging.

Available evidence suggests that these areas were not originally malarious and that the drainage difficulty was then not experienced at all.[39] But as time went on, they were becoming more waterlogged and so more malarious, and hence the height of the embankments had to be increased continuously to keep pace with the increasing height of the flood tides.

It may, perhaps, be interesting to note that when England had earlier faced a similar problem, they adopted a different solution. They were quick to reject the faulty suggestion offered by a Dutch engineer Vermuyden in 1611 that the sweet water channels from the interior be led to the sea face by artificial dug canals, excluding the tides by sluices with automatic doors. The English, however, later on adopted the right policy on the advice of another Dutch engineer Westerdyke and got rid of the difficulty. He advised them to remove altogether all obstructions, including sluice and weirs, with a view to introducing tides as much as possible into the interior of the country. He suggested the English to lower the beds of the rivers so that as much quantity of seawater as possible should enter at flow tide and come out at ebb tide.[40] This, Westerdyke argued, would make the river more navigable by clearing the beds by the scouring action of huge quantity of water going in and out at intervals. Besides, the sweet water river coming from the interior and mixing with salt water would diminish its salinity. Moreover, the rivers would get easy to the sea, thus ensuring prevention of flood. Finally, the healthiness of the place would be improved and the low lands would be filled up by silt brought by the tides. Nevertheless, the spirit of the old Vermuyden policy, which England had rejected more than 200 years ago for dealing with their fen lands, was pressed into service in the Lower Bengal.

RIVER DECAY AND SILTATION

Closely connected with the problem of embankment and obstructed drainage were the facts of river decay and siltation, which stemmed partly from long-term evolution of the environment, but largely from the impact of the 'development policy' of the colonial government. Under the early British rule, environmental conditions were progressively decaying in Bengal. In January 1863, Dr Elliot observed that the greatest sufferers had been the villagers on the banks of stagnant rivers filled with vegetation and weeds.[41] He noticed huge cultivation of bamboos and plantains in close proximity to houses, overcrowded owing to increase of population. Huts were huddled together in villages obstructing streets and drains. The best and the largest tanks, he complained, were gradually silting up, while trees often covered the smaller ones. Dr J. Sutherland, deputy inspector-general of Hospitals, Presidency Circle, argued in April 1868 that intensification of the epidemic was aided by bad ventilation.[42] In March 1868, Dr R. F. Thompson, civil assistant surgeon of Hooghly, reported that the epidemic was aggravated by impure drinking water, rank vegetation in the tanks and polluted surface water drainage.[43] Dr D. B. Smith observed: 'the worst village I have yet seen in the district (of Hooghly) is Mohunbatty. Here is a concentration of everything that is insanity. It is utterly unfit for human habitation'.[44]

Alarming insanitary condition was not unique to Mohunbatty. This was, in fact, a general condition for all the districts of Lower Bengal. During 1870–1873, Dr Jackson reported that the phenomenon of unhealthy conditions was prevalent throughout everywhere the fever broke out. He observed that the old decaying villages where 'the soil had become saturated with filth of age, where old ruined temples and pakka houses abound, and old polluted pakka tanks were found, were always the most severely attacked'. Moreover 'in all places' where the fever prevailed with 'special intensity' the water supply was exceptionally bad.[45]

Evidences of unhealthiness in the district of Murshidabad can be found in abundance in Colonel Gastrell's accounts. Gastrell wrote in 1860 that 'the district of Murshidabad cannot be called healthy. . . . No sooner does the Bhagirathi fail sufficiently low to allow the waters to drain off into it than sickness commences all along the river banks'.[46] It was this influx of jhil water that the villagers themselves used to attribute the sickness so prevalent before the cold reason had fairly set in. When to this was added the numerous half-burned human carcasses that were daily thrown into the river, which was then almost a chain of stagnant pools, there would be little cause to wonder at the sickness of those who habitually used this water for drinking and cooking purposes.[47]

Almost similar conditions prevailed in Jessore, Nadia, Howrah and elsewhere. The state of unhealthiness stemmed chiefly from the problem of impure water supply, siltation and death of rivers.[48] In Presidency Division, out of thirty-three villages examined, the average spleen rate was 46% in the village situated along a live river, while of thirty-eight villages the spleen rate was 64.5% in villages situated near a dead river.[49] In Jessore, the spleen rate was 44.5% in twenty-one villages, which were situated near moderate jungle. The spleen rate was in sixty-two villages situated adjacent to thick jungle.[50] In Nadia district, the average spleen rate was 37% in seven villages situated near moderate jungle, while in eighteen villages situated near thick jungle the average spleen rate was 63%.[51] In Murshidabad district, in eleven villages adjacent to live river the average spleen rate was 38.6% while it was 51.5% where the villages were situated along a dead river. In twenty villages situated near a bheel which was however annually flooded, the average spleen rate was 39%. But the fifteen villages situated near a bheel, not annually flooded, witnessed an average spleen rate of 57%.[52]

Were the districts in eastern part of Bengal relatively free from malaria? Ira Klein seems to suggest this.[53] Professor B. B. Chaudhuri has also argued that the general absence of fatal disease like the Burdwan fever along with other factors favoured the rapid growth of population there.[54] Closer examination of available evidence however does not seem to warrant this view. The eastern districts, it is true, witnessed a steadier growth of population, compared to the Western, Central and Northern Bengal. But whenever the situation was comparable, the results were almost the same.

In June 1869, W. G. Deane, deputy magistrate and deputy collector of Jessore, reported that the topographical character of a great portion of Jessore had been considerably modified.[55] Vast bheels were then turned into high meadows and deep watercourses had been obliterated.

The bheels started silting in 1860, and by the cold season of 1865 a most destructive fever broke out along the banks of the Naba Ganga, which ran to the south of the bheel. If one turns to the village in the direction of Kollea in the Narail subdivision, one can see that the same agency was at work with similar results. By June 1869, the Chitra was a dead stream, and for some years back the village for several miles around had suffered fearfully from epidemic fever. Deane argued that if enquiries were made, it would have appeared that wherever a bheel or watercourse had silted, fever had broken out in the neighbourhood.[56]

In fact, the nineteenth-century epidemic fever of Bengal had had its origin in Eastern Bengal itself. It broke out at Muhammadpur in Jessore district in 1824–1825, and thence it travelled westward to Nadia.[57] It broke out among a body of 500–700 convicts working on a road from Jessore to Dacca. In a short time, 150 of the prisoners died, and the officers in charge of them fled. The epidemic did not quit Muhammadpur for several years but seemed to disappear in 1843. However, it broke out again and ‘in the next two years, spread over the whole district'. After a temporary cessation, the fever broke out again in 1854–1856, and about this time it began to spread westward to Nadia and 24 Parganas.[58]

Since the 1891, fever of a less virulent type had been prevalent in Jessore and formed the subject of a special enquiry by the Drainage Committee in 1906–1907. The committee concluded that (i) the whole district of Jessore was extremely unhealthy; (ii) malarial fever prevailed extensively everywhere; (iii) by a rather arbitrary comparison, the thanas of Jhenida, Gaighata, Salikha and Bagharpara were the most malarious and (iv) the least malarious were the thanas of Barkalia, Lohagara, Kotchandpur and Gudkhali.[59] The enquiring officers attributed the prevalance of pervasive malarial fever in the district, 'to the great facilities afforded to the breeding of mosquitoes, chiefly by the presence of in and around the village of jungle, dirty tanks, ditches, marshes and canal water in every direction, and to a lesser degree, to the bheels and dead rivers.'[60]

In the early 1920s Dr C. A. Bentley noticed an extension of malaria in several districts of Eastern Bengal since the construction of some hundred miles of railways, and the districts of Dacca and Mymensing especially showed signs of being far more seriously affected than formerly. Tangail, Manikganj and the north of Faridpur district were areas of Eastern Bengal most seriously affected with malaria.[61] Narail, 22 miles off Jessore, was also affected with malaria around the year 1870. At Magura, fever broke out in November 1864. All these happened after the silting up of the *Jugni Bagni Beel*. The sickness was great for 8 miles below Magura.[62] It was particularly severe at Binodpur and the places between it and Magura. At Senhati, adjacent to Khulna, about one-fifth of the population were suffering from spleen disease in or around the same period. Dr Smith believed that this was due to bad water supply. The tanks were all in the most neglected state, particularly the *Kobiraj Pukur* and *Sarkarjer tank*.

There was only 2 feet of water in the former, while in the parts of the latter, Smith noticed, the vegetation was so thick that 'cattle can graze over it'. But still its waters were drawn by the villagers.[63] Moreover, some of the jungles had been cut down by the order of the deputy magistrate, but the waste had not been removed. The village had the river Chitra to the north of it, about 4 miles distant the Bhairab on the south and west, and the Altai the east, all tidal streams, but recently silted up. People complained that 'the water of our tanks is like black blood'.[64] Added to this general state of environmental decay were more crucial economic questions like agrarian condition, crop pattern, foodstuff and clothing. This brings us to still another causal incidence of fever in Bengal: poverty. And this requires a discursive shift and we need to recast our intellectual gaze to some new area.

POVERTY AND MALNUTRITION

I have argued elsewhere that malaria in Bengal is, in fact, a euphemism for malnutrition.[65] Malnutrition in Bengal arose primarily from agricultural decline. It may, however, sometimes seem difficult to determine whether agricultural decline and the consequent poverty led to the epidemic fever in Bengal or the vice versa. For many areas in Bengal showing signs of agricultural decline scarcely warrant any incidence of epidemic malaria. The situation is comparable to the Black Death of Europe in the fourteenth century. The bubonic plague, which during the epidemic years of 1348–1350, caused an initial loss of life of about 20%, was ascribed by many to poverty and squalor of English countryside. But historians are at a loss to explain why certain places and areas should have remained nearly free from infection.[66] So far as the malaria epidemic of Bengal is concerned, it is quite conceivable that the epidemic fever passed by a few remote district or habitation, whose isolation would protect them against the epidemic infection.

Speaking about the effect of embankments on agriculture in Burdwan and Hooghly, Dr Bentley argued in 1925 that the shutting out of the Damodar water on the agriculture of the districts brought out disastrous consequences, for 'the profits of the agricultural classes in this district (Hooghly) are less now than in 1860'.[67] The reduction of profits was accounted for by the decreasing fertility of the soil in those parts of the district, which were within the sphere of influence of the Damodar inundations. One important aspect of epidemic fever in Burdwan was that more often than not it was preceded or followed by flood or famine. Famine or scarcity means that a sizeable section of rural people would go without food, and flood means loss of food crops for the cultivators, which brings in starvation for those who could no longer fall back upon their means of subsistence. J. C. K. Peterson rightly observed that the deltaic portion of the district of Burdwan was more liable to famine as the people depended almost entirely upon the winter rice crop for their means of subsistence. The autumn rice crop could hardly compensate for a failure of this crop, which was cultivated on a comparatively small scale.[68]

During the period when epidemic fever was at its worst, Burdwan experienced two devastating famines, one in 1866 and another in 1874. Dr Elliot believed that the famine of 1866 was responsible for the fever epidemic in the district. In fact, the causal link between flood, famine and fever in Bengal was so entangled that it is difficult to engage them separately. This was best exemplified by the famine of 1874. The year 1872 was unfavourable in Burdwan. The rains commenced very late, and when it commenced, it was not evenly distributed throughout district.[69] As a result, the outturn of *aman* rice crop was very small. Again, the rains in 1873 in Burdwan were not as greatly deficient in quantity as they were unseasonable in distribution. The effects of the unseasonable rainfall on the harvest varied with the crops. The *aus* or early rice crop escaped injury. The late crops, however, suffered severally. The year 1874 thus found the district ravaged by the impact of two years of markedly adverse harvest. Not only were the material resources of the people depleted, but also their physical capacity to bear a strain was also markedly impaired. Distress had gradually been making way in April 1874.[70] As the year rolled on, the distress of people deepened. Food grain supply or famine relief by the government was notoriously poor. Some of the poorest people were reportedly eating grass seeds, and almost every house appeared to contain a larger or smaller group of lean and badly nourished persons.[71] The Burdwan famines of 1866 and 1874 are two exemplary instances that speak of people's prolong suffering from undernourishment.

Sometimes, scarcity was brought about not by famines, but by floods and droughts. During the famine of 1943–1944, flood in Burdwan and Hooghly districts on 17 July 1943, and again on 4–5 August, badly affected about 2,50,000 cultivators.[72] By the same year, there was a great flood in the river Subarnarekha, which brought great havoc to the people with the loss of ripe and ready-for-the-sickle *aus* paddy. About 100 villages of the area in Midnapur were totally washed away, and 10,000 people rendered homeless. Cholera broke out in the flooded area and death from starvation was unaccountable.[73]

Apart from flood, famine and the consequent impoverishment, there was also a remarkable deficient supply of vitamins and salt to the foodstuff of the common people. After 1813, when the monopoly of the English East India Company was thrown open, various other East India Companies, private traders, Armenians, Chinese and indigenous traders from all over the country collected to Calcutta, and the population of Calcutta was multiplied fast. The burden of food supply fell on the agriculturists of Bengal, particularly Burdwan, 'the granary of Bengal'. Rice, milk, chickens, goats, sheep and cows drawn from the adjacent districts were sent off to Calcutta.[74] The newly constructed railway network in the region facilitated the process. With the opening of the Suez Canal in 1869, this process accentuated further. British exports from India now took less time to reach England. Moreover, since the freight charges were now reduced by 30% per cubic ton, some new items also were added to the traditional British exports from India. This explains why the export of rice from Bengal and wheat from the U.P. and the Punjab increased enormously since 1869.[75]

The export of rice from Calcutta had, in fact, increased by 196% between 1873 and 1878. Estimates show that the rice trade with Calcutta was larger than that with the rest of province.[76] Bulk of these exports went to Ceylon, Singapore and particularly to Mauritius to feed the population there, originally indentured labourers for the local plantation industries.[77] The nature of this export trade was completely different from the export of high-quality rice from Bengal to the advanced markets of Europe, America and Japan, which had been determined by sheer laws of market.[78] The larger colonial interests of the British conditioned the export of common rice to the plantation areas. Nevertheless, all these phenomena had their impact on the general well-being of the people of the province. There did ensure a period of progressive undernourishment and malnutrition among the weaker section of Bengal.

The phenomenon of undernourishment and malnutrition did continue even in the opening decades of the twentieth century. Recent researches have emphasized the increasing impoverishment of Bengal peasantry during the entire colonial period.[79] The research of George Blyn on Indian agricultural statistics from 1893 to 1946 has revealed a truly staggering picture of stagnation or even decline.[80] The supplementary calculation of Amiya Bagchi reveals a similar pattern for productivity per acre for the period 1900–1905 to 1935–1940. The value of commercial crops per acre went up very slightly from Rs. 36.7 to Rs. 37.9, while that of food crops declined from Rs. 25.4 to Rs. 22.7, and of all crops from Rs. 27.6 to Rs. 26.3.[81] The severity of the blow to the cash position of the Bengal peasants can be guessed from an estimate given by the Bengal Jute Enquiry Committee Report in 1934 regarding the variations in purchasing power between 1920–1921 and 1932–1933.[82] According to these estimates, the total value of marketable crops in Bengal fell from an annual average of Rs. 724 million for the decades 1920–1921 to 1929–1930 to Rs. 327 million in 1932–1933, that is, a fall of more than 50%. On the other hand, monetary liabilities actually rose from Rs. 279 million to Rs. 283 million. This implied that the free purchasing power of the cultivators fell from Rs. 445 million to only Rs. 44 million, that is, a fall of 90%.[83]

All these indicate that the overall trend of food production per capita was declining in Greater Bengal over the first half of the twentieth century. This was in fact a part of the process of the agrarian crisis consequent upon the scale of primary accumulation unleashed in India. Worse still, right from the mid-1930s of the twentieth century, incipient famine condition prevailed in various parts of Bengal. The memorandum of the Bengal Provincial Kisan Sabha, for instance, goes on record to state: 'the joke in Bengal is that the Government has, by an executive order, abolished famine and substituted for it, when occasion arises, shortage'.[84]

Scarcity of food, malnutrition and a general state of impoverishment were further aggravated by another process of change in the structure of agriculture. With the increasing import of cheap cotton clothes by the British, Bengal cotton weavers were gradually thrown out of their traditional occupation and they took to cultivation whenever possible. This phenomenon resulted in increased pressure on land. Since the prices of paddy were much higher due to its export-oriented nature, the weavers took to the cultivation of paddy. The changeover to commercial crop and high-priced food grain like rice meant a shift away from poor man's food crops like jowar, bajra or pulses, and it often brought disaster in famine years. However, due to increased pressure on land for the cultivation of paddy, fallow lands, pastures and lands for growing green vegetables were converted into rice fields. Cattle found no grazing ground, and the result was that 'the cows could no longer be milched, and vegetables no longer grown'.[85]

Other important changes resulting in undernourishment can be noticed in decrease in fish of all kinds and the great increase in the prevalence of certain mammals, wild hog for example.[86] Both these changes were important from an economic point of view. The reduction of fish meant a decrease in food supply with adequate protection content, and the increase in wild hog meant a greater damage to crops during periods of scarcity. The most noticeable change in the flora and fauna of Bengal was, however, the lapsing of some of the cultivated or inhabited lands into jungle. It was particularly noticeable in places where population had declined.[87] There is, however, little statistical information about the changes in the proportion of cultivated and uncultivated land. However, Dr Bentley reported that prior to the epidemic fever, seven-eighths of the land in Burdwan was under cultivation, whereas the returns in 1922 showed only 47% of the cultivable areas as being cropped.[88] Successive collectors had reported a progressive shrinkage of the cultivated area in Nadia, and a loss of fertility and consequent agricultural deterioration had been noticed in many other districts of Central and Western Bengal and elsewhere. Thus, taking into consideration the broad fact that only 58% and 60% of the cultivable areas were brought under the plough in Central and Western Bengal, respectively, it would appear in view of the remarkable decay of population that something was enormously wrong with the colonial administration which helped diminish very seriously the food supply of the people.

CHANGES IN THE CROP PATTERN

When one examines the crops grown and the recent changes in the crop pattern under colonial rule, certain significant facts are brought to light. Before the advent of the British rule in Bengal, cotton and sugarcane were produced over a large tract of land. British textiles and sugar mills were unknown to the villagers. Excepting parts of Midnapur and Bankura, almost every household in Lower Bengal used to cultivate some amount of cotton and sugarcane for their own household consumption. These two crops used to take almost a year to ripe for harvest and required intensive irrigation for nearly eight to nine months. This meant that sugarcane and cotton cultivation demanded huge water and that large beels and ponds were exhausted of their water resources in the process. Fallen leaves in the ponds from the surrounding trees found no time to rot and the proliferation of mosquitoes was therefore unheard of.[89]

The introduction of British cotton goods and its penetration into the remote village markets, a process largely facilitated by the expansion of railway network and the establishment of sugar mills, changed the situation altogether. Cultivation of cotton was discouraged, as cheap imported cotton clothes were made available to the villagers in plenty. And introduction of sugar mills discouraged initiative for sugarcane cultivation meant for private consumption. These two factors worked in tandem to reduce the cultivation of the two water-consuming crops.[90] Instead of cotton and sugarcane, farmers now took to cultivate potatoes, which required less water, and village ponds, as a result, were seldom depleted, thereby providing ample provision for mosquito breeding.[91] Census reports record that there were as many as 1,23,245 villages in Bengal in 1911.[92] If one takes on an average fifteen irrigation tanks per village, one can argue that no less than a million and a half vegetated ponds had been created during the period under review.

The situation was made worse by the expansion of jute cultivation in Lower Bengal. The manufacture of jute was then the most important industry in the province, and the export of raw and manufactured jute was its most valuable commercial asset. By 1925, 60% of the jute grown in Bengal came from the less malarious eastern districts, and the supply of Burdwan and the Presidency Division constituted barely in 10%.[93] In terms of average, Bentley's study shows that the normal area under jute in Eastern Bengal in 1925 was 13,73,300 acres, compared to 3,53,000 acres in the Burdwan and Presidency Divisions.[94] But available figures of 1908 show that cultivation of jute in the Lower Bengal had expanded up to an area of 7,45,600 acres of land.[95] Jute was harvested along the months of September, October and November, and these three months were notoriously malarious. Jute plants were cut and submerged in the village ponds or in the *beels* and kept there for a month to rot. When the plants became quite rotten, they were taken up, the stalks were broken and the fibre came out. They were then washed out in the filthy and obnoxious water, a veritable breeding place for mosquitoes. Thus, expansion of jute cultivation brought in its trail proliferation of malaria. Contemporary literary tracts more often than not lamented over the extension of jute cultivation and its associated evil.[96]

CONCLUSION

The nature of recent research on epidemic malaria in colonial Bengal suggests that scholars, as it were, have exhausted all the conceivable areas of exploration about the functions of human agency in bringing about the epidemic. Some have, therefore, found it more worthwhile to look for the logic of its singularity in location while others have moved away from human to non-human agents for the causation of malarial fever in Bengal.[97] Admittedly, these works are important, and I have no profound quarrel with the preferential foundation of their alternative imaginations. Such discursive shifts are always welcome but we should not also disregard the multilayered texts of political economy of a colony.

Arguably, the predisposing causes of the epidemic emanated from the topography of the riverine areas of the province but the proximate causes stemmed largely from the colonial infrastructures – roads, railroads, ports, mines, plantations – which accelerated the process of environmental decay and accentuated the crisis. The consequences were arguably twofold. First, impeded drainage begot large number of stagnant pools and marshes, which provided congenial breeding grounds for mosquitoes. Second, loss of fertility of the soil due to cessation of inundation had diminished the amount of winter harvest, which meant starvation for a sizable section of the rural masses. The phenomena of reduced winter harvest and the consequent starvation can be studied against the background of an increasing export of rice from Lower Bengal, partly to the developing city of Calcutta but largely to the British colonies in South and Southeast Asia. Scarcity of food grains for rural consumption was further aggravated by an incentive to increased production of jute. Apart from the problem of ill health, which the retting of jute plants involved, far more alarming was the indication of a tendency for jute to displace the paddy.

The trend of declining quality and quantity of Bengali foodstuff had in fact dated from the first half of the nineteenth century. In 1910, David McCay, Bengal sanitary commissioner, reviewed researches on jail dietaries of the previous twenty-five years as well as the general health of the Bengali population at large.[98] McCay succeeded in establishing the fact that there had been a significant protein deficiency in the *dal-bhat* diet of the Bengalis. Worse still, McCay proved that apart from an inherent protein deficiency, the Bengalis could absorb only about two-thirds of the protein available in cereals. John Lindenbaum and others further enquired into this malabsorption syndrome in the 1930s and argued that a symptomatic disorder of the small intestine seriously interfered with the absorption of essential nutrients. This intestinal disorder was caused by infected water. Coming to the question of Bengal where pure drinking water was an evident luxury, one may conclude that there had been an overall decline in the general health conditions of the Bengalis. In such a state of chronic debilitation, malaria or any other disease was likely to have an epidemic dimension. Viewed in this light, epidemic malaria in Bengal was, in fact, a function of colonial maladministration.

NOTES

1. David Arnold, 'Cholera and Colonialism in British India', *Past and Present*, 113 (1986): 126.

2. Raja Digambar Mitra, *The Epidemic Fever in Bengal* (Kolkata: The Hindoo Patriot Press, 1873), 33.

3. Mitra, *The Epidemic Fever*, 32–33.

4. *Hindoo Patriot*, September 9, 1872, September 16, 1872.

5. Note of Col. J. E. T. Nicolls, Chief Engineer, Bengal, On the Effect of Roads and Railways on the General Drainage of the Country in Lower Bengal. Proceedings of the Government of Bengal (hereafter Progs. GOB), General Department (hereafter Gen. Dept.), Sanitation Branch (hereafter San Br.) March 1869. No. 17. p. 26. West Bengal State Archives (hereafter WBSA).

6. Note of Col. J. E. T. Nicolls.

7. W.W. Clemesha, 'Notes on the Influence of Railway Construction on Malaria', *Records of Malaria Survey of India*, 1, no. 2 (1917): 163.

8. Clemesha, 'Notes on the Influence', 164.

9. S.R. Christopher and C. A. Bentley, *Proceedings of the Indian Medical Congress,* (Bombay: no pub., 1909), 81.

10. P. Hehir, *Malaria in India* (Oxford: Oxford University Press, 1927), 46.

11. Karali Charan Ray, *Bange Malaria* (Basantapur: no pub., 1917).

12. Haridhan Bandyopadhyay, *Banglar Shatru* (Sodepur: no pub., 1924).

13. Daniel Klingensmith, 'Of "Ancient Irrigation" and Modern Dams: Orientalism, Nationalism and Water Policy in late Colonial Bengal, 1925–1947'. Working Paper, 2007.

14. Sir Williams Willcocks, *Ancient System of Irrigation in Bengal* (New Delhi: B. R. Pub. Corp., 1984). Reprint.

15. D'Souza, Rohan, 2010. 'Seeing like a River: The Bengal Presidency's Hydraulic Transition', in *Science and Society in India 1700–2000*, ed. Arun Bandopadhyay (New Delhi: Manohar, 2010), 171.

16. Willcocks, *Ancient System,* 26–27.

17. R.K. Mukherji, *The Changing Face of Bengal* (Kolkata: University of Calcutta, 1938), 212.

18. Kuntala Lahiti-Dutt, 'Negotiating Water Management in the Damodar Valley: Kolkata Hearing and the DVC', in *Water First: Issues and Challenges for nations and Communities in South Asia,* ed. Kuntala Lahiri-Dutt et al. (New Delhi: Sage India, 2008), 316–34.

19. C.A Bentley, *Malaria and Agriculture in Bengal* (Kolkata: Bengal Secretariat Book Depot, 1925), 102–103.

20. Ira Klein, 'Malaria and Mortality in Bengal, 1840–1921', *Indian Economic and Social History Review,* IX, no. 2 (1972):139.

21. *Records of the Malaria Survey of India*, 1930, 1, no.2 (1930):70.

22. *Records of the Malaria Survey*, 4–5.

23. Progs. GOB. Gen. Dept. March 1863, No: 108, p. 65. WBSA.

24. Progs. GOB. Gen. Dept. San. Br. May 1869, Nos. 11-12, pp. 9–12. WBSA.

25. From Baboo Joy Krishto Mookerjee and others, to the Hon'ble A. Eden, Secy to the GOB. (Dated 19th March 1869). Progs. GOB. Pol. Dept. San. Br. May 1869. No.12. p. 10. WBSA.

26. R. V. Cockerell's Report No: 42A, 29th January 1868. Para. 7.

27. Baboo Joy Kissen Mookherjee's Memorandum to the Hon'ble W. Grey, Lieutenant Governor of Bengal. Progs. GOB. May 1869. Pol. Dept. San. Br. No: 12, p. 10. WBSA.

28. Vide D. G. Crawford, *Hughli Medical Gazetteer* (Kolkata: Bengal Secretariat Press, 1903), 125.

29. Dr. D. B. Smith's Second Report dated 12th May 1870. Progs. GOB. Gen. Dept. San. Br. June, 1870. Nos: 10–12. pp. 7–23. WBSA.

30. Appendix to the Annual Report of the Sanitary Commission Bengal for the years 1873. Also Vide Crawford, *Hughli Medical,* 27.

31. Appendix to the Annual Report of the Sanitary Commission Bengal for the years 1873, para 376, 76.

32. Appendix to the Annual Report of the Sanitary Commission Bengal for the years 1873, 77.

33. Bentley, *Malaria and Agriculture,* 51.

34. Memorandum supplied by Baboo Digambar Mitra related to certain obstruction to the drainage of the epidemic districts. 'Report of the Commission appointed in 1864 to enquire into the nature and probable causes of the epidemic Fever in the districts of Hooghly, Burdwan, Nadia and the 24 Parganas'. Appendix II. Progs. GOB. Dept. April 1864, No. 23, p. 21, WBSA.

35. *Hindoo Patriot*, Sept. 9, 1872.

36. *Hindoo Patriot*. Sept. 9, 1872.

37. Ira Klein, 'Malaria and Mortality in Bengal, 1840–1921', *Indian Economic and Social History Review,* IX, no. 2 (1972):139.

38. Ira Klein, 'Malaria and Mortality', 149–50.

39. G. C. Chatterjee, *The Malaria Problem of the Tidal Zone in Bengal* (Kolkata: Central Anti-Malaria Co-Operative Society Ltd, 1935), 1–2.

40. G. C. Chatterjee, *The Malaria Problem*, 2.

41. Progs. GOB., March, 1863, Gen. Dept., No: 108. pp. 63–64. WBSA.

42. Report on the Epidemic Fever by J Sutherland, M. D., Deputy Inspector-General, Presidency Circle. No: 51, dated 13th April, 1868, Progs. GOB., Gen. Dept., San. Br. June 1868. No: 14. pp. 14–17. WBSA

43. Report of Dr. R. F. Thompson, Civil Assistant Surgeon of Hooghly. No: 34. March 17, 1868. Progs. GOB., Gen. Dept., San. Br., No. 14. pp. 17–19. WBSA.

44. Report of Dr. D.B. Smith, Sanitary Commissioner Bengal, to the Secy to the GOB. Progs. GOB. Judicial (hereafter Jud.) Dept. San. Br. March 1868. Para 25. WBSA.

45. Report on the Burdwan Fever by Dr. C. J. J. Jackson, Sanitary Commissioner, Bengal. Appendix to the *Annual Sanitary Report of 1873*, Para 376. pp. 77–79.

46. *Gastrell's Geographical and Statistical Account of the Murshidabad District,* 1860, Calcutta. Cited by L.S.S. O'Malley, *Bengal District Gazetteers, Murshidabad* (Kolkata: Bengal Secretariat Book Depot, 1914), 81–82.

47. *Col. Gastrell's Geographical and Statistical Account of the Murshidabad District.* 1860, Calcutta. Cited by L.S.S. O'Malley, *Bengal District Gazetteers, Murshidabad* (Kolkata: Bengal Secretariat Book Depot, 1914), 82.

48. O'Malley, L.S.S., *Bengal District Gazetteers, Jessore* (Kolkata: Bengal Secretariat Book Depot., 1912), 61–65. J.H.E. Garret, *Bengal District Gazetteers, Nadia* (Kolkata: Bengal Secretariat Book Depot., 1910), 62. L.S.S. O'Malley, 1909. *Bengal District Gazetteers, Howrah* (Kolkata: Bengal Secretariat Book Depot., 1909), 54, 76–77.

49. G. E. Stewart and A. H. Proctor ed., *Report of the Drainage Committee, Bengal* (Kolkata: Bengal Secretariat Press, 1907), Appendix I, XIII.

50. G. E. Stewart and A. H. Proctor, Appendix I, XXI.

51. G. E. Stewart and A. H. Proctor, 'Interim Report on the Nadia District', Feb. 1907, XXVII.

52. G. E. Stewart and A. H. Proctor, 'Interim Report on the Murshidabad District,' Feb. 1907. p. XXXV

53. Ira Klein, 'Malaria and Mortality', 143.

54. 'Agrarian Economy and Agrarian Relations in Bengal, 1859–1885' in *The History of Bengal, 1757–1905*, ed. N. K. Sinha (Kolkata: Calcutta University Press, 1967), 244–245.

55. W. G. Deane, Deputy Magistrate and Deputy Collector of Jessore, to the Magistrate of Nadia (dated 11th June, 1869). Progs. GOB. Pol. Dept. San – Dr. Feb. 1870. No: p. 21. WBSA.

56. W. G. Deane, Deputy Magistrate and Deputy Collector of Jessore, to the Magistrate of Nadia.

57. 'Report on the Epidemic Fever in parts of the Nuddea and Burdwan Division' by Dr J Elliot.

Supplement, *Calcutta Gazette.* 18th March, 1863. Also, in Progs. GOB. Dept. San. Br. March 1863. No: 108. p. 63. WBSA.

58. L.S.S. O'Malley, *Bengal District Gazetteers. Jessore* (Kolkata: Bengal Secretariat Book Depot., 1912), 61–62.

59. G. E. Stewart and A. H. Proctor, *Report of the Drainage Committee, Bengal*, Appendix I, XXI.

60. L.S.S. O'Malley, *Bengal District Gazetteers, Jessore* (Kolkata: Bengal Secretariat Book Depot, 1912), 64

61. C. A. Bentley, *Malaria and Agriculture*, 103.

62. D. B. Smith to W. H. Ryland, Officiating Assistant Secy to GOB (No. 147 dated Calcutta, the 29th Jan. 1870). Progs. GOB, Pol. Dept., San. Br, Feb 1870, No. 16. p. 15. WBSA.

63. D. B. Smith to W. H. Ryland, Officiating Assistant Secy to GOB (No. 147 dated Calcutta, the 29th Jan. 1870). Progs. GOB, Pol. Dept., San. Br, Feb 1870, No. 16, p. 16.

64. D. B. Smith to W. H. Ryland, Officiating Assistant Secy to GOB (No. 147 dated Calcutta, the 29th Jan. 1870). Progs. GOB, Pol. Dept., San. Br, Feb 1870, No. 16, p. 16.

65. Arabinda Samanta, *Malarial Fever in Colonial Bengal, 1820–1939: Social History of an Epidemic* (Kolkata: Firma KLM Pvt. Ltd, 2002).

66. E.E. Rich and C. H. Wilson, eds., *The Cambridge Economic History of Europe, IV, Chapter I* (New York: Cambridge University Press, 1967), 5–8.

67. C. A. Bentley, *Malaria and Agriculture*, 39–40.

68. J. C. K. Peterson, *Bengal District Gazetteers, Burdwan* (Kolkata: Bengal Secretariat Book Depot, 1910), 99–100.

69. A.P. MacDonnell, *Report on the Food Grain Supply and Statistical Review of the Relief Operations in the Distressed Districts of Behar and Bengal during the Famine of 1873–74* (Kolkata: Bengal Secretariat Press, 1876), 335.

70. MacDonnell, *Report on the Food Grain Supply*, 339.

71. MacDonnell, *Report on the Food Grain Supply*, 340.

72. Paul R. Greenough, *Prosperity and Misery in Modern Bengal: The Famine of 1943–44* (New York: Oxford University Press, 1982), 120.

73. Greenough, *Prosperity and Misery*, 159.

74. Nibaranchandra Bhattacharyay, *Bangalir Khadya O Pusti* (Kolkata: no pub., 1935), 42.

75. Sabyasachi Bhattacharyay, *Oupaniveshik Bharater Arthaniti* (Kolkata: Ananda Publishers, 1989), 51.

76. *Report on the Internal Trade of Bengal for the year 1876–77* (Kolkata: Bengal Secretariat Press, 1878), 24.

77. N. Mukherjee, 'Foreign and Inland Trade, 1883–1905' in ed. N.K. Sinha, *The History of Bengal, 1757–1905* (Kolkata: Calcutta University Press, 1967), 349.

78. Smriti Kumar Sarkar, 'The rice Milling Industry in Bengal, 1920–1950: A Case Study of the Impact of Mechanization on Rural Peasant Economy', *The Calcutta Historical Journal,* XIII. Nos. 1–2 (1988): 11.

79. Boudhayan Chattopadhyay, *Food Insecurity and the Social Environments* (Kolkata: K.P. Bagchi & Company, 1991).

80. George Blyn, *Agricultural Trends in India: 1891–1947. Output, Availability and Productivity* (Pennsylvania: University of Pennsylvania Press, 1966), 119f.

81. Amiya Bagchi, *Private Investment in India. 1900–1939* (Cambridge: Cambridge University Press, 1972), 95.

82. Vide M.M. Islam, *Bengal Agriculture, 1920–1946, A Quantitative Study* (Cambridge: Cambridge University Press, 1978), 110–111.

83. Chattopadhyay, *Food Insecurity*, 21.

84. Chattopadhyay, *Food Insecurity*, 33–34.

85. Bhattacharyay, *Bangalir Khadya*, 42–44.

86. Vide Bentley, *Indian Medical Gazette*, LVII (1922), 323.

87. Bentley, *Indian Medical Gazette*, LVII (1922), 324.

88. Bentley, *Indian Medical Gazette*, LVII (1922), 324.

89. Rejkrishna Mandal, *Malariar Karan o Pratikar* (Kolkata: no pub., 1908), 24.

90. Mandal, *Malariar Karan*, 24–25.

91. Mandal, *Malariar Karan*, 25.

92. *Census of India*, 1911, V, II, 2.

93. Bentley, *Malaria and Agriculture,* 57.

94. Bentley, *Malaria and Agriculture*, 59.
95. Mandal, *Malariar Karan*, 27.
96. Ray, *Bange Malaria*, 19.
97. Nandini Bhattacharya, 'The Logic of Location: Malaria Research in Colonial India, Darjeeling and Duars, 1900–30', *Medical History*, 55, no. 2, (2011): 182–202. Rohan Deb Roy, *Malarial Subjects: Empire, Medicine and Nonhumans in British India, 1820–1909* (Cambridge: Cambridge University Press, 2017).
98. Sanitary Commissioner, Bengal, *Investigation on Bengal jail Directories with some observations on the influence of the Directory on the Physical Development and well being on the people of Bengal* (Kolkata: Bengal Secretariat Press, 1910).

BIBLIOGRAPHY

Published Primary Sources

West Bengal State Archives, Calcutta

1. Proceedings of the Government of Bengal

Note of Col. J. E. T. Nicolls, Chief Engineer, Bengal, On the Effect of Roads and Railways on the General Drainage of the Country in Lower Bengal. Proceedings of the Government of Bengal (hereafter Progs. GOB), General Department (hereafter Gen. Dept.), Sanitation Branch (hereafter San Br.) March 1869. No. 17.

'Report on the Epidemic Fever' by J Sutherland, M. D., Deputy Inspector-General, Presidency Circle. No: 51, dated 13th April, 1868, Progs. GOB., Gen. Dept., San. Br. June 1868. No: 14.

Appendix to the Annual Report of the Sanitary Commission Bengal for the years 1873, para 376.

Baboo Joy Kissen Mookherjee's Memorandum to the Hon'ble W. Grey, Lieutenant Governor of Bengal. Progs. GOB. May 1869. Pol. Dept. San. Br. No: 12.

D. B. Smith to W. H. Ryland, Officiating Assistant Secy. to GOB (No. 147 dated Calcutta, the 29th Jan. 1870). Progs. GOB, Pol. Dept., San. Br, Feb 1870, No. 16.

D. B. Smith to W. H. Ryland, Officiating Assistant Secy. to GOB (No. 147 dated Calcutta, the 29th Jan. 1870). Progs. GOB, Pol. Dept., San. Br, Feb 1870, No. 16.

Dr. D. B. Smith's Second Report dated 12th May 1870. Progs. GOB. Gen. Dept. San. Br. June, 1870. Nos: 10–12.

From Baboo Joy Krishto Mookerjee and others, to the Hon'ble A. Eden, Secy. to the GOB. (Dated 19th March 1869). Progs. GOB. Pol. Dept. San. Br. May 1869. No.12. Memorandum supplied by Baboo Digambar Mitra related to certain obstruction to the drainage of the epidemic districts. 'Report of the Commission appointed in 1864 to enquire into the nature and probable causes of the epidemic Fever in the districts of Hooghly, Burdwan, Nadia and the 24 Parganas'. Appendix II. Progs. GOB. Dept. April 1864, No. 23.

Progs. GOB. Gen. Dept. March 1863, No: 108.

Progs. GOB. Gen. Dept. San. Br. May 1869, Nos. 11–12. Progs. GOB., March, 1863, Gen. Dept., No: 108.

Report of Dr. D.B. Smith, Sanitary Commissioner Bengal, to the Secy. to the GOB. Progs. GOB. Judicial (hereafter Jud.) Dept. San. Br. March 1868.

Report of Dr. R. F. Thompson, Civil Assistant Surgeon of Hooghly. No: 34. March 17, 1868. Progs. GOB., Gen. Dept., San. Br., No. 14.

Report on the Burdwan Fever by Dr. C. J. J. Jackson, Sanitary Commissioner, Bengal. Appendix to the *Annual Sanitary Report of 1873*, Para 376.

W. G. Deane, Deputy Magistrate and Deputy Collector of Jessore, to the Magistrate of Nadia (dated 11th June, 1869). Progs. GOB. Pol. Dept. San- Dr. Feb. 1870.

2. Official Reports

Elliot, Dr J. 'Report on the Epidemic Fever in parts of the Nuddea and Burdwan Division'. Supplement, *Calcutta Gazette*. 18th March, 1863.

Garret, J.H.E. *Bengal District Gazetteers, Nadia*. Kolkata: Bengal Secretariat Book Depot., 1910.

MacDonnell, A.P. *Report on the Food Grain Supply and Statistical Review of the Relief Operations in the Distressed Districts of Behar and Bengal during the Famine of 1873–74*. Kolkata: Bengal Secretariat Press, 1876.

O'Malley, L.S.S. *Bengal District Gazetteers, Jessore*. Kolkata: Bengal Secretariat Book Depot., 1912.

O'Malley, L.S.S. *Bengal District Gazetteers, Murshidabad*. Kolkata: Bengal Secretariat Book Depot, 1914.

O'Malley, L.S.S. *Bengal District Gazetteers, Howrah*. Kolkata: Bengal Secretariat Book Depot., 1909.

Peterson, J. C. K. *Bengal District Gazetteers, Burdwan*. Kolkata: Bengal Secretariat Book Depot, 1910.

Report on the Internal Trade of Bengal for the year 1876–77. Kolkata: Bengal Secretariat Press, 1878.

Sanitary Commissioner, Bengal. *Investigation on Bengal jail Directories with some observations on the influence of the Directory on the Physical Development and well-being on the people of Bengal*. Kolkata: Bengal Secretariat Press, 1910.

Stewart, G. E., and A. H. Proctor, ed. *Report of the Drainage Committee, Bengal*. Kolkata: Bengal Secretariat Press, 1907.

3. Periodicals

Hindoo Patriot, September 9, 1872, September 16, 1872.

Indian Medical Gazette, LVII.1922.

4. Contemporaneous Publications

Bandyopadhyay, Haridhan. *Banglar Shatru*. Sodepur: no pub., 1924.

Bentley, C.A. *Malaria and Agriculture in Bengal*. Kolkata: Bengal Secretariat Book Depot, 1925.

Bhattacharyay, Nibaranchandra. *Bangalir Khadya O Pusti*. Kolkata: no pub., 1935.

Chatterjee, G. C. *The Malaria Problem of the Tidal Zone in Bengal*. Kolkata: Central Anti-Malaria Co-Operative Society Ltd, 1935.

Christopher S.R., and C. A. Bentley. *Proceedings of the Indian Medical Congress*. Bombay: no pub., 1909.

Crawford, D. G. *Hughli Medical Gazetteer*. Kolkata: Bengal Secretariat Press, 1903.

Gastrell's Geographical and Statistical Account of the Murshidabad District. Kolkata: no pub. 1860.

Hehir, P. *Malaria in India*. Oxford: Oxford University Press, 1927.

Mandal, Rejkrishna. *Malariar Karan o Pratikar*. Kolkata: no pub., 1908.

Mitra, Raja Digambar. *The Epidemic Fever in Bengal*. Kolkata: The Hindoo Patriot Press, 1873.

Mukherji, R.K. *The Changing Face of Bengal*. Kolkata: University of Calcutta, 1938. Ray, Karali Charan. *Bange Malaria*. Basantapur: no pub., 1917.

Records of the Malaria Survey of India, vol.1, no.2, 1930.

Willcocks, Sir Williams. *Ancient System of Irrigation in Bengal*. New Delhi: B. R. Pub. Corp., 1930. (Reprint, 1984).

A. Secondary Sources

Arnold, David. 'Cholera and Colonialism in British India', *Past and Present*, no. 113, 1986.

Bagchi, Amiya. *Private Investment in India. 1900–1939*. Cambridge: Cambridge University Press, 1972.

Bhattacharya, Nandini. 'The Logic of Location: Malaria Research in Colonial India, Darjeeling and Duars, 1900–30', *Medical History*. 55, no. 2, 2011.

Bhattacharyay, Sabyasachi. *Oupaniveshik Bharater Arthaniti*. Kolkata: Ananda Publishers, 1989.

Blyn, George. *Agricultural Trends in India: 1891–1947. Output, Availability and Productivity*. Pennsylvania: University of Pennsylvania Press, 1966.

Chattopadhyay, Boudhayan. *Food Insecurity and the Social Environments*. Kolkata: K.P. Bagchi & Company, 1991.

Deb Roy, Rohan. *Malarial Subjects: Empire, Medicine and Nonhumans in British India, 1820–1909*. Cambridge: Cambridge University Press, 2017. Greenough, Paul R. *Prosperity and Misery in Modern Bengal: The Famine of 1943–44*. New York: Oxford University Press, 1982.

Islam, M.M. *Bengal Agriculture, 1920–1946, A Quantitative Study*. Cambridge: Cambridge University Press, 1978.

Klein, Ira. 'Malaria and Mortality in Bengal, 1840–1921', *Indian Economic and Social History Review*, vol. IX, no.2, 1972.

Klingensmith, Daniel. 'Of "Ancient Irrigation" and Modern Dams: Orientalism, Nationalism and Water Policy in late Colonial Bengal, 1925–1947'. Working Paper, 2007.

Lahiti-Dutt, Kuntala. 'Negotiating Water Management in the Damodar Valley: Kolkata Hearing and the DVC', in Kuntala Lahiri-Dutt et al. eds., *Water First: Issues and Challenges for nations and Communities in South Asia.* New Delhi: Sage India, 2008.

Mukherjee, N. 'Foreign and Inland Trade, 1883–1905' in ed. N.K. Sinha, *The History of Bengal, 1757–1905.* Kolkata: Calcutta University Press, 1967.

Rich, E.E., and C. H. Wilson, eds. *The Cambridge Economic History of Europe, IV, Chapter I.* New York: Cambridge University Press, 1967.

Rohan, D'Souza. 'Seeing like a River: The Bengal Presidency's Hydraulic Transition', in Arun Bandopadhyay ed. *Science and Society in India 1700–2000.* New Delhi: Manohar, 2010.

Samanta, Arabinda. *Malarial Fever in Colonial Bengal, 1820–1939: Social History of an Epidemic.* Kolkata: Firma KLM Pvt. Ltd, 2002.

Sarkar, Smriti Kumar. 'The rice Milling Industry in Bengal, 1920–1950: A Case study of the impact of Mechanization on rural peasant economy', *The Calcutta Historical Journal,* XIII. Nos. 1–2, 1988.

Sinha, N.K. ed. *The History of Bengal, 1757–1905.* Kolkata: Calcutta University Press, 1967.

Chapter 12

Contagious Labour and Epidemics in Colonial India and South Africa

Jacob Steere-Williams

Their race and their labour were inscribed onto their very names. These were not the names their Xhosa parents gave them but names *given to them* by British colonial officials. As African men who likely could not read or write, the traces of their past are indelibly left in routine archival files: contract records, monthly reports, dismissals, mortality lists and the occasional photograph. "British medical officers christened these men, we can only presume irreverently," names like 'Bubo', 'Swaartbooi' ('black boy' in Afrikaans), 'Contact' and 'Jim Crow'.[1] The latter name, which reappears in British colonial records in South Africa around 1900, is particularly revealing of the ways that transatlantic networks of racial thought were mapped onto indigenous bodies in the late nineteenth and early twentieth century.[2] But why were these African men named in this way in colonial records, and what do such often overlooked naming practices tell us about the intersection of colonial history and the history of public health?

As the names 'Bubo' and 'Contact' suggest, these men were named after their labour practices in the fight against bubonic plague. In 1894, plague erupted out of China, devastating Hong Kong; from there, it spread in pandemic waves around the world.[3] Lasting until the late 1950s, the Third Plague Pandemic accounted for anywhere from 12 to 15 million deaths, centralized in India and China. But the pandemic left endemic ripples across the globe, imprinting a lasting impact on modern systems of public health. It struck the British-occupied Cape Colony in 1900, during the height of the South African War, leading to some of the most destructive ecological, environmental and social changes in South African history.[4] The British colonial government employed hundreds, if not thousands, of African men in the first two decades of the twentieth century in an all-out assault against plague. These men did the bulk of both dangerous and routine public health labour during the Third

Plague Pandemic; they were 'labourers', 'gangers', 'cleansing staff', 'disinfecting staff' and 'rat catchers'. Central in the fight against plague, they faced unparalleled daily dangers to their health and to the health of their families. The stories of these labourers have been largely kept out of the historical record.[5]

The outbreak of plague worldwide came at a time of unprecedented European intrusion and expansion into East Asia, Southeast Asia and Africa, a heightened period of 'New Imperialism'.[6] The late nineteenth century was also a time of immense change in Western public health and medical science, which saw both laboratory-based bacteriology and field-based epidemiology at their respective heights of cultural authority as the bastions of surveillance in the modern state.[7] By 1900, the causative organisms had been cultured and isolated for tuberculosis (by Robert Koch in 1882), cholera (by Koch again in 1883), typhoid fever (by Karl Eberth in 1880) and bubonic plague (by Alexandre Yersin and Shibasaburo Kitasato in 1894). On a parallel track, epidemiologists by 1900 had unravelled the major pathways by which many infectious diseases spread, learning that cholera and typhoid are communicated via food and water, and that plague is spread, as Pasteurian doctor Paul-Louis Simond demonstrated in 1898, via a rat-flea connection.[8]

But clarity about the origin, cause and spread of infectious disease – in other words about germ theories – in this period, rarely translated easily into day-to-day germ practices.[9] As numerous scholars have shown, British public health officials instituted racialized public health measures, many of which targeted the supposed pathogenicity of Indian and African bodies.[10] This chapter, focusing on anti-pandemic labour, moves us beyond the European rhetoric of indigenous bodies as unique foci and spreaders of disease, by examining the immediate and lasting health threats placed upon indigenous labourers as a result of the British colonial system of public health. In the late nineteenth and early twentieth century, British colonial officials blamed indigenous peoples for the spread of infectious diseases such as plague and typhoid fever, and also charged Indians and Africans with the bulk of anti-epidemic labour. This racialized colonial hygienic logic opened the door for unique forms of anti-colonial resistance from Indians and Africans, as Poonam Bala and David Arnold have shown, but it also put indigenous peoples at unique health risks.[11] My interest in this chapter, in other words, is on the racialized, gendered and spatial politics of colonial public health. When plague struck British colonial port cities in the late nineteenth and early twentieth century, where an individual lived, and where and how they worked, very much impacted the extent to which they would be exposed to disease-causing microorganisms. The place and labour of indigenous Indians and Africans, in the broader configuration of imperial policy, also determined who British colonial officials blamed for the spread of an epidemic, where in an urban space anti-epidemic techniques would target, and who would undertake such dangerous work.

Thinking about labour in colonial locations in the first decades of the acceptance of the germ theory is an important window into the racialization and gendered nature of public health work. Randall Packard's *White Plague, Black Labor* goes some way in framing how mining practices and the demand for African labour led to differential health outcomes, specifically chronic ailments such as tuberculosis, between colonizer and colonized in South Africa.[12] And yet, the exigencies of a pandemic of bubonic plague in the years around 1900 produced very different kind of 'work' for the empire, and a different set of health consequences for indigenous people. Examining anti-pandemic labour necessitates that we ask who was doing the labour of public health work in the fight against plague? What were they actually doing? Why were they chosen? What was the impact of this work on indigenous populations, on the health landscape and environment, and on the politics of imperialism?

Central to the broader aims of this volume, examining anti-pandemic labour in colonial South Africa and India reveals the complex ways that European imperialism and colonial public health strategies reified the racial logic that indigenous peoples were 'diseased', by placing indigenous people at the front lines of anti-epidemic control.[13] In responding to the Third Plague Pandemic, for example, British colonial officials routinely argued, in theoretical articles and in monthly and annual reports, that Indians and Africans were 'more susceptible' to plague than Europeans.[14] But here, as in other contemporary examples, epidemiology and vital statistics reinforced the racial logic of colonialism.[15] Buried beneath the framing of indigenous peoples as 'diseased' was the reality that in responding to serious health threats such as plague, cholera, and typhoid, Indians and Africans were at the front lines of public health work. Coupled with structural inequalities in housing and urban segregation, increased transmission rates for infectious disease among indigenous peoples was the by-product of colonial public health. And, as the case studies of India and Africa demonstrate during the Third Plague Pandemic, the lasting impact was immense; colonial officials displaced indigenous peoples in urban centres in an attempt to stamp out the so-called hiding places of plague, leading to long-term health inequalities that lasted far beyond the pressures of an epidemic.

This chapter focuses on two aspects of race, place and health in exploring anti-epidemic labour in colonial South Africa and India. Part one examines how African labourers came into close contact with plague during the Third Plague Pandemic, disinfecting urban spaces, destructing homes, managing disinfecting machines and catching rats. Part two shows how conservancy work in British cantonments in India, in the fight against another deadly infectious disease, typhoid fever, fell into the hands of low-caste coolie labourers, who handled and destructed European excreta in an attempt to remake Indian spaces hygienic and sanitary in the minds of colonial officials. These anti-epidemic measures put indigenous labourers into close contact with the dangerous media that spread infectious disease with fatal results for indigenous communities. By focusing on the actual practices of anti-epidemic control, I show how labour, race and colonialism intersected, causing lasting demographic impacts on the Global South. The combination of racialized policies, commercial projects and indigenous labour enforced throughout the age of British imperialism opened new in-person contact points for the introduction of disease, often spawning into epidemiological disasters in the colonized world (Samanta, Ahmed and Dey in this volume).

While the voices of indigenous labourers have often been silenced in the archives, by looking at unique archival material on the day-to-day activities of labouring people, this chapter recasts and illuminates how the structure and logic of British imperialism put groups of indigenous labourers at greater risks for suffering from and dying of infectious disease.[16] I argue, in line with the broader aim of this volume, that the racialized organization of imperial public health work and the imagining of indigenous urban spaces as dangerous and unclean were factors in spreading infectious diseases around the globe in the late nineteenth and early twentieth century.[17] At the same time, however, I also show the complicated ways that putting indigenous labourers in charge of anti-epidemic work provided an opportunity to critique the colonial project of what Ruth Rogaski has called 'hygienic modernity'.[18]

PLAGUE WORK IN THE CAPE COLONY

On 5 March 1900, at 7:00 a.m. the SS *Kilburn* with a crew of thirty-two landed at the Cape Town docks in Table Bay. The ship had arrived from Rosario, Argentina, having departed there on 15 February, carrying forage grain that the British government had purchased to feed military horses during the South African War. Table Bay dock workers noted that three crew members were sick, and the acting port health officer, Dr Manikus, confirmed with the *Kilburn*'s acting chief officer that 'a few cases of plague' were on the ship. Manikus further learned that the British captain of the vessel, Robert Valder, had already died of plague en route, his dead body still on board.[19] Alfred John Gregory, Cape Town's Medical Officer of Health (MOH), came at once and recognized the three sick sailors as well-marked cases of bubonic plague. He withdrew fluid from the buboes of all three sick individuals on the ship, inoculating the sickest man with a 40 c.c. dose of Yersin's anti-plague serum and returned to his office, ordering the ship and crew to a makeshift quarantine 90 miles north at Saldanha Bay, to be closely watched day and night by police guards. Laboratory evidence confirmed all three were positive cases of bubonic plague, and for further precautions Gregory ordered that the body of the *Kilburn*'s dead captain be wrapped in sheets soaked with carbolic acid and buried in an iron coffin at Saldanha Bay. Gregory quickly wrote to the commissioner at Robben Island, asking for the assistance of the newly arrived Irish bacteriologist, James Alexander Mitchell, who at the time was in charge of leprosy research on the island.[20] Mitchell was quickly transferred to watch over the quarantine at Saldanha Bay and to disinfect the ship and its contents and inoculate the entire crew. Upon setting up the *Kilburn* at Saldanha Bay, Gregory was cautiously optimistic that 'no danger to the Colony should arise from the presence of these cases, as I think that our measures should be efficacious in preventing any spread'.[21] But his hopes were dashed, and as the medical officer at one of the British Empire's most coveted ports, a fulcrum between the Atlantic and Indian Oceans, Gregory knew he had a potentially explosive public health crisis on his hands.

And for a while it seemed like the Cape Colony might be spared the plague – newspapers reported that Gregory had acted decisively with regard to plague on the SS *Kilburn* – by November, plague cases popped up in King William's Town, among Africans living at Izeli in the Izinyoka compound 8 miles outside of the town. In February 1901, plague broke out in Cape Town. The first reported case, of an African dock worker who lived in District Six, set off a widespread panic in the city. By March, there were 150 cases and 60 deaths, and by June, 700 cases and 326 deaths. When the epidemic waned in the fall, there were over 800 cases and 400 dead.[22] Officials reported more cases among 'Native Kaffirs', the British derogatory slang for indigenous Africans, and 'coloureds', a term reserved for immigrant labourers from various parts of Southeast Asia. But as soon as plague died down in Cape Town in late 1901, it exploded from port city to port city in the Cape Colony, in King William's Town, East London and Port Elizabeth, with cases lingering for over a decade, and plague reaching endemic levels in South Africa.

William John Ritchie Simpson was the chief architect of anti-plague measures in the Cape Colony. Simpson worked as the health officer in Calcutta for over a decade and was keenly active in British hygienic networks.[23] He was well informed, for example, of when Kitasato and Yersin identified *Yersinia pestis* as the causative organism for plague in 1894, and when Paul Louis-Simond, working at the important port city of Karachi (Figure 12.1), linked the flea-rat-human zoonotic connection with plague in 1898.[24] When plague exploded in India, Simpson orchestrated one of the most extreme and intrusive public health approaches anywhere in the British Empire, defining the ways in which the Third Plague Pandemic provided what David Arnold calls an unheralded 'attack on the body'.[25]

Throughout Indian cities in the 1890s, British colonial officials such as Simpson mobilized massive public health efforts to fight plague, targeting Indian urban environments, Indian homes and Indian bodies. During the Third Plague Pandemic, millions of Indians were evicted from their homes, expelled to segregation, also called 'health' camps, and disinfected, sometimes in vats of dangerous and caustic carbolic acid.[26] At the centre of anti-plague measures in colonial India were so-called gangs of 'coolie' labourers, who did the routine and dangerous work of handling plague corpses, disinfecting, fumigating, whitewashing and sometimes destroying Indian homes. Anti-plague measures in India were a mix of bacteriological specificity and racialized imperial action. As plague waned in India, Simpson headed back to Britain, where he co-founded the London School of Hygiene and Tropical Medicine, and taught Hygiene at King's College. He believed in 1898 that he was done with colonial public health. But an explosion of typhoid fever during the South African War drew him back into the imperial fray.

In 1900, Britain's parliament sent a royal commission to enquire about the massive typhoid deaths, sending three distinguished doctors: military epidemiologist James Lane Notter, pathologist David Bruce and the tropical hygienist William Simpson. The three spent a year travelling from field hospital to field hospital in the Transvaal and Orange Free State, trying to unravel the cause of the typhoid outbreak. It was arduous work and the three spent more time bickering with one another rather than sorting out the spread of the disease.[27] But when it was clear in early 1901 that plague was erupting

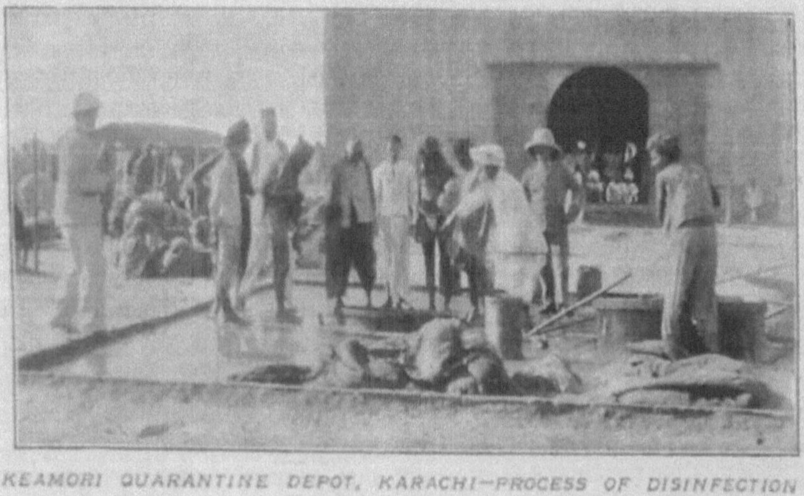

KEAMORI QUARANTINE DEPOT, KARACHI—PROCESS OF DISINFECTION
Photo by Mr. J. H. C. Kelly

Figure 12.1 Keamori Quarantine Depot, 1898. *Source*: Wellcome Library, RAMC.

in the Cape Colony, the colonial secretary ordered Simpson to travel to Cape Town and the MOH for the Cape Colony, John Gregory.

Simpson, a self-stylist expert on plague, set to work immediately with a vision for a central anti-plague response and public health administration. He was committed, as Echenberg notes, to the late Victorian racial logic that indigenous Indians and Africans were inferior and the central source of spreading plague. Simpson advised the colonial secretary, T.L. Graham, to enact a portion of British law, the Public Health Amendment Act of 1897, which provided colonial officials – with aid from the local police force – sweeping powers to enter homes at any time of day, inspect and if necessary forcibly remove inhabitants who were suspected of having plague or were in houses which were deemed 'unfit for human habitation'.[28] It allowed officials to disinfect people, their clothes and their houses. It even granted officers the ability to destroy houses if deemed necessary. Simpson arranged a special Plague Administration Board, with John Gregory as its administrative head and plague officers in each of the major port cities in the colony. Each officer raised a mini public health army, starting in Cape Town, and quickly got to work.

Simpson organized a methodical approach and a detailed recording system, even designing a form medical officers and local doctors should use each time they discovered a case of plague. The form included the date and address of plague cases, the number of rats found and destroyed, and, importantly, the type of public health action taken, whether cleansing, disinfecting or destroying a house. 'The disease should be attacked in a systematic and precise manner', Simpson warned, 'and not in a haphazard fashion'.[29] Simpson's anti-plague approach centred not on a bacteriological solution – colonial officers did receive samples of Haffkine's anti-plague inoculation, but results were not conclusive – but on an epidemiological one.[30] For Simpson and Gregory, mapping was a key tool in visualizing where plague cases had occurred, where infestations of rats were located and where general filthiness prevailed. Gregory, more even handed and mild mannered than Simpson, was nonetheless adamant that a systematic approach should guide the anti-plague work in the colony. He and Simpson worked together with a local surveyor to produce an incredible epidemiological plague map of the city, marking a red dog on a yellow square for houses infected with plague cases, a yellow square alone for houses infected with plague-infected animals but with no plague cases and a red dot alone for locations where a plague corpse was found but whose residence was unknown (Figure 12.2).[31]

Key to the entire anti-plague public health scheme in Cape Town, and later in other cities in the Cape Colony, was an infrastructure of African workers to carry out the actual work of cleansing, rat catching and disinfecting the

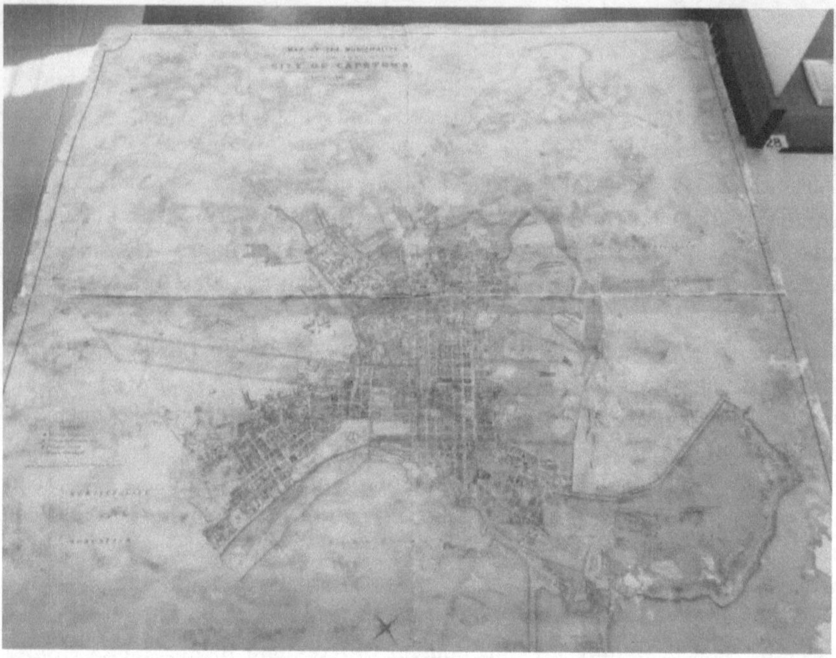

Figure 12.2 Plague Map of Cape Town, 1900. *Source*: Western Cape Archives, MOH.

urban environment. Gregory first hired two European doctors, J. B. Collie, supervise a disinfecting staff who would target specific areas known to harbour plague, and H. L. Creed to oversee a cleansing staff to generally cleanse the city. In three days Collie and Creed had assembled a 'Disinfecting Corps' and 'Cleansing Corps', 'intended to deal with houses not known to be infected with Plague, & generally to cleanse the City of Cape Town and to deal with "suspected" cases of plague or plague-prone areas'.[32] Worried that both crews needed further supervision, the British colonial secretary called upon E. N. Jackson, superintendent to the Breakwater Convict Station, to inspect and report on the disinfection process, and generally to use police force to uphold the anti-plague measures.[33] Police were a key arm of the public health approach of removing indigenous Africans from their urban homes, sending them to a racially segregated plague camp and cleansing and disinfecting their empty homes, illustrated in a contemporary 1901 image in *The Graphic* (Figure 12.3).

The cleansing and disinfecting officers in Cape Town recruited 100 African labourers at wages of three pennies a day, a small European staff and asked for 'volunteers' from among the male convicts at Robben Island. They offered convicts one day off their sentence for each day on plague duty, six pennies per day wages and 'indulgences in the shape of Coffee and Tobacco'. Over 400 convicts 'immediately volunteered', and he hired 280 of them.

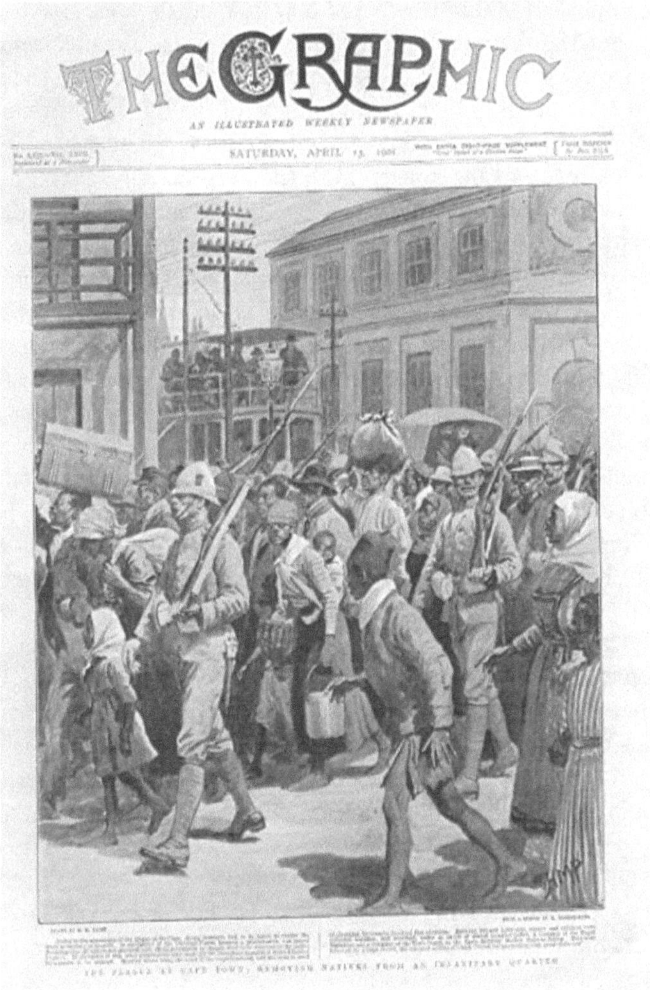

Figure 12.3 'The Plague at Cape Town'. *Source*: *The Graphic*, 13 April 1901.

Gregory and Simpson ordered the labourers first to District Six, which Simpson in a private memo called a 'centre of Plague'.[34] Using the racial epidemiological logic of diseased Africans living in diseased environments, he argued that cases of plague in other areas of town probably originated from District Six. Simpson recommend that cleansing and disinfection labourers be directed to killing rats, removing floor boards, disinfecting entire houses, pouring disinfectant down rat runs and removing inhabitants to either plague eviction camps or sheltering them temporarily outside their homes in mobile iron huts.[35] Creed's team posted 19,000 plague handbills throughout the city:

19,000 in English, 4,900 in Dutch and 600 in Yiddish (none in African languages). From March until the end of June 1901, Creed's team cleansed over 600 houses throughout the city, concentrated in District Six. They caught over 2,000 rats and used over 2,300 gallons of disinfectants to the cost of £3,500. 'No words can', Creed noted in his report, 'paint the indescribable filth in which many of the houses were found to be. On several occasions my men, on entering a room that had been closed for two or three days were overpowered by the foul air within, and in three instances men were dragged out of these dens by their companions in an asphyxiated condition'.[36] And, 'that the danger was real', Creed continued in his memo to Gregory, 'may be gathered from the attached return of cases of Plague which occurred amongst my Staff', eight cases and four deaths, 'in every case the contagion was traced to the work upon which they were engaged'.[37]

This intensive work continued in Cape Town until late June, when plague cases dwindled in the city, and thousands of Africans had been removed to the eviction camp. The racial logic of anti-plague labour continued, however. William Stoney, assistant director of the Plague Administration, wrote to Gregory in June 1901 to say that white labourers should be reduced; 'I am of the opinion', he noted in a confidential letter, 'that we should make more use of the convicts and native labour . . . to complete the necessary repairs in some of the Plague infected houses, in order that we may get up to date with all the work as speedily as possible'.[38] This logic was both economic and racial. British officials complained that there was constant turnover in the disinfecting and cleansing staff, causing 'a very large increase of clerical labour'.[39] Europeans employed by plague officials earned anywhere from seven to fifteen shillings a day. And although plague cases decreased within the city of Cape Town, plague continued to inflict pain and misery on the wider Cape Colony, with cases appearing in King William's Town, Port Elizabeth and Durban. The anti-plague measures in those provincial colonial cities mirrored what had occurred in Cape Town. Looking at the extensive archival files from this period, it is clear that the bulk of all British colonial expenditure on plague was spent on indigenous African labour and on disinfectants.

In one month alone, for example, in Port Elizabeth, D. C. Rees, the plague officer, noted in his report to Gregory, of the £1,600 spent on anti-plague work, £1,100 was spent on disinfection labour costs. Taken together with the cost of disinfectants – typically phenyl or crude carbolic acid – which were imported from Britain and Germany (Figure 12.4), and the bulk of anti-plague measures revolved around disinfection, where gangs of labourers would use pump sprayers inside and outside of buildings. When houses were deemed 'unfit for human habitation', they were simply destroyed.

There were a handful of complaints made by Africans about the intrusive, destructive and dehumanizing anti-plague measures, but none were taken seriously by British plague officials.[40] Even Europeans who complained often did not get much traction. In Port Elizabeth, for example, in 1905 teams of plague labourers destroyed Arthur Clarence Reed's property, a housing building that he rented to over a hundred Africans (Figure 12.5). Reed's building was deemed dangerous, filthy and rat infested. After his property was destroyed he sued the Port Elizabeth Town Council, and the case went as far as the Supreme Court. But the judge ruled in favour of the plague officials, noting 'the Council owed a duty to the public to leave no stone unturned to check the ravages of the disease'.[41]

And for several years throughout the Cape Colony that is precisely what plague officials did; leave no stone unturned. The work became routinized, with gangs focusing on homes and buildings deemed unfit for habitation, and on foodstuffs such as cereals, grains, and forage. Labourers dipped sacks in disinfectant and dried them in the open sun in hopes of thwarting both rats and plague bacilli. As one plague official noted, 'many thousands of bags' have been 'dealt with in this way. This method is believed not only to effectively destroy any infection in the sacks, but also render sacks of grain so dealt with obnoxious to rodents.'[42]

As one plague officer reported: 'Closed spaces in Stores and buildings have been explored, and stacks of timber have been raised . . . rat holes and burrows have been disinfected and cemented, cover for rodents has been cleared

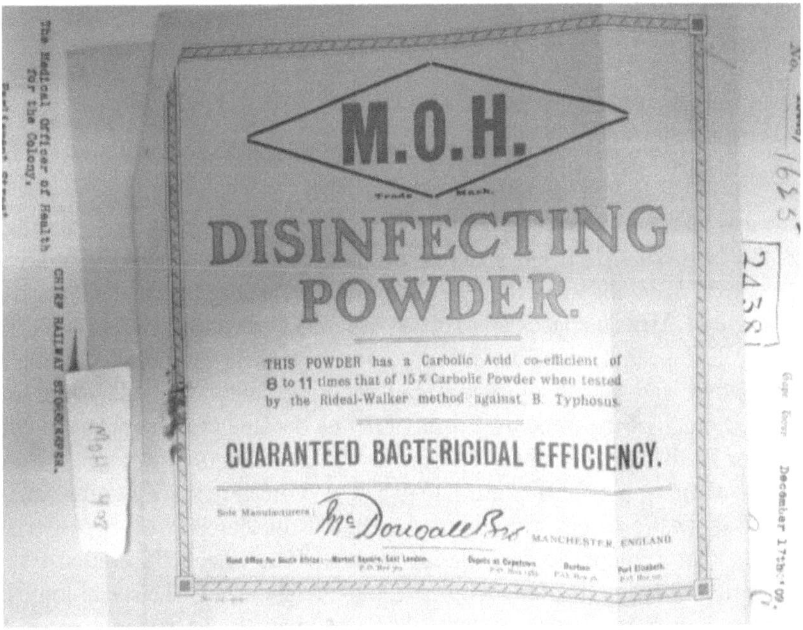

Figure 12.4 Advertisement for MOH Disinfecting Powder. *Source*: Western Cape Archives, MOH/403.

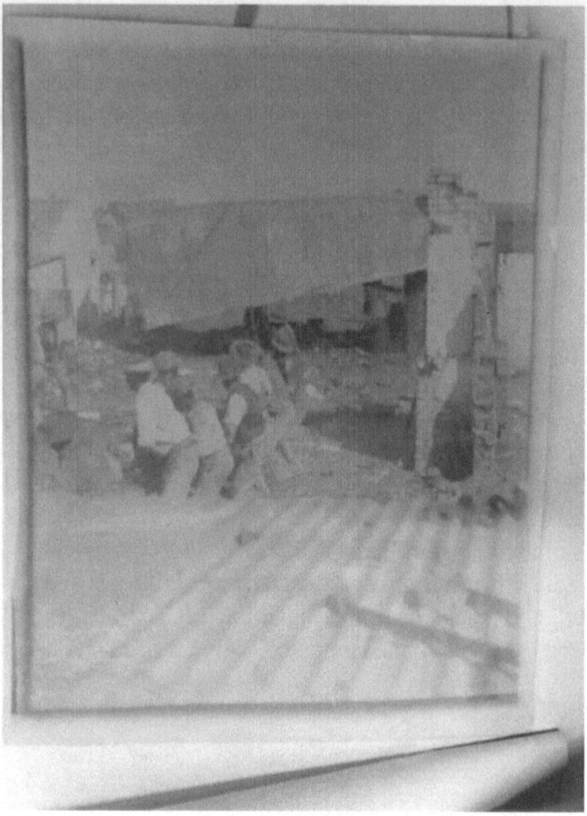

Figure 12.5 Destruction of Reed's Property, Port Elizabeth. *Source*: Western Cape Archives, MOH/4.

away and nesting and excreta destroyed . . . the work has been very carefully and thoroughly carried out, and that no pains have been spared to make it successful'. More than anything plague proved an excuse to remake the urban landscape of African spaces that British officials were attempting to turn into sanitary European ones. The fear of plague kept this whitewashed colonial dream alive, and the newly discovered zoonotic pathway of plague in rats provided much of the impetus. From 1901 rats became the canary in the coal mine for British plague officials. Even in months when there were no plague cases in humans, plague officials had gangs of African labourers daily intruding into domestic spaces, ripping up floorboards in search of plague-infected rats. Another epidemiological plague map, at Port Elizabeth, demonstrates the overlap between the dangers of anti-plague labour and the racial logic of British colonialism. British officials there, the map shows, ordered gangs of labourers to target specific 'foci', or 'centres' of infection, hand-circled in blue, and to work in concentric rings outward.

Most striking about maps (Figure 12.6) like this produced during the Third Plague Pandemic is the extent to which, while they provide a unique spatial perspective of the labour involved in public health work fighting plague, they decorporealize the actual work itself. Even the qualitative reports by British officials fail to humanize the labour involved, the labourers themselves or the imminent dangers attendant to plague work. Perhaps the process of giving African gang workers names like 'bubo', 'contact' or 'Jim Crow' was part of that dehumanization process as well.

That in India and South Africa, British officials relied on indigenous men to do anti-epidemic work should give us some pause as well, though much can be said the same of disinfection work in Britain, where MOHs hired poor, urban and immigrant men to do the dangerous and routine work of clearing and disinfecting urban centres. The gendered choices tell us a great deal, as well, especially coupled with their overlay onto contemporary racial categorizations, about the conception of some types of public health work in the post-bacteriological age as manly work. Often British officials spoke of hiring physically fit men and firing labourers who could not meet the colonial demands of such physical labour.

Although we know indigenous women engaged in public health work as well, often as washerwomen, their voices and stories are almost silent. This

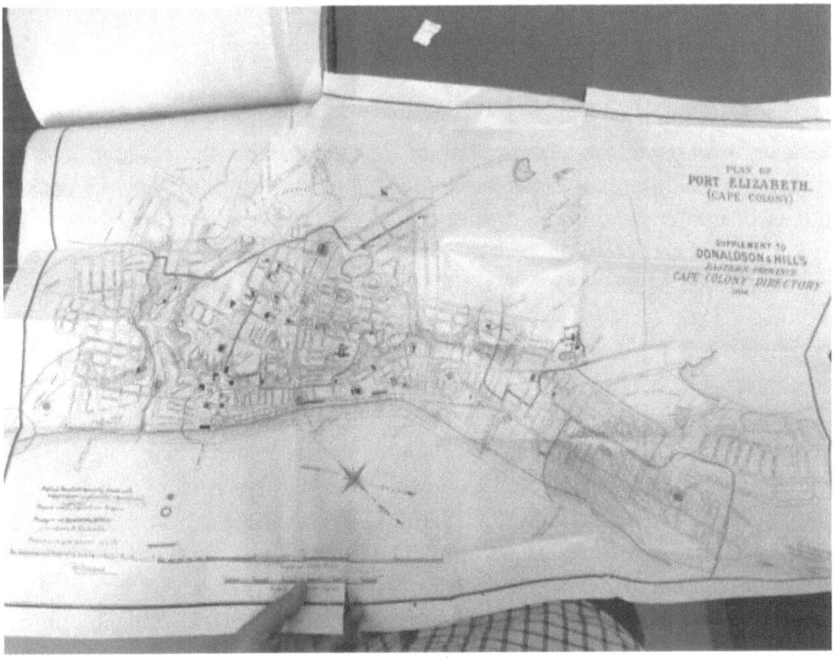

Figure 12.6 Plague Map, Port Elizabeth, 1905. *Source*: Western Cape Archives, MOH/4.

should tell us something as well about how the germ theory not only restructured urban environments, but also gendered stereotypes of who was fit and proper to do certain types of public health work.

The Third Plague Pandemic engendered fear and panic, as Robert Peckham has argued, not just from its high case fatality, but also the pandemic's disruption of imperial control, expansion and trade.[43] Plague control became, as Christos Lynteris argues, 'the prototype of all human pandemics', entangling colonial, economic and scientific discourses.[44] In colonial South Africa, anti-plague legislation set the stage for later apartheid practices of urban segregation, and thus represents one of the most important parts of global history. It is difficult, if not impossible, to tell how many Africans died either directly from plague labour or indirectly through familial networks. What is clear is that Africans disproportionately died from plague, and that their health outcomes as a result of anti-plague work, particularly the attempt to remake the urban environment, had lasting impacts. As much as the expediency and fear of a pandemic of plague drove intrusive and destructive colonial public health measures that negatively impacted indigenous populations, everyday disease threats did as well. Chief among them in a different part of the British Empire, in India, was the threat to imperial stability posed by a food-and-water borne, faecal-oral disease, typhoid fever.

EXCREMENTAL OBSESSIONS

There was a long gestation of excremental obsession in England stretching back to at least mid-nineteenth century. It began within the nascent field of epidemiology, in arguing long before the laboratory discovery of the causal agents of cholera and typhoid, that the two diseases were primarily spread by air, water and clothing contaminated with the faecal discharges of sick patients. Chief Medical Officer of the Privy Council, John Simon, for example, in an 1866 Cholera Memorandum, noted that 'excrement-sodden earth, excrement-reeking air, excrement-tainted water, these are for us the causes of cholera'.[45] This was the view taken up by E. D. Dickson and Edward Goodeve, British representatives at the 1867 Cholera Conference at Constantinople, who warned that the 'chief source of the malady' was discharges, which needed to be disinfected to destroy the 'cholera poison'.[46] Recurrent cholera threats to England in the 1870s, 1880s and 1890s were framed in a similar way, with a series of governmental memos warning that '*All matters which the patient discharges from his stomach and bowels are infective*'. But more than the excremental threat of cholera was the faecal-stained, annual reality of typhoid. William Budd went as far in a famous phrase to call the sewer drain an extension of the intestine, a powerful graph between the individual body and the body politic. Annual reports by England's MOHs during this period show the range and sheer doggedness of sanitary activities that localized on excreta – disinfecting human and animal faeces, and things that came into contact with faeces, took up an enormous amount of time in the everyday practices of Victorian public health.

But the practices of disinfection were haphazard at best at this time, with debates over the relative merits of steam versus dry heat technologies, the Washington Lyon over the Thresh disinfector, alongside the use of a bevy of chemical disinfectants.[47] The post-bacteriological age wrought an explosion of experimental research on disinfection, particularly after Emanuel Klein, A. C. Houston and Sidney Martin proved in a series of novel experiments that *Bacillus typhosus* and *Vibrio cholera* could live for extended periods in excreta discarded in normal garden soil: in other words, the ecological life of germs. The story of how disinfection took hold in practice, however uneven, in England is taken up in Graham Mooney's recent *Intrusive Interventions*. We know far less about how disinfection efforts targeted excrement across the British Empire in the decades that followed the germ theory.

If we look across the British imperial spaces in the late nineteenth and early twentieth century, what we find at first mirrors Warwick Anderson's argument about American health officers' attempts at hygienic modernity in the Philippines: British public health officials were concerned with the pathogenicity of Indian and African bodies.[48] Addressing the Indian Medical Congress at Calcutta in 1894, for example, English physician and editor of the *British Medical Journal*, Ernest Hart, quipped that cholera is 'a filth disease, carried by dirty people to dirty places, and there spread by dirt and the use of dirty water'.[49] It is clear that Hart's fear was not about white English bodies in the tropics, but Indian ones.

But beyond the rhetoric of filthy indigenous Indians or Africans, British medics were obsessed, sine qua non, over their own excrement. More specifically, at the filthy habits of British soldiers. It seems that before the promiscuous body of the Indian or African could come under the sanitary gaze of Western public health, the space of the cantonment and the field hospital, the body of the white male soldier and the objects of Western excreta all had to first be managed. But as I suggest here, the spatial and corporeal sanitary management of white geographies and white bodies was through black and brown labour.

Charles Melville, professor of Hygiene at the Royal Army Medical College (RAMC), impressed 'on every young officer going to India that, as regards disease prevention, the removal of excreta is infinitely the most important question that he will have to face'.[50] It was a view echoed by RAMC officers like R. J. Blackham, who noted that 'the disposal of sewage is a burning sanitary question of the hour in all quarters of the globe'. 'Conservancy is *the* most important matter', Blackham argued, to 'the health of British troops'.[51] Melville went as far as to lay out an entire spatial thinking, that 'with every yard that the excreta are removed from the vicinity of barracks the danger diminishes in inverse ratio to the square distance'.[52] Melville's was a well-versed Manichaean dichotomy between the sanitary cantonment and the filthy village bazaar. J. B. Hamilton, statistical superintendent for the Government of India, and later health officer in South Africa, put it quite succinctly, stating that, 'outside the cantonment limits India is exceedingly foul . . . the sanitary position of our troops in India is – they reside in 'oases of cleanliness surrounded by deserts of filth'.[53] Thus articulated, the problem was twofold. British sanitary officers first had to bound the sanitary oasis of the western cantonment, and second, they had to carefully navigate how British troops entered the Orientalist wilderness of the unsanitary desert of the village bazaar. It was a fascinating imagined geography. In reality transferring between both spaces was a complex mix of people, animals, things, and, very materially, of excrement. Beyond the rhetoric, the cantonment and bazaar were permeable colonial enclaves, to borrow a phrase from Nandini Bhattacharya.[54]

There was a kind of self-fulfilling, circular logic to British ideas of excrement, mapped onto conceptualizations of racial hierarchy, the body and the body politic. The rhetoric was often on Indian excrement, but the reality was the fear and proximity to British excrement. Consider the remarks of William Ewart, who in 1905 lectured IMS officers departing for India to focus on a regime he called the 'hygiene of the bowel', the need for 'intestinal sanitation'.[55] His was a focus exclusively on white British bodies.

One way to parse out the rhetoric versus the reality of excrement is thinking through the politics of labour in public health work. Take, for example, the massively popular handbook from William Alex Muirhead, *Practical Tropical Sanitation*, whose frontispiece is an interesting depiction of the rhetoric of early twentieth century colonial public health, a striking vision of hygienic modernity.

Key within the chart, 'The Bridge of Health' (Figure 12.7), was a division of labour at the bottom, where the excrement lives, and where indigenous 'sanitary labourers' were key. British cantonments in India employed legions of low-caste Indian 'sweepers', otherwise called 'conservancy men' or 'conservancy coolies' (although women were also employed in the work) who did the everyday practices of excrement removal and control. Florence Nightingale went as far as to call Indian conservancy sweepers 'human drain-pipes', which Charles Melville later agreed in 1912 was 'his proper function, and should be his only function'.[56]

There were three central ways of dealing with excrement in British cantonments in India around 1900: burying, burning or sterilizing. The most common was the Dry Earth pail system. Latrines were fitted with pails (only sometimes

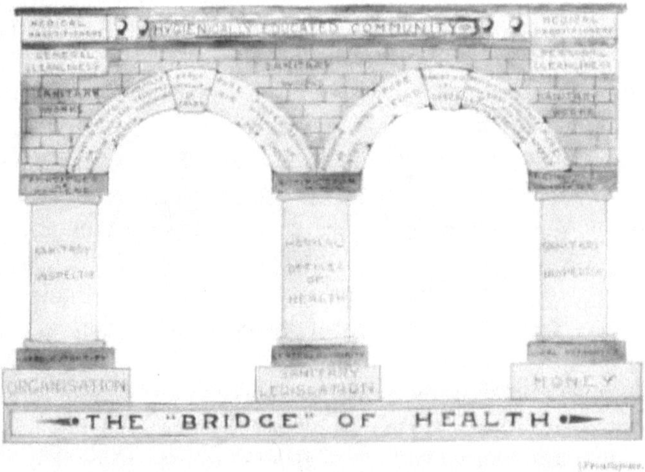

Figure 12.7 The 'Bridge' of Health. *Source*: William Alex Muirhead, Practical Tropical Sanitation (London: John Murray, 1914).

lidded), into which excrement dropped, then a layer of dry earth was used to cover faeces. Twice a day a corps of labourers collected pails, dumped them in a horse-drawn or hand-drawn Crawley cart, and brought the fetid sludge outside of the cantonment and emptied it into trenches. Some trenches were only a few yards outside of the cantonment, but other stations reported that their 'fecal trenching grounds' (actually their name) were a mile away. The most popular trench system was called the Allahabad System, designed by RAMC Majors A. C. Williams and D. J. Meagher, which relied on shallow trenches: rectangular in shape, 16 × 5 feet – depth of 3 inches – capacity of 60 gallons each, what a typical Crowley cart could hold – conservancy sweepers would spread the excreta over the trench, then cover it with earth. After a few weeks the trench could be cultivated – again too by conservancy labourers, to make tobacco or sugarcane. Seen as a form of colonial resistance, through indigenous labour British excrement could be turned into the sweet fruits of colonial commodities.

While it was the most common method of dealing with cantonment excrement, by the first decade of the twentieth century trenching was coming into criticism, as dangerous and inefficient; heavy rain might wash away excrement into water sources, and shallow trenches were the veritable homes of flies and other animals. There was rarely concern on the part of British colonial officials that Indian labourers were coming into direct contact with the dangerous media of spreading faecal-oral diseases such as cholera and typhoid. In 1898, after numerous outbreaks of typhoid at Dagshai were said to be due to the shallow trench system, the colonial Government of India made orders to disinfect and burn the entire site and abandon it for a year.

Those RAMC and IMS officials against the trench system argued that it required too numerous Indian sweepers who, other than cost, many British officers felt, could not be trusted. Patrick Hehir, director of Medical Services in Burma, noted that the 'jolting of the carts' caused 'excreta to assume a viscid glutinous form' and spill from the sides of the cart, leaving faecal deposits throughout camp – ready to spring the next outbreak of typhoid, dysentery or cholera.[57]

Here we run into a fascinating conceptualization of the Indian sweeper. For all of their doing, of keeping cantonments sanitary 'oases', sweepers were demonstrably feared by British medics. RAMC officer Bruce Skinner opined that 'every detail of the scavenger's work must be watched'.[58] There was a particularly vocal British fear of what happens at night, of Indian sweepers doing unsanitary handling of British excrement in the dark. Hehir, for example, noted that 'the darkness offers temptations to the workmen to deposit excreta in places not intended for the purpose'. And so, the night-soil men became in British India 'day-soil' men, with officers like Hehir insisting that 'all removal of excreta should be carried out during the day time when it can be properly supervised and its defects observed'.[59] And the fear of what happens at night in spreading disease was not just fixated on Indian bodies. In reality, it was often the night-time mishaps of British troops in cantonments. A recurring theme in RAMC and IMS reports was the late night, often drunken urination onto the ground by British troops. In other words, it was not just 'promiscuous' Indian defecators, to borrow Anderson's phrase, which rarely comes up in British army records from this time, but rather promiscuous British micturators, particularly after A. C. Houston's 1900 discovery of high concentrations of *B. typhosus* in the urine of sick typhoid patients.

But for all its critics the trench system had its advocates. Indian Army Cantonment inspector H. B. Thornhill recommended the Allahabad System for all cantonments except those in the hill stations: 'let this method be given a full, searching, and extended trial', he trumpeted, 'and then call in the biological expert with his microscope and cultivating tubes to do his best'.[60] One alternative to the dry-earth, trenching system that emerged was the so-called wet system – where a pint of carbolic acid or perchloride of mercury was kept in the latrine pails, refilled by sweepers twice a day. RAMC officer in the Punjab, L. W. Harrison, believed the wet system could be implemented by soldiers better than sweepers: British men were ordered to 'drench' their stools after every evacuation using a spoon and kerosene pail full of disinfectant.[61]

By 1905, some medical officers were even incorporating sterilization machines to assist in the excremental-elimination system. RAMC officer

Glenn Allen, at Punjab, oversaw a system that many cantonments adopted. It used the wet system, but had sweepers empty latrine pails into an excreta sterilizer, where the contents were steamed at 60 degrees Celsius for 30 minutes.[62] From there a team of sweepers took the 'sterilized' excrement to the trenches.

The most popular alternative to the trenching system was incineration – a potent phallic throne of hygienic modernity that promised complete excrement elimination. There were a host of incinerators: open patterns like Raitt's incinerator, named after cantonment magistrate at Rawalpindi, and closed style incinerators like the Sialkot. The Sialkot, for example, promised a capacity to destroy in one day the excreta of 100 men, leaving behind a small pile of fine ash, a Phoenix-like transformation. Incineration advocates, and there were many – by 1910 over half of all cantonments had an incinerator – promised a reduced need for sweepers and Crowley carts – those visible nuisances of the so-called unhygienic past. Incinerators were placed next to latrines, where a smaller group of conservancy sweepers could quickly transfer pails to fire. It was an inversion to Melville's earlier spatial geography that excrement distancing kept men safe. The incinerator kept the matter close and in the open.

But here too there were objections to incineration: the first was fuel; coal or wood was widely recognized as the best option, but it was expensive and difficult to come by at many stations. Stable litter or bazaar garbage was also used, but troops complained of nauseating smells and obnoxious smoke. And even though incineration promised a cost-savings in the manual labour of scavenging, it reified the role of the Indian sweeper as excremental expert: 'the gravest of all the defects in this method', Lukis and Blackham's *Tropical Hygiene for Anglo-Indians and Indians* noted, 'is that whilst in the other systems the sweeper is important, in the practice of incineration he stands supreme, and the whole of the conservancy arrangements of a community depends on the good-will and behavior of the sweepers'.[63] For all of the focus on the Indian sweeper, or conservancy 'coolie' as the bastion of hygienic control in the cantonment, there was little colonial reflection on the health costs of such public health labour. This is not entirely surprising, but deserves close historical scrutiny, as the long-term impact of colonialism in India continues to shape the incidence of food- and water-borne diseases such as cholera, typhoid and dysentery.

CONCLUSION

J. B. Hamilton, statistical superintendent for the Government of India, grandstanded in 1890 that it was up to the 'civilized nation, England, to teach the backward nations of the East the value of cleanliness and the theory of germs'.[64] That rhetoric fits neatly into what scholars have said about the pathologization of indigenous bodies and that public health was tool of empire. But the rhetoric does not squarely match the reality if we centralize the labour and geography of thinking public health work in the colonies. Burning, burying and disinfecting excrement was inexorably about British anxieties of their own filth-producing capabilities, which had to be handled, managed and sanitized by indigenous experts – who in British hierarchical terms were low-caste Indians. These excremental obsessions reveal the spatial and racial logic of public health, and no doubt set the stage for more overt attacks on colonized bodies, for example, as seen during the Third Plague Pandemic. But the racialized labour of public health work in the colonies also has a great deal to tell us about the long-term impacts of colonial public health in the Global South, particularly the systemic problems of housing, food and infectious diseases that have 'disappeared' from the Western world.

NOTES

1. See, for example, R.J. Dick to John Gregory, "List of Men Employed on Town Plague Staff, King William's Town," dated 15 August 1903. Western Cape Archives and Records Service, South Africa, MOH/18. For a broader account of British colonial naming practices put upon indigenous peoples, see Clare Anderson, *Subaltern Lives: Biographies of Colonialism in the Indian Ocean World, 1790–1920* (Cambridge: Cambridge University Press, 2012).
2. On the connection between racial theory and practice in South Africa and the American South, see John C. Cell, *The Highest Stage of White Supremacy: The Origins of Segregation in South Africa and the American South* (Cambridge: Cambridge University Press, 1982) and George Fredrickson, *White Supremacy: A Comparative Study in American & South African History* (Oxford: Oxford University Press, 1981).
3. Robert Peckham, *Epidemics in Modern Asia* (Cambridge: Cambridge University Press, 2016), especially Chapter 1.
4. Maynard Swanson has suggested that the colonial response to plague in South Africa set the stage for urban segregation during the Apartheid era. See M. Swanson, "'The Sanitation Syndrome': Bubonic Plague and Urban Native Policy in the Cape Colony, 1900–1909," *Journal of African History* 18:3 (1977), 387–410.
5. The few scholarly works on the Third Plague Pandemic and the British colonial response have focused on printed sources, rather than the voluminous archival files. See, for example, Myron Echenberg, *Plague Ports: The Global Urban Impact of Bubonic Plague, 1894–1901* (New York: New York University Press, 2007), Chapter 10.
6. For a brief overview of the characterization of 'New Imperialism,' see, for example, Antionette Burton, *The Trouble with Empire: Challenges to Modern British Imperialism* (Oxford: Oxford University Press, 2015), and Tony Ballantyne,

Entanglements of Empire: Missionaries, Maori, and the Question of the Body (Durham: Duke University Press, 2014).

7. Tom Crook, "Sanitary Inspection and the Public Sphere in Late Victorian and Edwardian Britain: A Case Study in Liberal Governance," *Social History* 32:4 (2007), 369–393. See also, Dorothy Porter, *Health, Civilization and the State: A History of Public Health from Ancient to Modern Times* (London: Routledge, 1999), Chapter 8.

8. On unravelling the epidemiology of typhoid in the late Victorian period, see Jacob Steere-Williams, *The Filth Disease; Typhoid Fever and the Practices of Epidemiology in Victorian England* (Rochester: University of Rochester Press, 2020). Simond's discovery was not widely accepted for about a decade. See Marc Simond, Margaret L. Godley, and Pierre D.E. Mouriquand, "Paul-Louis Simond and His Discovery of Plague Transmission by Rat Fleas: A Centenary," *Journal of the Royal Society of Medicine,* 91, no. 2 (February, 1998), 101–104.

9. The now classic account of nineteenth-century debates around germ theories is Michael Worboys, *Spreading Germs: Disease Theories and Medical Practice in Britain, 1865–1900* (Cambridge: Cambridge University Press, 2000). An important contribution to the way that germ theories were put into practice in British colonial locations is Pratik Chakrabarti, *Bacteriology in British India: Laboratory Medicine and the Tropics* (Rochester: University of Rochester Press, 2017).

10. David Arnold, *Colonizing the Body: State Medicine and Epidemic Disease in Nineteenth Century India* (Berkeley: University of California Press, 1994); Megan Vaughn, *Curing Their Ills: Colonial Power and African Illness* (Cambridge: Polity Press, 1991); Daniel Gorman, *Imperial Citizenship: Empire and the Question of Belonging* (Manchester: Manchester University Press, 2006); Diana Heath, *Purifying Empire: Obscenity and the Politics of Moral Regulation in Britain, India, and Australia* (New York: Cambridge University Press, 2010).

11. Poonam Bala, *Contesting Colonial Authority: Medicine and Indigenous Responses in Nineteenth and Twentieth Century India* (Plymouth: Lexington Books, 2012). David Arnold, *Colonizing the Body.*

12. Randall Packard, *White Plague, Black Labor: Tuberculosis and the Political Economy of Health and Disease in South Africa* (Berkeley: University of California Press, 1989).

13. On the broader ways that indigenous peoples were seen as 'diseased' within the framework of the British Empire, see Suman Seth, *Difference and Disease: Medicine, Race, and the Eighteenth-Century British Empire* (Cambridge: Cambridge University Press, 2018).

14. In a 1904 memo, for example, John Gregory, MOH for Cape Town, recorded that indigenous Africans were 45.19% mortality from plague, which Europeans only had, by comparison, at 24.94% mortality. See John Gregory, "The Present State of Plague in the Colony," 25th inst. 1904 (no month listed). Western Cape Archives and Records Service, South Africa. MOH/21.

15. Mark Harrison, "Science and the British Empire," *Isis* 96 (2005), 56–63; Daniel Headrick, *The Tools of Empire: Technology and European Imperialism in the Nineteenth Century* (Oxford: Oxford University Press, 1981).

16. Tracey Banivanua Mar makes a similar argument about examining the archival silences of indentured women in Queensland. See Tracey Banivanua Mar, "The Contours of Agency: Women's Work, Race, and Queenland's Indentured Labor Trade," in Carol Williams (ed.) *Indigenous Women and Work: From Labor to Activism* (Urbana: University of Illinois Press, 2012), Chapter 4.

17. Antoinette Burton, *Archive Stories: Facts, Fictions, and the Writing of History* (Durham: Duke University Press, 2005); J.J. Ghaddar and Michelle Caswell, "To Go Beyond: Towards a Decolonial Archival Praxis," *Archival Science* 19 (2019), 71–85.

18. Ruth Rogaski, *Hygienic Modernity: Meanings of Health and Disease in Treaty-Port China* (Berkeley: University of California Press, 2015).

19. A.J. Gregory, "Bubonic Plague on Steamship 'Kilburn,'" dated 7 March 1900. Western Cape Archives and Records Service, South Africa, MOH/42.

20. A.J. Gregory, "Bubonic Plague on Steamship 'Kilburn,'" dated 7 March 1900. Western Cape Archives and Records Service, South Africa, MOH/42.

21. A.J. Gregory, "Bubonic Plague on Steamship 'Kilburn,'" dated 7 March 1900. Western Cape Archives and Records Service, South Africa, MOH/42

22. Anon., "The Plague: Prevalence of the Disease," *British Medical Journal* (15 June 1901), 1514.

23. R.A. Baker and R.A. Bayliss, "William John Ritchie Simpson (1855–1931): Public Health and Tropical Medicine," *Medical History* 31;4 (1987), 450–465. On Simpson's work on plague on the Gold Coast, see Ryan Johnson, "*Mantsemei,* Interpreters, and the Successful Eradication of Plague: The 1908 Plague Epidemic in Colonial Accra," in Ryan Johnson and Amna Khalid (eds.) *Public Health in the British Empire* (New York: Routledge, 2012), Chapter 7. On Simpson's plague work in China, see Carola Anne Benedict, *Bubonic Plague in Nineteenth Century China* (Stanford: Stanford University Press, 1996); on Simpson's plague work in India, see I.J. Catanch, "Plague and the Tensions of Empire: India, 1896–1918," in David Arnold (ed.) *Imperial Medicine and Indigenous Societies* (Manchester: Manchester University Press, 1991), Chapter 7.

24. Echenberg argues that Simpson did not fully accept Simond's rat-flea theory until the late 1900s. See Echenberg, *Plague Ports,* 70.

25. Arnold, *Colonizing the Body.* Mary P. Sutphen, "Not What but Where: Bubonic Plague and the Reception of Germ Theories in Hong Kong and Calcutta, 1894–1897", *Journal of the History of Medicine and Allied Sciences,* 52:1 (January 1997), 81–113; Srilata Chatterjee, "Plague and Politics in Bengal, 1896 to 1898," *Proceedings of the Indian History Congress,* 66 (2005–2006), 1194–1201. On Simpson's controversial stand on bacteriology, see Christos Lynteris, "Pestis Minor; The History of a Contested Plague Pathology," *Bulletin of the History of Medicine,* 93;1 (Spring 2019), 55–81.

26. Jacob Steere-Williams, "Coolie Control: State Surveillance and the Labour of Disinfection Across the Late Victorian British Empire," in Robert Heynen and Emily van der Meulen (eds.) *Surveillance States: Transnational Histories* (Toronto: University of Toronto Press, 2019), Chapter 2.

27. Jacob Steere-Williams, *The Filth Disease,* Chapter 5.

28. "Regulations Framed under Part 15 of The Public Health Amendment Act, 1897," Government Notice-No.269, 1901. Western Cape Archives and Records Service, South Africa, MOH/11.

29. W.J. Simpson to T.L. Graham, dated 15 May 1901. Western Cape Archives and Records Service, South Africa, MOH/42.

30. Early reports in Cape Town were that nine of the thirteen persons first inoculated died. W.J. Simpson to A.J. Gregory, dated 4 May 1901. Western Cape Archives and Records Service, South Africa, MOH/42

31. Plague Administration Form, titled "Summary of Daily Record of Work Done," Western Cape Archives and Records Service, South Africa, MOH/42

32. Letter from H.L. Creed to Colonial Secretary, Western Cape Archives and Records Service, South Africa, MOH/2.

33. Fred Whitham to E.N. Jackson, "Inspecting of Cleansing and Disinfecting Staffs," dated 3 June 1901. Western Cape Archives and Records Service, South Africa, MOH/42.

34. W.J. Simpson to F. Graham, dated 18 May 1901. Western Cape Archives and Records Service, South Africa, MOH/42.

35. H.L. Creed, "Report on the Cleansing Operations," dated 26 September 1901. Western Cape Archives and Records Service, South Africa. MOH/27.

36. H.L. Creed, "Report on the Cleansing Operations," dated 26 September 1901. Western Cape and Records Service, South Africa. MOH/27.

37. H.L. Creed, "Report on the Cleansing Operations," dated 26 September 1901. Western Cape Archives and Records Service, South Africa. MOH/27.

38. William Stoney to John Gregory, dated 12 June 1901. Western Cape Archives and Records Service, South Africa. MOH/23.

39. R.J. Dick to John Gregory, dated 15 August 1903. Western Cape Archives and Records Service, South Africa. MOH/11.

40. See, for example, Western Cape Archives and Records Service, MOH/260.

41. "Supreme Court," *Cape Times* (7 March 1905), newspaper clipping, Western Cape Archives and Records Service MOH/4.

42. T.D. Mitchell, "Systematic Cleansing Scheme: Port Elizabeth," page 6. dated 2 April 1905. Western Cape Archives and Records Service, MOH/4.

43. Robert Peckham, "Infective Economies: Empire, Panic, and the Business of Disease," *Journal of Imperial and Commonwealth History* 2 (2013), 211–237.

44. Christos Lynteris, *Ethnographic Plague: Configuring Disease at the Chinese-Russian Frontier* (London: Palgrave, 2016), 2.

45. John Simon, *Annual Report of the Medical Officer of the Privy Council for 1866* (London: Eyre and Spottiswoode, 1867).

46. *Dispatch from Her Majesty's Ambassador at Constantinople, with Documents, Presented at both Houses of Parliament* (London: Eyre and Spottiswoode, 1868).

47. On debates over technologies of disinfection in England and Wales, see Graham Mooney, *Intrusive Interventions: Public Health, Domestic Space, and Infectious Disease Surveillance, 1840–1914* (Rochester: University of Rochester Press, 2015).

48. Warwick Anderson, *Colonial Pathologies: American Tropical Medicine, Race, and Hygiene in the Philippines* (Durham: Duke University Press, 2006).

49. Ernest Hart, "Cholera: Where it Comes From and How it is Propagated," *British Medical Journal* (1 July 1893), 1.

50. Charles Melville, *Military Hygiene and Sanitation* (London: Edward Arnold, 1912), 209.

51. R.J. Blackham, "The Goux System and its Application to India," *Journal of the Royal Army Medical Corps,* 6 (1906), 662.

52. Melville, *Military Hygiene and Sanitation,* 209.

53. J.B. Hamilton, "Enteric Fever in India," *British Medical Journal* 1553 (4 October 1890), 788

54. Nandini Bhattacharya, *Contagion and Enclaves: Tropical Medicine in Colonial India* (Liverpool: Liverpool University Press, 2012).

55. William Ewart, "The Principles of Treatment of Typhoid Fever," *British Medical Journal,* vol.2 no.2345 (9 December 1905), 1501–1507, 1502.

56. Melville, *Military Hygiene and Sanitation,* 222.

57. Patrick Hehir, *Prevention of Disease and Inefficiency* (Allahabad: Pioneer Press, 1911), 284.

58. Bruce Skinner, "Incineration of Human-Excreta: Further Observations," *Journal of the Royal Army Medical Corps* (January 1911), 41.

59. Hehir, *Prevention of Disease and Inefficiency,* 265.

60. H.B. Thornhill, "Disposal of Excremental Matter in Cantonments," Wellcome Archives, WC270.

61. Captain L.W. Harrison, RAMC, "Continuous as Opposed to Intermittent Latrine Disinfection," 1906, 4. Wellcome Archives, WC270.

62. Glenn Allen, "The Thermal Death Point of Pathogenic Bacteria and the Portable (Army) Excreta Steriliser," *BMJ Military Health,* 7 (1906), 633–635.

63. C.P. Lukis and R.J. Blackham, *Tropical Hygiene for Anglo-Indians and Indians* (Calcutta: Thacker and Spink, 1914), 177

64. J.B. Hamilton, "Enteric Fever in India," 788.

BIBLIOGRAPHY

Archival collections

Wellcome Archives, London.
Western Cape Archives and Records Service, Cape Town, South Africa.

Published sources

Anderson, Clare. *Subaltern Lives: Biographies of Colonialism in the Indian Ocean World, 1790-1920* (Cambridge: Cambridge University Press, 2012).

Anderson, Warwick. *Colonial Pathologies: American Tropical Medicine, Race, and Hygiene in the Philippines* (Durham: Duke University Press, 2006).

Allen, Glenn. "The Thermal Death Point of Pathogenic Bacteria and the Portable (Army) Excreta Steriliser," *BMJ Military Health,* 7 (1906), 633–635.

Anon. "The Plague: Prevalence of the Disease," *British Medical Journal* (15 June 1901), 1514.

Arnold, David. *Colonizing the Body: State Medicine and Epidemic Disease in Nineteenth Century India* (Berkeley: University of California Press, 1994).

Baker, R.A. and R. A. Bayliss. "William John Ritchie Simpson (1855–1931): Public Health and Tropical Medicine," *Medical History* 31:4 (1987), 450–465.

Bala, Poonam. *Contesting Colonial Authority: Medicine and Indigenous Responses in Nineteenth and Twentieth Century India* (Plymouth: Lexington Books, 2012).

Ballantyne, Tony. *Entanglements of Empire: Missionaries, Maori, and the Question of the Body* (Durham: Duke University Press, 2014).

Benedict, Carola Anne. *Bubonic Plague in Nineteenth Century China* (Stanford: Stanford University Press, 1996).

Bhattacharya, Nandini. *Contagion and Enclaves: Tropical Medicine in Colonial India* (Liverpool: Liverpool University Press, 2012).

Blackham, R.J. "The Goux System and its Application to India," *Journal of the Royal Army Medical Corps,* 6 (1906), 662.

Burton, Antoinette. *Archive Stories: Facts, Fictions, and the Writing of History* (Durham: Duke University Press, 2005).

Burton, Antionette. *The Trouble with Empire: Challenges to Modern British Imperialism* (Oxford: Oxford University Press, 2015).

Catanch, I.J. "Plague and the Tensions of Empire: India, 1896–1918," in David Arnold (ed.) *Imperial Medicine and Indigenous Societies* (Manchester: Manchester University Press, 1991), Chapter 7.

Cell, John C. *The Highest Stage of White Supremacy: The Origins of Segregation in South Africa and the American South* (Cambridge: Cambridge University Press, 1982).

Chakrabarti, Pratik. *Bacteriology in British India: Laboratory Medicine and the Tropics* (Rochester: University of Rochester Press, 2017).

Chatterjee, Srilata. "Plague and Politics in Bengal, 1896 to 1898," *Proceedings of the Indian History Congress,* 66 (2005–2006), 1194–1201.

Crook, Tom. "Sanitary Inspection and the Public Sphere in Late Victorian and Edwardian Britain: A Case Study in Liberal Governance," *Social History* 32:4 (2007), 369–393.

Dispatch from Her Majesty's Ambassador at Constantinople, with Documents, Presented at both Houses of Parliament (London: Eyre and Spottiswoode, 1868).

Echenberg, Myron. *Plague Ports: The Global Urban Impact of Bubonic Plague, 1894–1901* (New York: New York University Press, 2007).

Ewart, William. "The Principles of Treatment of Typhoid Fever," *British Medical Journal,* 2:2345 (9 December 1905), 1501–1507.

Fredrickson, George. *White Supremacy: A Comparative Study in American & South African History* (Oxford: Oxford University Press, 1981).

Ghaddar, J.J., and Michelle Caswell. "To Go Beyond: Towards a Decolonial Archival Praxis," *Archival Science* 19 (2019), 71–85.

Gorman, Daniel. *Imperial Citizenship: Empire and the Question of Belonging* (Manchester: Manchester University Press, 2006).

Hamilton, J.B. "Enteric Fever in India," *British Medical Journal* 1553 (4 October 1890), 788.

Harrison, Mark. "Science and the British Empire," *Isis* 96 (2005), 56–63.

Hart, Ernest. "Cholera: Where it Comes From and How it is Propagated," *British Medical Journal* (1 July 1893), 1

Headrick, Daniel. *The Tools of Empire: Technology and European Imperialism in the Nineteenth Century* (Oxford: Oxford University Press, 1981).

Heath, Diana. *Purifying Empire: Obscenity and the Politics of Moral Regulation in Britain, India, and Australia* (New York: Cambridge University Press, 2010).

Hehir, Patrick. *Prevention of Disease and Inefficiency* (Allahabad: Pioneer Press, 1911).

Johnson, Ryan. "*Mantsemei*, Interpreters, and the Successful Eradication of Plague: The 1908 Plague Epidemic in Colonial Accra," in Ryan Johnson and Amna Khalid (eds.) *Public Health in the British Empire* (New York: Routledge, 2012), Chapter 7.

Lukis, C.P., and R.J. Blackham. *Tropical Hygiene for Anglo-Indians and Indians* (Calcutta: Thacker and Spink, 1914),

Lynteris, Christos. *Ethnographic Plague: Configuring Disease at the Chinese-Russian Frontier* (London: Palgrave, 2016).

Lynteris, Christos. "Pestis Minor; The History of a Contested Plague Pathology," *Bulletin of the History of Medicine,* 93:1 (Spring 2019), 55–81.

Mar, Tracey Banivanua. "The Contours of Agency: Women's Work, Race, and Queenland's Indentured Labor Trade," in Carol Williams (ed.) *Indigenous Women and Work: From Labor to Activism* (Urbana: University of Illinois Press, 2012), Chapter 4.

Melville, Charles. *Military Hygiene and Sanitation* (London: Edward Arnold, 1912).

Mooney, Graham. *Intrusive Interventions: Public Health, Domestic Space, and Infectious Disease Surveillance, 1840–1914* (Rochester: University of Rochester Press, 2015).

Packard, Randall. *White Plague, Black Labor: Tuberculosis and the Political Economy of Health and Disease in South Africa* (Berkeley: University of California Press, 1989).

Peckham, Robert. *Epidemics in Modern Asia* (Cambridge: Cambridge University Press, 2016).

Peckham, Robert. "Infective Economies: Empire, Panic, and the Business of Disease," *Journal of Imperial and Commonwealth History* 2 (2013), 211–237.

Porter, Dorothy, ed. *Health, Civilization and the State: A History of Public Health From Ancient to Modern Times* (London: Routledge, 1999).

Rogaski, Ruth. *Hygienic Modernity: Meanings of Health and Disease in Treaty-Port China* (Berkeley: University of California Press, 2015).

Seth, Suman. *Difference and Disease: Medicine, Race, and the Eighteenth-Century British Empire* (Cambridge: Cambridge University Press, 2018).

Simon, John. *Annual Report of the Medical Officer of the Privy Council for 1866* (London: Eyre and Spottiswoode, 1867).

Simond, M., Margaret L. Godley, and Pierre D. E. Mouriquand. "Paul-Louis Simond and His Discovery of Plague Transmission by Rat Fleas: A Centenary," *Journal of the Royal Society of Medicine*, 91:2 (February, 1998), 101–104.

Skinner, Bruce. "Incineration of Human-Excreta: Further Observations," *Journal of the Royal Army Medical Corps* (January 1911), 41.

Steere-Williams, Jacob. *The Filth Disease; Typhoid Fever and the Practices of Epidemiology in Victorian England* (Rochester: University of Rochester Press, 2020).

Steere-Williams, Jacob. "Coolie Control: State Surveillance and the Labour of Disinfection Across the Late Victorian British Empire," in Robert Heynen and Emily van der Meulen (eds.), *Surveillance States: Transnational Histories* (Toronto: University of Toronto Press, 2019), Chapter 2.

Sutphen, Mary P. "Not What but Where: Bubonic Plague and the Reception of Germ Theories in Hong Kong and Calcutta, 1894–1897", *Journal of the History of Medicine and Allied Sciences,* 52:1 (January 1997), 81–113.

Swanson, Maynard. "'The Sanitation Syndrome': Bubonic Plague and Urban Native Policy in the Cape Colony, 1900–1909," *Journal of African History* 18:3 (1977), 387–410.

Vaughn, Megan. *Curing Their Ills: Colonial Power and African Illness* (Cambridge: Polity Press, 1991).

Worboys, Michael. *Spreading Germs: Disease Theories and Medical Practice in Britain, 1865–1900* (Cambridge: Cambridge University Press, 2000).

Chapter 13

Epidemics and the Indigenous Tribes

Sub-Himalayan Bengal and the Jungle Mahals (ca. 1860–1930)

Sahara Ahmed

It often happens that the effects upon the actual labour forces and the neighbouring native populations may pass unnoticed and unrecorded, only the outbreak of disease among Europeans attracting attention; but there can be little doubt that were such cases investigated it would be found that the infection of Europeans, troops and well-to-do natives was only a concomitant and a result of a vastly greater amount of malaria among the poorer population, and especially among the labour force itself.[1]

Diseases were never associated only with ill health. In fact, dominant ideologies and religious beliefs have, across time, always had a major impact in shaping the meanings of diseases and the manner in which they originate and circulate.[2] Unlike its urban counterpart, cholera was primarily a disease of the countryside. Cholera symbolized rural vulnerability in the face of illiteracy, poverty, filth and underdevelopment.[3] Numerous literary representations of diseases like leprosy or tuberculosis signified human misery associated with industrialization and the spread of urbanization in India.[4] Hence, the notion of 'social construction' of diseases has unravelled numerous accounts of it, myriad perspectives of coping with the same and strategies of prevention adopted particularly in the West. In case of the Duars in Jalpaiguri, the obsessive interest of the planters to keep the costs of production low induced decreased expenses on health and sanitation of the workers.[5] Paucity of proper medical and sanitary facilities was often justified by recourse to stereotypes of culture of the worker.[6] They were thought to be averse to any kind of treatment. Malaria was found to have taken its greatest toll along with cholera and smallpox.[7] It was observed that an incredibly high death rate was complemented by a diminished birth rate.[8] The report further corroborated that 'hidden immigration' too was found to be the reason behind a decrease in population.[9] Facts were distorted to justify stereotypes. The real reason, however, lay elsewhere. It was found that absence of mandatory registration had caused the anomalies in figures.[10] The worker was relevant as long as he rendered his services. His sickness or death entailed no moral responsibilities. Hence, 'social construction' of the diseases has unveiled morbidities, mortalities and the ability to cope with them across various sections of the society in Bengal. The literature on the social history of diseases has been proliferating in India since it has witnessed some of the worst epidemics. This has also unleashed a genre of regional-level studies on the social history of diseases. Since they were recurrent visitors and could strike specific regions with epidemic vengeance. Nuanced responses of a society are evident from this burgeoning literature – the urban middle class, the rural gentry, the intelligentsia, the print world, village medical practitioners, pilgrims and the indigenous people. They also were active participants in the rising national consciousness and anti-colonial sentiments as seen in India (Bala in this volume). The ultimate category (i.e. the indigenous people) incorporated the rural masses, primarily the settled sedentary agriculturalists sans the indigenous tribes. Dearth of information induced by certain omissions and commissions had led to flawed documentation regarding the impact of diseases on indigenous tribes. Certain preconceived notions garnered support from various echelons of colonial rule. For instance, the issue of 'racial immunity' informed colonial discourse considerably. The proponents of this theory offered three arguments to substantiate it: Firstly, there prevailed a consensus on the matter among historical observers of the disease.[11] Secondly, it was observed that patterns of lethality during yellow fever epidemics emphasized the issue of racial immunity and thirdly, a certain heritable resistance to malaria had supposedly had no serious impact within the population.[12] Likewise a similar resistance to yellow fever had developed too.[13] This belief has been corroborated by some researches: Kenneth Kiple's work, for instance, subscribed to the view that genetic immunity played a leading role among the Africans and their descendants against the spread of yellow fever.[14] Others like Todd Savitt, J. R. McNeill, K. David Patterson and J. A. Carrigan argued that black people were naturally resistant to the worst effects of the disease.[15] Philip Curtin acknowledged the existence of a generic immunity but emphasized the significance of increased exposure to the disease during childhood in acquiring immunity and as a corollary its mildness.[16] A prevalent assumption was that certain communities acquired immunity as opposed to others and were distinctly identified as more 'vigorous' races.[17] For instance, the Santhals, in particular, were regarded a sturdy race impervious to the diseases that visited Bengal with punitive rage as opposed to the Nepalese.

Other indigenous tribes like the Meches and Rabhas of Sub-Himalayan Bengal were 'found' to be immune to 'malarious' fevers (viz., malaria, blackwater fever and influenza).[18] Despite the prevailing ambiguities this assumption of immunity or partial immunity to malaria continued to inform British Indian medical discourse throughout the nineteenth century.[19] This again had some discrete features from the earlier nineteenth-century ideas of racial immunity to fever.[20] In a similar vein both David Rennie and E. T. Dalton had subscribed to the view that Meches, indigenous tribes of the Duars, were peculiarly immune to the fevers.[21] They corroborated that racial immunity and acclimatization theories were pari passu at work. Hence a link was established between the two, ascribing equal importance to the latter, that is, specific locales.[22] These three factors acting in unison, namely, racial immunity, location and fever, gained prominence in the twentieth century with the inception of malaria research.[23] Koch harped upon 'acquired immunity' to justify the absence of prophylaxis for the entire population.[24]

Several theories have been posited to explain the phenomenon of epidemic diseases that wreaked havoc in the nineteenth and twentieth centuries. The ecological equilibrium or ecology-environmentalism and disease paradigm advocated by Sheldon Watts and Ira Klein is significant on many counts.[25] Sheldon Watts too has linked disease and political economy and made commercialization of agriculture responsible for it.[26] The location-specific perspective or the disease being peculiar to a locale had informed colonial discourse considerably.[27] Some have preconceived notions of a denser jungle eliciting a more endemic disease and precipitating a more febrile atmosphere.[28] The veracity of the theory of racial immunity of the indigenous tribal population to the diseases that were endemic to specific locales and the vulnerability of the new settlers to the same need perusal. Perhaps it was a condition for validation of colonial rule or a ploy to reduce expenses in health care for the 'jungle tribes'[29] and are arguments that need further explication. Nationalist critiques have identified colonial 'modernization' policies for the rapid propagation of the diseases in assuming epidemic proportions.[30] Accounts of missionary doctors need perusal since often they are reminiscent of contrary details. Coupled with this, the pertinent question of a disease exacerbating the effects of another induced by an enhanced vulnerability of the members of a particular tribe is evident in some accounts and poses several questions which could illuminate their perspective of the disease. Oral accounts of the indigenous tribes and their experiences or memoirs of their forefathers might unravel untold insights of the epidemics.

THE ECOLOGY-ENVIRONMENTAL PARADIGM

The first wave of cholera epidemic in Bengal was witnessed in 1817 and malaria in the 1820s, their causations induced major surveys and investigations.[31] Although the cause of malaria and the manner of its transmission remained unknown until the end of the nineteenth century, colonial medical and topographical texts repeatedly identified 'fever' as a primary attribute of the Indian environment.[32] An initial concern for European health quickly merged into discussions of the destructive impact of malarial fever on the indigenous population, especially in Bengal.

James Taylor gave graphic descriptions of the effect of floods on the environs of Dhaka.[33] Observation and experience emboldened some physicians to try to identify those regions of India where malaria appeared particularly prevalent and severe. These obviously included marshy or waterlogged areas and 'low jungles' like the Terai, but also almost anywhere where tropical heat and moisture combined such as Lower Bengal, Assam and the canal tracts of northern India.[34] Even though the precise cause of malaria remained obscure it was believed that forest clearance helped to remove the disease and 'open up' forest and tribal areas to outside settlement and agricultural colonization would lead to its eradication.[35] In advocating such a policy for the eastern forests of the Central Provinces in 1871, Captain J. Forsyth argued that the obstacle of malaria would persist only so long as the country continues to be 'uncleared'.[36] He cited examples of Wynad, Assam and Cachar as other standing instances of the successful occupation of malarious countries by the help of European enterprise. In 1914, Major W. H. Kenrick, IMS, published a detailed report on malaria in the Central Provinces.[37] At the time, nearly 40% of the province was still forested, particularly in the hills and these were identified as the most malarious. Endemic malaria was so closely associated with forests that, in Kenrick's mind, the term 'jungle fever' though obsolete in some ways remained strikingly opposite. He subscribed to the concept that the denser the jungle, the higher the endemicity; the greater the extent of cultivation, the lower the incidence of malaria.[38] Increase in acreage was triggered by an enhanced revenue demand often impinging upon forest land, and the atmosphere of the Duars and neighbouring districts has been described as 'dank', 'febrile' and 'salubrious' in most colonial accounts.[39]

The earliest reference to diseases in colonial repertoire for the Duars was in the *Itineraire* of Hooker. Hooker had lamented that,

> More beautiful sites for fine mansions could not well be and it is difficult to suppose so lovely a country should be so malarious as it is before and after the rains excessive best probably diffusing the miasma from small stagnant surfaces.[40]

The opening up of the forests was initiated in the 1860s in the Duars and in the mountainous tracts of the Himalayas. A process akin to this was noticed in the Jungle Mahals too. Dense forests covered with heavy undergrowth and intermittent marshy lands were soon transformed into 'managed landscapes'. Allured by commercial prospects the landscapes were soon dotted with lush tea gardens of both sal and teak plantations in both northern and southern Bengal. The opening up of the 'country' was further accelerated by the inauguration of the railways, the Ajoy-Sainthia and Sainthia-Tinpahar Railway Lines in 1860, the Bengal Nagpur Railway Lines in 1898 and the Northern Bengal Railway Line in 1874.

One needs to harp on the fact that even after these human interventions on nature, the diseases prevalent in the regions did not change its character in the early twentieth century or even in the latter half. A first-hand report on the common diseases of Jalpaiguri (included diarrhoea, dysentery, goitre, spleen, cholera and malarial fever) has been found in Sunder's report.[41] J. A. Milligan, the settlement officer of Jalpaiguri, J. F. Gruning and H. B. Rowney have also recorded the severity of the fatal diseases of Jalpaiguri and its neighbouring districts in the first quarter of the twentieth century, especially malaria.[42] The Malaria Commission of the Royal Society visited the Duars region in 1901 and found that 'the malaria indemnity of Duars was extraordinarily high and that black-water fever was common in that locality'.[43] C. A. Bentley's report on the contrary categorizes another aspect, 'the human factor', which negates the prioritization of environmental factors as a possible reason behind the causation of malaria.[44] Bentley elaborates upon Koch's three-tier analysis of villages with no malaria, villages with malaria confined to children and finally villages with malaria among children and some adults.[45] It is the third category that seemed to be the most vulnerable as the population appeared to be fluctuating with the influx of 'non-immune immigrants'.[46] It is this 'human factor' that according to Bentley had added 'fresh fuel to the already glowing fire', where a few anopheles mosquitoes had found human carriers of the disease.

> This factor, which when it sets temporarily, is capable of producing epidemic malaria and when long continued must give rise to an endemicity.[47]

Moreover, Bentley's investigations unravelled that 'non-immune immigrants' did not constitute the whole of the 'human factor' in malaria.

It is unnecessary to go further into this question beyond stating that among aboriginal tribes and certain poverty-stricken communities in India, a very high endemic index of malaria may frequently be found, depending apparently upon the general squalor, the hand-to-mouth existence and other conditions associated with low social status. The way in which such economic conditions influenced malaria seems to be bringing about relapses and state of continued infection.[48]

> Ross in computing the probable time during which infection may remain in the body capable at any time of being stimulated into activity by the action of depressing influences, fixes the period in British troops at about six months.

In this case he was dealing with Europeans, originally healthy, picked men, well-fed, well housed and under constant medical supervision. But, when we consider natives, often originally possessed of poor physique and little stamina, living under conditions of depression, privation and hardship pushed to the extreme, it is obvious that these form a soil far more suitable for the continued existence of malaria, and the problem therefore becomes an entirely different one.[49]

This according to the investigating team was known as the 'residual infection factor'. An emaciated, poverty-stricken people were far more vulnerable to the disease than others. 'Physiological misery' had rendered a huge number of people susceptible to the disease and hence the number of infected persons among the coolies or labour camps increased at a rapid pace.

> But in labour camps both factors we have described act together in the fullest intensity, and we can recognise a new state of affairs in the appearance of a system of vicious cycles always producing the same result, namely, the extraordinary exaltation of malaria.[50]

Similarly in the Jungle Mahals the diseases most commonly met with in the district were malarial fevers, dysentery, diarrhoea, influenza, cholera, smallpox and skin diseases. Malarial fevers were prevalent before and after the rains, and were especially common in the low-lying country bordering the Ganges and in the Damin-i-koh portion of the Godda and Pakaur subdivisions.[51] In localities, the drainage being defective, the land is apt to become waterlogged and stagnant, water collected in hollows and depressions. The type most commonly met with is intermittent fever, but remittent cases were fairly numerous at the close of the rainy season.

Eruptive fevers, such as smallpox, measles and chickenpox, were endemic throughout the Santhal Parganas, Garbeta, Fulkusuma, Barabhum, Banjabhum and Dalbhum, and sometimes became epidemic during the months preceding the rains. Epidemics of cholera broke out from time to time beginning with the hot weather and ending with the rains. In the Santhal Parganas, Rajmahal, Godda and Deoghar suffered most and two worst epidemics on record were those of 1897 and 1906.[52] The first outbreak of plague occurred in 1901 in Sahibganj in the Santhal Parganas.[53] Influenza had appeared in epidemic form in the late nineteenth and twentieth centuries.

A. K. Jameson's Settlement Report corroborates Dr Bentley's initial assumptions that the embankings had led to water logging and had exacerbated the malarial fevers.[54] Hence the two theories, the environmental perspective or the ecology-environmental and disease paradigm and the miasmatic theory (one can infer that malaria was derived simply from the words mal air) that the colonial records are replete with, in unison blamed the environment and the indigenous population of Bengal and their unhealthy habits for the propagation of the diseases. These prevalent theories may have partial veracity but proved inconclusive.

THE MYTH OF TRIBAL IMMUNITY

A common belief among the colonial fathers was that despite the rapid propagation of the diseases like malarial fever it was not a serious problem for the indigenous/tribal communities of the Duars region (like the Meches, Totos, Rabhas and Dhimals) or the Jungle Mahals (like the Santhals, Mundas, Oraons, Birhors and Lodhas) since they developed a level of immunity to these endemic diseases which often became epidemic. However, other common diseases such as goitre, dysentery and diarrhoea of Sub-Himalayan Bengal were equally serious for the inhabitants including the Rajbanshis and others.[55]

J. F. Gruning, D. H. E Sunders, J. W. Milligan and others maintained that Jalpaiguri and its neighbouring districts, situated to the south of the Darjeeling Terai and the Bhutan hills, were well known to be unhealthy.[56] In eight out of the ten years ending 1901, it figured among the six districts with the highest mortality from fever in the province of Bengal, and malaria was prevalent all the year round and its intensity was felt during and after the rains. The mean ratio of births for the ten years from 1893 to 1902 was 31.31 per 1,000 and of deaths 31.74 per 1,000. The figures for 1907 were births 39.72 and deaths 34.33 per 1,000.[57] The improvement was inaccurate due to lack of registrations in the Duars region. In eight out of the ten years ending 1901, it figured among the six districts with the highest mortality from fever in the province of Bengal and malaria was prevalent all the year round and its intensity was felt during and after the rains. Thus, the mean ratio of births, as mentioned above remained more or less similar.[58] A slight improvement for births and deaths was observed in 1907.[59] Apparent paucity of registrations in the Duars region contributed to this inaccurate improvement.[60]

The test of the malarial intensity of any region is the percentage of children from two to ten years of age who have malarial parasites in their blood. The figure representing this percentage is termed the malarial endemicity index or shortly the endemic index.[61] Hence the endemic index of the district shows a fairly high percentage as ascertained in 1901 from 16% in Jalpaiguri to a high of 72% in Nagrakata in the Duars.[62] Subsequently in 1907, on further investigation, it was found that even these figures were incorrect and the situation was grossly underestimated and the true endemic indices were 10–20% higher.[63] This also indicated the level of risk at which the immigrant population was exposed since their main concern was the Europeans and the plantations.

Gruning and Rennie mention that the Rajbanshis and Meches were relatively immune to the fever.[64] However, contradictorily he maintains that infantile mortality was very high.[65] The existence of a sturdy people in such a deadly region can only be explained, according to him, as the survival of the fittest. Those who have survived acquired immunity after suffering repeated infections in childhood.[66]

An interpretation akin to this was noticed for the Central Provinces. In 1914, Major W. H. Kendrick posited that, although the 'dark-skinned aborigines' were themselves apparently immune to serious infections, they acted as serious carriers and spread the infection among more vulnerable groups and the new settlers especially suffered.[67] If this is to be applied to the Duars it should be understood that the indigenous were spared of the scourge, the new settlers who fell prey to the disease were the Europeans and the tea plantation labourers, the Santhals, Oraons and Mundas from Chota Nagpur.[68] Gruning's, Sunder's and Milligan's reports corroborate that the disease spread to the tea labour camps bordering the forests affecting entire camps while sparing others and the indigenous tribes like the Meches, Totos, Rabhas and Rajbanshis who were immune to the disease.[69]

For the Jungle Mahals (the present Jungle Mahals area corresponds to the three districts of Bankura, Purulia and West Midnapur),[70] O'Malley, Hunter and others indicated that mortality from fevers in the Santhal Parganas was less than in other districts of Bengal: from 1892 to 1904 the death rate was above 20 per mile in four years. However, in each of the succeeding three years, the death rate was as high as 25 per mile. The number of reported deaths in Birbhum District from fever alone in 1872 was a staggering 12,906 persons. A report purported that

> fever also was very prevalent in some parts of the district and particularly in villages situated south east of Suri and bordering on Burdwan. No reports as to the extent to which the disease prevailed have been submitted by the police.[71]

Once again this brings us to the issue of lack of regular registration of births and deaths for the indigenous tribes. Several accounts maintain that the Santhals in particular escaped the terrible scourge because of their strong physique and healthy habits. While others maintain that,

> If we bear this in mind we shall realise at once the reality of immunity in malaria. The aborigine harbours large number of the malaria parasite in his blood when in childhood but is in high degree tolerant of its presence and immune to its effects.[72]

Hence the presence of children with enlarged spleens suffered during their childhoods and developed a certain level of immunity later on. Such an interpretation is riddled with contradictions. On the one hand, it harps on racial immunity and on the other it admits the vulnerability of the children of the same tribe.

For the Duars, the contradictions are starker. Since the colonial records claim that the indigenous people were somewhat immune to the disease but the new settlers were the most vulnerable. The new settlers included the Europeans, the tea garden labourers, largely from Chota Nagpur area comprising the Santhals, Oraons and Mundas.[73] Subsequently, it follows that the same people were immune to the disease in Chota Nagpur but became vulnerable on reaching the Duars.

In a similar vein, David Hardiman argues that the drawback with this argument was that even in the supposedly 'healthy' tracts of the areas of South Gujarat that adjoined the Arabian Sea and had no forests was an area in which high-caste landowners carried on commercial agriculture with *adivasis* making up most of the agricultural labour force (working either as bonded labourers or indebted tenants) – the health of the adivasis was not noticeably better than that of their counterparts in the forest zones.[74]

This was a fate suffered by such people elsewhere in India. P. O. Bodding, a missionary ethnographer whose wife was a doctor, carried out a detailed study of the health and therapeutic practices of the Santal (Santhal) adivasis of eastern India in the early twentieth century.[75] He noted that they suffered from most diseases found in India at that time. He was told by his Santal informants that they had not suffered from syphilis, tuberculosis or leprosy before the middle of the nineteenth century. Although he felt that this was perhaps an exaggeration, he suggested that their former isolation may have protected them from many infections. By the twentieth century, however, all of the three above-mentioned diseases had become widespread in the community. The most prevalent maladies of all were malaria, then skin diseases, bowel complaints such as dysentery, eye diseases, pneumonia and rheumatism. They also suffered badly in epidemics, fearing cholera and smallpox in particular.

All of this suggests that the indigenous population of the region were particularly vulnerable to epidemics. Colonial records maintain that cholera was seen throughout the years in nineteenth- and twentieth-century Bengal. Gruning's observations on Jalpaiguri and its neighbouring districts have been corroborated by W.W. Hunter, L.S.S. O'Malley and the Sanitary

Commissioners' report attest that many streams and wells might have been contaminated which may have reduced flow, or dried up, rendering its epidemic. The two worst epidemics on record for the Santhal Parganas was in 1897 when 7,107 or 4 per mile of the population died and of 1906 when the number of deaths was 6,160 persons or 3.4 per mile.[76] The mortality rate for tribal population of Jalpaiguri was 2.36% of the total mortality of the district.[77] The worst affected tracts were the Falakata and Alipur tahsils and the reason for this was a considerable Mech population who were infected.

The epidemic affected large portions of the Falakata and Alipur tahsils as well. The disease spread at a rapid pace amongst the Mech population who became more susceptible owing to their nomadic habits. The two worst epidemics on record for the Santhal Parganas were in 1897 when 7,107 or 4 per mile of the population died and of 1906 when the number of deaths was 6,160 persons or 3.4 per mile.[78] The mortality rate for tribal population of Jalpaiguri was 2.36% of the total mortality of the district.[79] Cholera occasionally appeared in an epidemic form. It prevailed throughout the area in 1865, especially among a gang of prisoners from Rangpur jail who were engaged in building barracks for troops at Jalpesh.

In April 1869, cholera broke out in the eastern and western parts of the district. The district spread northwards from Cooch Behar, which it had previously ravaged and also from Rangpur and Purnea districts, where it was virulent. It advanced into the Duars, attacking all sexes, ages and castes alike, and sparing few. The disease followed the main line of road appearing at Titalia and Siliguri. It also occurred in the south of Jalpaiguri town. Sporadic cases were also there in the northern tracts.

It subsided with the coming of the rains in May. This was followed by another scourge in 1872 and lasted from April to November. Milligan further corroborated that, the figures of mortality in the jail showed that out of a daily average of 61.26 prisoners, twenty deaths from cholera occurred within thirty-five days.[80] In 1885–1886, mortality owing to fever was 23.71 per mile (i.e. thousand) and in 1886–1888, it was 31.01 per mile, being the worst in Bengal.[81] Gruning further elaborated that they don't bury their corpses like other races but throw them into the nearest streams and flee to the forests, polluting the streams with bodies. As a result, the streams get polluted and infect the people who use the stream water living along the forest tracts. The Duars Labour Act was passed in 1912 with an aim to alleviate their conditions.[82]

Milligan opined that the period 1906–1916 sanitation was a major problem for Jalpaiguri and the neighbouring districts. In 1924–1925, the highest death rate from cholera (2.5 per 1,000) was reported.[83] Charitable dispensaries were operational though few in number. The Meches and other tribes, however, had either fled or the services never reached them. The system of registration of mortality for some selected urban and rural areas was introduced under the Bengal Births and Deaths Registration Act (Act IV of 1873). However, this was mainly confined to the urban areas and at a limited scale in the rural areas.

> The inhabitants are generally dull looking with their pale faces, enlarged abdomen and emaciated limbs and their health on the whole giving proof of it being below par.[84]

Women were generally in worse health than men. The connection between malaria, an enlarged spleen, and anaemia was pointed out by missionary doctors working in the tract in 1926. They called this 'malarial anaemia', but more recent investigations in this area have discovered that there is widespread sickle-cell anaemia among the adivasis.[85] While providing some protection against malaria, it is also very debilitating. There is also a close connection between female nutritional anaemia and maternal and foetal morbidity and mortality. An Indian anthropologist who carried out research in the area in the late 1920s remarked on the very high infant mortality rate in the adivasi village that he studied – with 52.7% of all deaths there being of children under five. 24.4% of all children failed to survive to their fifth birthday.[86]

This all left the adivasis of this region particularly vulnerable to epidemic disease. Their poverty, poor sanitation, diet and water supply, and the chronic malaria that sapped their energy and undermined their immune system, along with – at that time – an undiagnosed sickle-cell anaemia, all made them particularly susceptible when influenza swept their villages in 1918. To compound this, the colonial state failed to provide any welfare for these people, and in particular any meaningful health care or guidance and leadership, and aid from civil society organizations was poorly developed and only able to have a small impact. The adivasis were largely left alone to suffer, and so traumatic was their experience that to this day they still, in those hill and forest villages, remember that terrible time of ma¯nmodi, a fever that assumed epidemic proportions as recounted by some older members of the tribe.[87] One can presume that the dreadful fever was akin to the great influenza epidemic of 1918 and was computed to have happened around the same time.

ORAL TESTIMONIES

Some oral accounts testified to the sufferings of the indigenous tribes and most of these substantiated and acknowledged the contributions of the missionaries in helping them to recuperate from some fatal illnesses instead of government agencies. Late Lalit Iswarary, a Mech resident of Alipurduar district, Thana Baro Daldali, was initially staying in a mission school near Mahakalguri in 1944 where he studied till the eighth standard. As a child he witnessed a cholera epidemic in his village. He recounted those missionaries wearing masks and gloves would enter every household and clean the garbage dumped carelessly and the water collected in pots from a nearby stream. They would attend to the sick by tendering medicines and made this an everyday practice and even involved children from the missionary school to develop the spirit of service to the sick and needy.[88] On another instance Debki Gabur, age seventy-three, a Mech resident of Alipurduar district, had witnessed the spread of *Kala Azar* (blackwater fever) popularly known as *Bhaluk Jar* or Bear Fever and how the ordinary folks ran after the bear who was an itinerant performer. Others even bartered goods to acquire hair of the bear and wore it in pendants around their necks as defence mechanisms against the disease. He further reminisces that poor people gathered in queues in front of the missionary houses for medicines.

In another account late Angasree Basumata, first Mech woman to be recruited as a teacher in Mahakalguri Mission School in the year 1948, was born in Shamuktala village in Alipurduar district.[89] Trained as a teacher from Calcutta she began spreading the message of social welfare and awareness about public health in the neighbouring villages for which she was shunned by her own community. With the active support of Mrs MacFarlane, she organized a women's missionary association to improve women's health, family welfare, child health coupled with a Christian Welfare Mission which encouraged schooling for young girls.[90]

Late Manaisree Narjinari was a well-known Mech *kaviraj* (physician) from Kamakhyaguri.[91] People from far and wide approached him for treatment. He recounted that numerous villages were affected by diseases like *Kala Azar* (blackwater fever), typhoid fever, malaria and jaundice. His personal experiences in treating the affected with barks of trees, leaves, remains of animal bones or skin to relieve pain constitute first-hand accounts of an indigenous medicine man.

CHARITABLE ORGANIZATIONS AT WORK

Missionary accounts are replete with the significance of 'healing' accounts during the epidemics particularly due to the disdain of the governmental agencies for the 'jungle folk'. Popularly known as the 'Church sappers and miners' and this epithet was earned by medical missions as a mark of honour for the services.[92] Mr MacFarlane recounted the experiences of a fortnight spent among the plague-stricken villagers, when 'thick gloom settled down over the whole place':

> Their sentiments towards the mission at that time underwent a complete change. At first it was viewed with deep suspicion. Now they began to come in twenties and thirties for medicines. We were welcome to their houses, and allowed to read and pray where no one would have permitted us to enter.[93]

The account further maintained that another powerful obstacle to the missionary is the gross superstitions of heathenism.[94] As the preachers moved about, they found restrictions being imposed upon them by the 'spirits of the mountains' as illness was commonly associated with possession by spirits.[95] Apart from the routine proceedings, the medical mission believed that its philanthropic gestures had earned the faith of the common people, since they had watched Mr Sutherland nursing a 'native' brother back to good health from the throes of death. Besides they also watched Dr. Ponder nursing the sick in hospital. In such instances, they noticed the enormity of the missionary message of spreading love. From the beginning each preacher, whether Scottish or Indian, happened to be a medical missionary.[96]

The government showed some confidence in the mission by giving a house and a grant of money to build the hospital, and Dr Ponder's assistant, a native Christian doctor, was also approved and the St Andrews Young Men's Guild agreed to pay his salary. Initially during the course of 1894, Dr Ponder was supported by the Woman's Guild.[97] With commendable promptitude and liberality, the Woman's Guild provided the means necessary not only for repairing but improving the hospital.[98]

In the course of his report for 1900, Dr MacDonald speaks of smallpox as raging Sikkim and the foothills and of the excellent services rendered by the Rev. Mr Macara in carrying out a vaccination campaign. In addition, it also mentions an epidemic of cholera in the months of May and June 'which carried off its victims in most cases in a few hours'. It was especially heartening to see the spirit displayed by those who were on duty in the hospital:

> The sights around were such as would smite the hearts of even less simple folks. But during those dark days the quiet look of determination on every face, and the snatches of hushed conversation indicated a resolve to die rather than forsake their Christian duty.[99]
>
> A fellow worker lamented the death of Nurse Campbell who fell prey to the disease. She was the one we could least have spared; but during the epidemic of typhoid she had exhausted herself nursing others, and had no strength left to fight the fever for herself.[100]

In the Santhal Parganas there were two railway dispensaries and four dispensaries maintained by missions, of whom the best attended were said to be those of the Church Missionary Society and the Indian Home Mission to the Santhals.[101] The missionaries also treated the sick both at the mission stations and in the villages. The missionary accounts unravel that the Santhals who used to regard a dispensary as the abode of the devils and would not accept European treatment attended them in fair numbers, provided the civil hospital assistant in charge was kind and sympathetic.[102]

Out of the public charitable dispensaries in the year 1908, the oldest was at Deoghar which was opened in 1864 and was maintained by private subscriptions, a municipal grant and a government contribution. It was located in a substantial *pucca* building for the treatment of paupers and infectious diseases and separate accommodation for relatives of patients akin to 'isolation' being practiced in the present context. In 1865, the dispensaries were established at the subdivisional headquarters of Dumka, Rajmahal and Godda. The Dumka Hospital is contained in a stone building and has a similar arrangement like the Deoghar dispensary.[103] In 1900, the zamindar of Lakhanpur, Rai Bahadur Sitab Chand Laha, had added a small cottage hospital with two wards for women. The Rajmahal Dispensary was a gift of the East Indian Railway Company. Godda had a substantial building with outhouses for the treatment of pauper and infectious patients.[104] In 1893, a dispensary was opened at Katikund and in 1897 another was opened at Bario, both in the Damin-i-koh.[105] These dispensaries were maintained by the Santhals who paid one *anna* per house annually, the government providing the services of civil hospital assistants. In 1898, a dispensary was opened at the subdivisional headquarters of Pakaur.[106] The raja had hitherto kept up a public dispensary, but villagers of low caste were not encouraged to attend it for fear that they might carry contagion to the inmates of the palace, hence this philanthropic gesture proved inconsistent with the high ideals of charity one espoused. As compensation, the raja made over a building erected for an institute near the *kachchari* for the new hospital subsequently. Next year another dispensary was opened by at Asanbani, the building and stock being the grant of Mr Maling Grant, and a private dispensary was initiated at Madhupur by Babu Balai Chand Dutt.[107]

Interestingly, in both the regions under the purview of this study, the government endeavours for health care were desultory and philanthropic organizations like zamindars, Christian missionaries and individuals in a private capacity contributed towards the partial well-being of these indigenous tribes. Often that too appeared insufficient. Hence the medicine men/women practitioners of traditional medicine retained a position of paramount importance in the tribal villages. In the absence of vaccinations and medication, people took recourse to traditional/folk medicines.

THE IMPACT OF VARIOUS FEVERS

Certain accounts attest that areas where a substantial section of the population had suffered infections from a disease like cholera, 'malarious fevers' often became susceptible to other diseases. Although a direct connection between the diseases could not be established, instances of one exacerbating the other disease cannot be ruled out. It was inquired as to why the Burdwan Division should have a consistently increasing number of lepers.[108] It was further reiterated that the general prevalence of leprosy over Lower and Eastern Bengal and Burma seemed to be a major concern and issue to be investigated. One persistent feature that these districts had in common was the perennial existence of cholera and fever.[109] Regions where cholera was endemic must have had certain definite yet unknown factors that rendered the disease its recurrent feature. H. W. Bellew maintained that,

> Certain regions and tracts of country in India which bear a striking general similarity in respect to the main features of their physical aspects and climatic characteristics are much more favourable to the development of the epidemic activity of cholera than other regions and tracts of country in India which differ from them very essentially in the characteristic features of their physiography and meteorology as well also in point of density of population. In the former class of regions or tracts of country cholera is found to be more or less always active at all times and seasons, and is consequently, although subject to regularly recurring periods of epidemic intensity, considered an endemic disease in such regions or tracts of country. In the other class of regions or tracts of country cholera is not found to be always active at all times and seasons. On the contrary, in these areas it prevails only in seasons of periodically recurring general epidemic diffusion of the disease, and consequently cholera in these regions and tracts of country is considered only an occasional visitor and an epidemic disease.[110]

A comparative study of the leper distribution maps with the cholera map further substantiates this argument. It was observed that the districts of Burdwan, Beerbhoom, Midnapore, Murshidabad, Darjeeling, Jalpaiguri, Rungpore, Sylhet and Cachar, in which leprosy was predominantly prevalent, were all situated in the area of endemic cholera.[111] Moreover, the report also purported that a famine immediately before the census may possibly disturb the uniformity of ratios.[112] Hence generally, in those districts which, on account of the endemic appearance of cholera, were categorized as the unhealthiest in India, leprosy was found to be primarily prevalent in them and vice versa.[113] The report further maintained that a causal connection between leprosy and cholera was not hinted at but it does not rule out the possibility of one disease having a deleterious effect on the common people and sapped the vitality of the population in entirety.[114]

It was also investigated that poverty and diseases had a distinct connect. As Bentley's report purported that,

> Experience seems to show that, in a community composed of malaria-stricken subjects in a state of physiological poverty and exposed to hardship and privation, infection diminishes very slowly, even in the absence of anopheles, and, in these circumstances, the presence of very few anopheles seems to be quite sufficient to keep up the maximum degree of parasite infestation.[115]

The influx of a large section of immigrant labour into the labour camps had a debilitating effect on the *coolies* in the labour camps. Sick people arrived in the camps from the works,

> For nothing is so unsettling as sickness, and, as malaria in the labour camps increases, many members of families decimated by these diseases endeavour to reach their homes often under conditions of great hardship.[116]

This was further illustrated by in a case referred to in another connection in a report on *Kala Azar*,

> A coolie woman, aged 19, from the Assam-Bengal Railway (then under construction) was admitted to the Nowgong dispensary during the rainy season of 1890 suffering from marked anaemia and dropsy of the feat and face. The history of illness was that she got on all right until her father died, after which she lived with another coolie girl, and according to her story she only received about one rupee a month from the contactor (probably minimum living allowances vide Chapter V1) and was consequently unable to feed herself properly. She soon became ill and she did not improve she left the works and 'begged her way into Nowgong, living on what she could pick.' (The clauses in parentheses are ours)[117]

Gruning too maintained that a particular fever rendered one vulnerable to another. As he pithily stated, 'among disease conditions resulting from the universal intensity of malaria throughout the Duars, none is more striking than black water fever which is exceedingly common among Europeans and natives'.[118] It was also found that only drug in use for malarial fevers was quinine and was often distributed in sugar-coated pills to popularize it. He further mentioned that cholera was a recurrent disease and the increasing mortalities had an incapacitating effect on the population. The tribal population infected by these diseases often disposed of the corpses in the nearby streams and were shunned by the governmental agencies for their unhygienic practices.[119] For the Jungle Mahals, Harry Timbres too lamented that large sections of the population succumbed to various fevers that often occurred simultaneously.[120]

CONCLUSION

The ecology, environmentalism and disease paradigm alone would not suffice an explanation for the phenomenon of epidemics except that the diseases, specifically malarial fevers, were as old as civilization. This paradigm was further emphasized by the location specificity of diseases which informed colonial discourses and that certain diseases were germane to particular locales. This, however, proves inadequate in explaining why certain anophelines are not carriers of malaria in the dense jungles of the Terai while some were in the urban areas. Hence 'denser the jungle the more malarious it is' lacks substantial evidence. Besides, parts of the Jungle Mahals were not 'dank' and 'febrile' but had experienced bouts of the epidemics. The nationalist critique of it had blamed colonial modernization projects for the epidemics. The 'opening up' of the country with the building of roads, railways and embankments had rendered an endemic disease assume epidemic proportions is tenable but should be supplemented with other viable arguments.

The epidemics, it should be borne in mind, occurred in waves, both malaria and cholera and often simultaneously or alternatively beginning in 1817 and continued till the early half of the twentieth century. As a corollary one cannot rule out the possibility of one infection rendering the individual more vulnerable to the other. Often the adults among some of these indigenous tribes were asymptomatic carriers of the diseases and were capable of spreading the infection. It was also often difficult to differentiate between one type of fever from another. Influenza and malarial fevers, as it were collectively known, assumed a virulent form and with the kind of health care facilities available it was often left undetected. Till date there is a persistence of 'unknown' fevers. Doctors and scientists too are unable to gauge and are often left to speculate.

The indigenous tribes were indubitably the victims of the scourges that became epidemic, and the issue of tribal immunity appears fallacious and was probably a ploy by the colonial authorities to avoid huge expenses on health care. They were contented with offering palliatives rather than preventive measures. Besides, they often wanted to avoid direct contact with them for their nomadic nature and nurtured a dislike for them for their shifting cultivation habits. In fact, there was never a consensus among medical observers that black immunity to yellow fever actually existed, the evidence from epidemics indicates that in fact it did not, and the analogy to the very real and well-documented evolutionary consequences of endemic malaria is not apt. As there is no evidence supporting the belief of black immunity to yellow fever or malaria in case of the indigenous people of the Duars and the Jungle Mahals, one needs to consider discarding such speculations. It is probable that racial immunity arguments were also put forth as a precondition to validate colonial rule.

NOTES

1. S.R. Christophers and C.A. Bently, *Malaria in the Duars*. Simla, 1911, 5.
2. Burton Cleetus, Tropics of Disease: Epidemics in Colonial India, *Economic and Political Weekly* 55, no. 21 (May, 2020): 2349.
3. Cleetus, "Tropics of Disease," 2349. Diseases like malaria, cholera and other fevers that became epidemic and appeared in waves found its representations in vernacular literature, novels, short stories and journals. Diseases were associated with poverty, social injustice, paucity of trained doctors and social ostracism. Bengali novelist Sarat Chandra Chattopadhyay had given vivid descriptions of the misery associated with the diseases in his novels *Ramer Sumati* (1914), *Pandit Mashay* (1917), *Srikanto* (1917–1933, in 4 parts) and *Palli Samaj* (1916).
4. Rabindranath Tagore's depiction of the disdain and social ostracism associated with tuberculosis in the death of Bali's husband in his novel, *Chokher Bali* (1903).
5. Subhajyoti Ray, *Transformations on the Bengal Frontier, 1765–1948*. London: Routledge Curzon Press, 2002, 89.
6. Ray, "Transformations on the Bengal Frontier," 89.
7. Christophers, Bently "Malaria in the Duars," 7.
8. Ray, "Transformations on the Bengal Frontier," 90.
9. Christophers, Bentley "Malaria in the Duars," 8.
10. Duars Planters Association Report, 1920, 116.
11. Kenneth F.Kiple, *The Caribbean Slave: A Biological History*. Cambridge: Cambridge University Press, 1984. See also James Johnson, *The Influence of Tropical Climates on European Constitutions*, London: Mottleyand Harrison, 1818 and Philip D. Curtin, "Epidemiology and the slave trade." *Political Science Quarterly* 83, no. 2 (1968): 190–216.
12. Ann Jo Carrigan, "Yellow fever: Scourge of the South," in Todd L. Savitt and James Harvey Young (eds.), *Disease and Distinctiveness* in the American South. Knoxville: University of Tennessee Press, 1978, 55–78.
13. Kenneth F.Kiple, "*The Carribean Slave*," 43.
14. McNeill, J. R. (1999) "Ecology, epidemics and empires: Environmental change and the geopolitics of tropical America, 1600–1825." *Environment and History* 5, no. 2 (1999): 175–84.
15. David K. Patterson, "Yellowfever epidemics and mortality in theUnited States, 1693–1905." *Social Science and Medicine* 34 no. 8 (1992): 855–65.

16. Philip D.Curtin "Epidemiology and the slave trade," *Political Science Quarterly* 83 (2): 190–216.

17. Christophers, Bentley, "Malaria in the Duars," 8–9.

18. J.F.Gruning, *Jalpaiguri*, Allahabad: The Pioneer, 1911. See also H.B. Rowney, *The Wild Tribes of India*, London: Thos de la Rue & Co., 1882.

19. David Field Rennie, *Bhotan and the Story of the Dooar War*. London: J. Murray, 1866, 347–48.

20. David Field Rennie, Bhotan and the Story of the Dooar War, 348.

21. E.T. Dalton, *Descriptive Ethnology of Bengal*, Kolkata: Government of Bengal, Council of Asiatic Society of Bengal, 1872, 138.

22. Nandini Bhattacharya, "The Logic of Location: Malaria Research in Colonial India, Darjeeling and Duars, 1900–30," *Medical History*, 55 (2011): 183–202.

23. Second Report of the German Colonial Office, "Professor Koch's Investigations on Malaria," *The German Medical Journal*, March 07 (1931): 325.

24. David Field Rennie, Bhotan and the Story of the Dooar War, 349.

25. Ira Klein, "Death in India: 1871–1921," *Journal of Asian Studies,* no. 32 (1973):639–59. See also Mark Harrison, Public Health in British India: Anglo-Indian Preventive Medicine, 1859–1914, Cambridge: Cambridge University Press, 1994, 164 and Poonam Bala, "Nationalizing Medicine: The Changing Paradigm of Ayurveda in India," in Poonam Bala ed., *Contesting Colonial Authority, Medicine and Indigenous Responses in Nineteenth and Twentieth Century India*. New Delhi: Primus Books, reprint, 2016, 1–12, originally published by Lanham MD: Lexington Books, 2012.

26. Sheldon Watts, "British Development Policies and Malaria in India 1897–c.1929," *Past and Present* 165 (1999): 141–81.

27. Nandini Bhattacharya, "The Logic of Location," 184.

28. David Arnold, Disease Resistance and India's Ecological Frontier, 1770–1947, in Biswamoy Pati ed., *Issues in Modern Indian History for Sumit Sarkar*. New Delhi: Popular Prakasan, 2000, 55.

29. W.M. Fraser, *The Recollections of a Tea Planter*. London: Tea and Rubber Mail, 1935, 83. Fraser opined during his sojourns that this "typical jungle folk" had no "right or title to the land" but before he approached the government with an application, the indigenous tribes were evicted. B.G. Karlsson, *Contested Belonging: An Indigenous People's Struggle for Forest Identity in Sub Himalayan Bengal*. Stockholm: Lund University Press, 1997, 93.

30. Arabinda Samanta, *Malarial Fever in Colonial Bengal: Social History of an Epidemic, 1820–1939*. Kolkata: Firma KLM, 2002; Sandeep Sinha, *Public Health Policy and the Indian Public: Bengal 1850–1920*. Kolkata: Vision Publications, 1998.

31. W.W.Hunter, *The Annals of Rural Bengal,* London: Smith Elder and Co., 1868, 10. See also L.S.S.O. Malley, *Santhal Parganas*, Bengal District Gazetteers, Kolkata: Bengal Secretariat Book Depot, 1909 and Mark Harrison, "A Question of Locality: The Identity of Cholera in British India, 1860–1890," in David Arnold, ed., *Warm Climates and Western Medicine*. Amsterdam: Rodopi, 1996, 133–59.

32. Partho Dutta, "Raynald Martin's Medical Topography (1837): The emergence of Public Health in Calcutta," in Biswamoy Pati and Mark Harrison, ed., *The Social History of Health and Medicine*. New Delhi: Primus Books, 2011, 15.

33. James Taylor, *A Sketch of the Topography and Statistics of Dacca*. Dacca: Huttman, 1840, 10.

34. David Arnold, "Disease Resistance and India's Ecological Frontier, 1770–1947," in Biswamoy Pati ed., *Issues in Modern Indian History for Sumit Sarkar*. New Delhi: Popular Prakasan, 2000, 77-90.

35. David Arnold, "Disease Resistance," 77. See also Annual Report of the Calcutta School of Tropical Medicine Institute of Hygiene and the Carmichael Hospital for Tropical Diseases (1924), Kolkata (1925), 22.

36. David Arnold, "Disease Resistance," 78. See also "Some Malarial Problems in Bengal," *Indian Medical Gazette*, 48 (1913): 112–13.

37. C. Strickland and K.L. Chowdhury, *Blackwater Fever and Malaria in the Darjeeling Terai*, Kolkata: India Tea Association, 1931, 33.

38. Nandini Bhattacharya, "The Logic of Location," 184.

39. L.S.S. O'Malley, *Bengal District Gazetteer: Darjeeling*. Kolkata: The Bengal Secretariat Book Depot, 1907, 53.

40. J.D. Hooker, *The Himalayan Journals*. London: John Murray, 1854, 20.

41. D.H.E. Sunder, *Survey and Settlement of the Western Duars in the Jalpaiguri District, 1889–95*. Kolkata: Bengal Secretariat Book Depot, 1895, 45.

42. J.A. Milligan, *Final Report on the Survey and Settlement Operations in the Jalpaiguri District, 1906–1917*. Kolkata: Bengal Sesretariat Press, 1919, 23. See also J.F. Gruning, *Jalpaiguri*. Allahabad: The Pioneer, 1911 and H.B. Rowney, *The Wild Tribes of India*. London: Thos de la Rue & Co., 1882.

43. "A Preliminary Report of the Royal Society Malaria Commission," *Indian Medical Gazette*, 37 (1947): 101–2.

44. Christophers,Bentley, "Malaria in the Duars," 7.

45. S.P. James, "Malaria in India," Scientific Memoirs by Officers of the Medical and Sanitary Department of the Government of India, New Series no. 2, Kolkata: Periodical Publications, 1902, 76.

46. Christophers, Bentley, "Malaria in the Duars," 8.

47. Christophers, Bentley, "Malaria in the Duars," 8.

48. Ronald Ross and L.J. Bruce-Chwatt, *The Great Malaria Problem and Its Solution: From the Memoirs of Ronald Ross*. London: The Keynes Press, 1988, 194.

49. Ross .Bruce-Chwatt, "The Great Malaria Problem," 194.

50. Christophers and Bentley, "Malaria in the Duars," 9, See also Ira Klein, "Development and Death: Reinterpreting Malaria, Economics and Ecology in British India," *Indian Economic and Social History Review,* 38 (2001): 147–79.

51. L.S.S. O'Malley, Santhal Parganas, Bengal District Gazetteers, *op.cit.*, 184. See also *Cholera in India:* 1862–1881, Bengal Province, Review. Kolkata: Bengal Secretariat Press, 1884, 10.

52. A.K. Jameson, *Final Report on the Survey and Settlement Operations in the District of Midnapore, 1911–1917*. Kolkata: Bengal Secretariat Press, 1911, 13.

53. L.S.S. O'Malley, *Santhal Parganas*, 185.

54. *Report of the Malaria Survey of the Jalpaiguri Duars*. Kolkata: Bengal Government Press, 1926, vii. See also S.R. Christophers, *Enquiry on Malaria, Blackwater Fever and Anchylostomiasis in Singhbhum: Preliminary Investigation into the*

Conditions on the Bengal Iron Company's Mines at Manharpur. Patna: Superintendent, Government Printing, Bihar and Orissa, 1923, 25.

55. *Report of the Malaria Survey of the Jalpaiguri Duars*. Kolkata: Bengal Government Press, 1926, vii.

56. J.A.Milligan, Final Report on the Survey and Settlement Operations,:15 See also J.F.Gruning, Jalpaiguri: 47 and H.B.Rowney, The Wild Tribes of India:65.

57. Kumud Ranjan Biwas, *West Bengal District Gazetteers, Jalpaiguri*. Kolkata: Bengal District Gazetteers, 1999, 278.

58. Subhajyoti Ray, *Transformations on the Bengal Frontier*, 79. See also Charu Chandra Sanyal, *The Meches and the Totos: Two Sub-Himalayan Tribes of North Bengal Darjeeling:* University of North Bengal, 1973, 17 and J.F. Gruning, Jalpaiguri, 48.

59. Kumud Ranjan Biwas, *West Bengal District Gazetteers*, Jalpaiguri, 278.

60. J.F.Gruning, Jalpaiguri, 48. See also Asok Mitra, *The Tribes and Castes of West Bengal*. Alipore: West Bengal Government Press, 1953, 224.

61. David Field Rennie, *Bhotan and the Story of the Dooar War*. London: J. Murray, 1866, 347–48.

62. J.F. Gruning, Jalpaiguri, 47. Mark Harrison, ""Hot Beds of Disease": *Malaria and Civilization in Nineteenth-Century British India*," *Parassitologia*, 40, no. 1–2 (1998): 11–18.

63. J.F.Gruning, Jalpaiguri, 49.

64. David Field Rennie, *Bhotan and the Story of the Dooar War*. Lodon: Pilgrims Publisher, 347.

65. K.S. Chattopadhyay, *Report on the Santhals of Bengal*. Kolkata: Bengal Secretariat Press, 1947, 22. See also David Arnold, ""An Ancient Race Outworn": Malaria and Race in Colonial India, 1860–1930," in Waltraud Ernst and Bernard Harris ed., *Race, Science and Medicine*. London: Routledge, 1999, 123–43.

66. *Annual Reports of the Dooars Planters' Association 1908–1948*. Kolkata: Bengal Secretariat Press, 1949.

67. Charles J. Jackson, *Report of the Sanitary Commission for Bengal*. Kolkata: Central Press Company, 1873, 22–23. See also Ira Klein, "Development and Death: Reinterpreting Malaria, Economics and Ecology in British India," *Indian Economic and Social History Review*, no. 38 (2001): 147–79.

68. J.A. Milligan, *Final Report on the Survey and Settlement Operations in the Jalpaiguri District, 1906–1917*. Kolkata: Bengal Secretariat Press, 1919, 25. See also J.F. Gruning, Jalpaiguri, 48 and H.B. Rowney, *The Wild Tribes of India*, 112.

69. *Annual Report of the Director of Public Health Bengal, 1920*. Kolkata: Bengal Secretariat Press, 1922, 14.

70. Implicit in the name, "Jungle Mahals" itself is a land shrouded in mystery and ambiguity. The effect of mainstream political changes was thus never felt in the Jungle Mahals till the advent of the British. It is the land of the Santhals, Bhumij and Kurmi (Mahato), Sabar, Koda, Munda, Hadi, Dom, Bagdi, Goala and Sadgope. Environment shaped the religious beliefs of these people who mainly worshipped the forces of nature.

71. *Annual Report of the Director of Public Health, Bengal, 1923, 105, no.51, 1923*. Kolkata: Superintendent Government Printing Press, 1925, 79.

72. *Annual Report of the Director of Public Health, Bengal, 1925*. Kolkata: Superintendent Government Printing Press, 1926, 60.

73. *Annual Report for the Director of Public Health, Bengal, 1926*. Kolkata, 1927, 43–44.

74. David Hardiman, "Influenza Epidemic of 1918 and the Adivasis of Western India," *Social History of Medicine* 25, no. 3 (2012): 644–664.

75. P. O. Bodding, *Studies in Santal Medicine and Connected Folklore*. Kolkata: The Asiatic Society, 1986 reprint—1st pub. in 3 parts, 1925–40,:142–3.

76. Chittabrata Palit, *Six Lectures on Santhal Society*. Kolkata: Corpus Research Institute, 2009, 59 and Suchibrata Sen, *Birbhum, Malaria and Harry Timbres, A Social History of Health and Medicine in a Colonial Bengal District*. Kolkata, 2015.

77. S.R. Christophers, "The Mechanism of Immunity against Malaria in Communities Living under Hyper-Endemic Conditions," *Indian Journal of Medical Research*, 12 (1924): 273–94.

78. Report of the Malaria Survey of the Jalpaiguri Duars, Kolkata: Bengal Government Press, 1926. See also Mark Harrison, *Climates and Constitutions: Health, Race, Environment and British Imperialism in India, 1600–1850*. Oxford: Oxford University Press, 1999.

79. J.A.Milligan, "Final Report on the Survey and Settlement Operations in the Jalpaiguri District, 1906–1917," 27.

80. J.A.Milligan, "Final Report on the Survey and Settlement Operations," 28.

81. "Jungle and Malaria in Bengal," *Indian Medical Gazette*, No. 63, 1939, 639.

82. C.A. Bentley, *Malaria and Agriculture in Bengal: How to Reduce Malaria in Bengal by Irrigation*. Kolkata: Bengal Secretariat Book Depot, 1925.

83. *Cholera in India: 1862–1881*, Bengal Province Review, Bengal Secretariat Press (1884).

84. David Field Rennie, "Bhotan and the Story of the Dooar War," 347. See also Warwick Anderson, "Immunities of Empire: Race, Disease, and the New Tropical Medicine, 1900–1920," *Bulletin of the History of Medicine*, no. 70 (1996): 94–118.

85. David Hardiman, "Influenza Epidemic of 1918 and the Adivasis of Western India," 644–664.

86. J.F. Gruning, Jalpaiguri, 48.

87. David Hardiman, "Influenza Epidemic of 1918 and the Adivasis of Western India," 663.

88. Oral testimony given by late Lalit Iswarary (passed away on 4 March 2014). He had the opportunity of working with the Christian missionary doctors. I am grateful to Dr Santana Mochchary for interviewing him on my behalf.

89. Oral testimony given by Debki Gabur, age seventy-three. I am grateful to Dr Santana Mochchary for interviewing her on my behalf.

90. Oral Testimony given by late Angasree Basumta (passed away in 2016). I am grateful to Dr Santana Mochchary for interviewing her on my behalf.

91. Oral Testimony given by Manaisree Narjinari (passed away in 2016). I am grateful to Dr. Santana Mochchary for interviewing him on my behalf.

92. J.A. Graham, *On the Threshold of Three Closed Lands, The Guild Outpost in the Eastern Himalayas*, London: R & R Clark Ltd, 1897, 74.

93. J.A. Graham, *On the Threshold of Three Closed Lands*, 76.

94. J.A. Graham, *On the Threshold of Three closed Lands*, 76.
95. J. A. Graham, 77.
96. D.G. Manuel, *A Gladdening River, Twenty-five Years' Guild Influence among the Himalayas*. London: A & C Black, 1914, 171. See also D.V. Rege, *Labour Investigation Committee: Report on an Enquiry into Conditions of Labour in Plantations in India*. New Delhi: Manager of Publications, 1946, 91.
97. D.G. Manuel, *A Gladdening River*, 172.
98. D.G. Manuel, *A Gladdening River*. 173.
99. D.G. Manuel, *A Gladdening River*, 175.
100. Report of the Sanitary Commissioner for Bengal, 1904. Kolkata: Bengal Secretariat Press, 1905.
101. L.S.S. O'Malley, *Santhal Parganas*, 186.
102. L.S.S. O'Malley, *Santhal Parganas*, 187.
103. H. Beveridge, Sahibganj and Rajmahal, *Calcutta Review*, XCVI (1893): 71.
104. L.S.S. O'Malley, Santhal Parganas, Bengal District Gazetteers, *op.cit.*, 186. See also R. Carstairs, *Harma's Village*. Puknuria, 1935, 251.
105. L.S.S. O'Malley, *Santhal Parganas*, 187.
106. H. Macpherson, *Final Report on the Survey and Settlement Operations in the District of Santhal Parganas, 1898–1907*. Kolkata: Bengal Secretariat Press, 1909, 37–38.
107. L.S.S. O'Malley, *Santhal Parganas*, 188.
108. L.S.S. O'Malley, *Santhal Parganas*, 188.
109. *Report of the Leprosy Commission in India*, 1890–91, Kolkata: Printed by the Superintendent of Government Printing Press, 1892, 95.
110. Report of the Leprosy Commission, London. 96.
111. H.W. Bellew, *History of Cholera in India from 1862–1881*. Kolkata: Bengal Secretariat Press, 1882, 773.
112. Report of the Leprosy Commission, 96.
113. Report of the Leprosy Commission, 96.
114. Report of the Leprosy Commission, 97.
115. Bentley Christophers, *Malaria in the Duars*, 10.
116. Bentley Christophers, *Malaria in the Duars*, 11.
117. Bentley Christophers, *Malaria in the Duars*, 12.
118. J. F. Gruning, Jalpaiguri, 48.
119. J. F. Gruning, Jalpaiguri, 49.
120. J. F. Gruning, Jalpaiguri, 49.

BIBLIOGRAPHY

Primary Sources

Printed Reports/Survey and Settlement Reports/Gazetteers/Medical Gazettes

Annual Report of the Director of Public Health Bengal, 1920. Kolkata: Bengal Secretariat Press, 1922.

Annual Report of the Director of Public Health, Bengal, 1923, 105, no.51, 1923. Kolkata: Superintendent Government Printing Press, 1925.

Annual Report of the Director of Public Health, Bengal, 1925. Kolkata: Superintendent Government Printing Press, 1926.

Annual Report for the Director of Public Health, Bengal, 1926. Kolkata, 1927.

Annual Reports of the Dooars Planters' Association 1908–1948. Kolkata: Bengal Secretariat Press, 1949.

'A Preliminary Report of the Royal Society Malaria Commission', *Indian Medical Gazette*, 37 (1947): 101–102.

Beveridge, H. "Sahibganj and Rajmahal", *Calcutta Review*, XCVI (1893):71.

Biwas, Kumud Ranjan. *West Bengal District Gazetteers, Jalpaiguri*. Kolkata: Bengal District Gazetteers, 1999.

Chattopadhyay, K.S. *Report on the Santhals of Bengal*. Kolkata: Bengal Secretariat Press, 1947.

Cholera in India: 1862–1881, *Bengal Province, Review*. Kolkata: Bengal Secretariat Press, 1884.

Christophers, S.R. *Enquiry on Malaria, Blackwater Fever and Anchylostomiasis in Singhbhum: Preliminary Investigation into the Conditions on the Bengal Iron Company's Mines at Manharpur*. Patna: Superintendent, Government Printing, Bihar and Orissa, 1923.

Christophers, S.R, and C.A. Bently. *Malaria in the Duars*. Simla 1911.

Gruning, J.F. *Jalpaiguri*. Allahabad: The Pioneer, 1911.

Jackson, Charles J. *Report of the Sanitary Commission for Bengal*. Kolkata, Central Press Company, 1873.

Jameson, A.K. *Final Report on the Survey and Settlement Operations in the District of Midnapore, 1911–1917*. Kolkata: Bengal Secretariat Press, 1911.

'Jungle and Malaria in Bengal'. *Indian Medical Gazette,* No. 63, 1939, 639.

Macpherson, H. *Final Report on the Survey and Settlement Operations in the District of Santhal Parganas, 1898–1907*. Kolkata: Bengal Secretariat Press, 1909.

Milligan, J.A. *Final Report on the Survey and Settlement Operations in the Jalpaiguri District, 1906–1917*. Kolkata: Bengal Secretariat Press, 1919, 23.

O' Malley, L.S.S. *Santhal Parganas*, Bengal District Gazetteers. Kolkata: Bengal Secretariat Book Depot, 1909.

Report of the Leprosy Commission in India, 1890–91. Kolkata: Printed by the Superintendent of Government Printing Press, 1892.

Report of the Malaria Survey of the Jalpaiguri Duars. Kolkata: Bengal Government Press, (1926).

Second Report of the German Colonial Office. "Professor Koch's Investigations on Malaria". *The German Medical Journal*, March 07 (1931): 325.

Sunder, D.H.E. *Survey and Settlement of the Western Duars in the Jalpaiguri District, 1889–95*. Kolkata: Bengal Secretariat Book Depot, 1895.

Secondary Sources

Books/Articles

Arnold, David. "An Ancient Race Outworn": Malaria and Race in Colonial India, 1860–1930', in Waltraud Ernst and Bernard Harris ed., *Race, Science and*

Medicine, London: Routledge, 1999.

Arnold, David. "Disease Resistance and India's Ecological Frontier, 1770–1947", in Biswamoy Pati ed. *Issues in Modern Indian History for Sumit Sarkar*. New Delhi: Popular Prakasan 2000.

Bala, Poonam, ed. *Contesting Colonial Authority, Medicine and Indigenous Responses in Nineteenth and Twentieth Century India*. New Delhi, Primus Books, reprint, 2016, 1–12, originally published by Lanham MD: Lexington Books, 2012.

Bellew, H.W. *History of Cholera in India from 1862–1881*. Kolkata: Bengal Secretariat Press, 1882.

Bhattacharya, Nandini. "The Logic of Location: Malaria Research in Colonial India, Darjeeling and Duars, 1900–30", *Medical History*, 55 (2011): 183–202.

Bodding, P.O. *Studies in Santal Medicine and Connected Folklore*. Kolkata: The Asiatic Society, 1986 reprint-1st pub. in 3 parts, 1925–40.

Carrigan, Ann Jo. "Yellow fever: Scourge of the South," in Todd L. Savitt and James Harvey Young, eds. *Disease and Distinctiveness in the American South*. Knoxville: University of Tennessee Press, 1978, 55–78.

Cleetus, Burton. "Tropics of Disease: Epidemics in Colonial India", *Economic and Political Weekly* 55, no. 21 (May 2020): 2349.

Curtin, Philip D. "Epidemiology and the Slave Trade", *Political Science Quarterly* 83, no. 2 (1968): 190–216.

Dalton, E.T. *Descriptive Ethnology of Bengal*. Kolkata: Government of Bengal, Council of Asiatic Society of Bengal, 1872, 138.

Dutta, Partho. "Raynald Martin's Medical Topography (1837): The Emergence of Public Health in Calcutta", in Biswamoy Pati and Mark Harrison ed. *The Social History of Health and Medicine*. New Delhi: Primus Books, 2011.

Fraser, W.M. *The Recollections of a Tea Planter*. London: Tea and Rubber Mail, 1935.

Graham, J.A. *On the Threshold of Three Closed Lands, The Guild Outpost in the Eastern Himalayas,* London: London: R & R Clark Ltd, 1897.

Hardiman, David. "Influenza Epidemic of 1918 and the Adivasis of Western India", *Social History of Medicine* 25, no. 3 (August 2012): 644 664.

Harrison, Mark. *Public Health in British India: Anglo-Indian Preventive Medicine, 1859–1914,* Cambridge: Cambridge University Press, 1994.

Harrison, Mark. 'A Question of Locality: The Identity of Cholera in British India, 1860–1890', in David Arnold, ed. *Warm Climates and Western Medicine*, Amsterdam: Rodopi, 1996.

Harrison, Mark. *Climates and Constitutions: Health, Race, Environment and British Imperialism in India, 1600–1850.* Oxford: Oxford University Press, 1999.

Hooker, J.D. *The Himalayan Journals*. London: John Murray, 1854.

Johnson, James. *The Influence of Tropical Climates on European Constitutions*. London: Mottley and Harrison, 1818.

Karlsson, B.G. *Contested Belonging: An Indigenous People's Struggle for Forest Identity in Sub Himalayan Bengal*. Stockholm: Lund University Press, 1997.

Kiple, Kenneth F. *The Caribbean Slave: A Biological History*. Cambridge: Cambridge University Press, 1984.

Klein, Ira. "Death in India: 1871–1921", *Journal of Asian Studies,* no. 32 (1973): 639–59.

Manuel, D.G. *A Gladdening River, Twenty-Five Years' Guild Influence among the Himalayas*. London: A & C Black, 1914.

Mitra, Asok. *The Tribes and Castes of West Bengal Alipore*: West Bengal Government Press, 1953.

McNeill, J. R. "Ecology, Epidemics and Empires: Environmental Change and the Geopolitics of Tropical America, 1600–1825." *Environment and History* 5, no. 2 (1999): 175–84.

Patterson, David K. "Yellow Fever Epidemics and Mortality in the United States, 1693–1905." *Social Science and Medicine* 34, no. 8 (1992): 855–65.

Palit, Chittabrata. *Six Lectures on Santhal Society*, Kolkata: Corpus Research Institute, 2009.

Ray, Subhajyoti. *Transformations on the Bengal Frontier, 1765–1948*. London: Routledge Curzon Press, 2002, 89.

Rege, D.V. *Labour Investigation Committee: Report on an Enquiry into Conditions of Labour in Plantations in India,* Delhi: Manager of Publications, 1946.

Rennie, David Field. *Bhotan and the Story of the Dooar War*. London: J. Murray, 1866, 347–48.

Rowney, H.B. *The Wild Tribes of India*. London: Thos de la Rue & Co., 1882.

Ross, Ronald and L. J. Bruce-Chwatt. *The Great Malaria Problem and Its Solution: From the Memoirs of Ronald Ross*. London: The Keynes Press, 1988.

Samanta, Arabinda. *Malarial Fever in Colonial Bengal: Social History of an Epidemic, 1820–1939*, Kolkata: Firma KLM, (2002).

Sanyal, Charu, Chandra. *The Meches and the Totos: Two Sub-Himalayan Tribes of North Bengal Darjeeling*. University of North Bengal, 1973.

Sen, Suchibrata. *Birbhum, Malaria and Harry Timbres, A Social History of Health and Medicine in a colonial Bengal district,* Kolkata: 2015.

Sinha, Sandeep. *Public Health Policy and the Indian Public: Bengal 1850–1920*. Kolkata: Vision Publications, 1998.

Strickland, C., and K. L. Chowdhury. *Blackwater Fever and Malaria in the Darjeeling Terai*, Kolkata: India Tea Association, 1931.

Taylor, James. *A Sketch of the topography and statistics of Dacca*. Dacca: Huttman, 1840.

Oral Testimonies

Oral testimony by late Lalit Iswarary. Oral testimony by Debki Gabur, age 73.
Oral testimony by late Angasree Basumta. Oral Testimony by Manaisree Narjinari.

Chapter 14

A Cinderella Disease

Colonialism and the Spread of Tuberculosis

Suvankar Dey

> It is Atua, the Great Sprit, coming into them, and eating up their inside; for the patient can feel those parts gradually go away, and then they became weaker and weaker till no more is left; after which the Sprit sends them to the Happy Islands.
>
> —Augustus Early, *Narrative of a Residence in New Zealand* (1832)

The great Maori statesman of the time and chief of the Great Bay Island, Ruartara, sailed for London in 1814, in order to export wheat to Port Jackson (Sydney) in exchange for hoes, axes, spades, sugar and tea. However, his journey aboard was not happy, for he returned home with tuberculosis. One of his political opponents Hongi Hika went to Britain to bring muskets and armour and was similarly contracted with chest disease, but he recovered. From the first half of the nineteenth century, tuberculosis became one of the leading causes of death among the Maori population in New Zealand. Of the worst few pathogens that Captain James Cook (1728–1779) had brought to New Zealand, the most devastating was tubercular disease (in which even three of his crew members had died on their first visit) and 'there was such an abundance of respiratory diseases for the next two decades and after that it is not helpful to try to draw lines between the alleged end of one epidemic and the beginning of the next'. Innocent superstitious indigenous people were terrified of this completely unknown new disease. Even in 1939, this 'curse of the New Zealand race' was responsible for 22% of Maori deaths.

One of the most important features of British imperial expansion was that of 'bacteriological genocide' of indigenous people and creation of a 'new disease environment' in the colonies. According to Emmanuel Le Roy Ladurie, the 'Microbian unification of the world' took place between 1300 and 1650, mainly due to the destructive European imperialism, forced land grabbing, unequal trade and travel.[1] This unprecedented success of European imperialism had been in many cases been determined by pathogens, especially by the massive epidemiological destruction in the America, Australia and New Zealand.[2] In this process, medical historians saw disease as a power. To them, the success of European conquest was not only dependent on advancement of military strength but also on their innate immunity to different deadly diseases. For Europeans, the emergence of these new disease environments often provided possibilities for expansion, for instance, in North and South America, the South Pacific and South Africa.[3] In the New World, decisive role played by smallpox, mumps, whooping cough, dengue, tuberculosis and scarlet fever had accelerated empire building with the help of state-supported annexation and armed violence. Crosby argued 'biological expansion' of European powers over a longer period of time resulted in devastating effects on flora, fauna and the indigenous communities.[4] Within 100–150 years after the 'invasion' of America by Columbus in 1492, about 80–90% of the Native American population and 8 million of the native Taino inhabitants of Hispaniola Island were completely disseminated by unknown diseases.[5]

Since the time of Colombian exchange, thanks to the imperial expansion, epidemic changed its basic form and left long-term impact on indigenous society and its people. The present chapter will discuss the causes of spread of tuberculosis in British colonies from various points of historical context. It will also try to explore how the definition of tuberculosis had changed drastically as a result of the industrialization, brutal advent of commercial capital, urbanization and rise of industrial development in the British colonies. In addition to this, it will also attempt to find answers to some of the questions such as – how did white men saw this disease and how they explained its aetiology in the context of native environment? Last but not the least, how Indian medical community and educated middle class understood tuberculosis with focusing on the growth and evolution of this disease in Indian subcontinent.

Over the past few decades, from the imperialist point of context, a number of historians have discussed both globally and locally about the profound consequences of diseases on different parts of the world.[6] With a few exceptions, there has been little discussion of tuberculosis from a global perspective compared to other diseases.[7] Mark Harrison and Michael Worboys argued tuberculosis remained a 'Cinderella Disease' as compared to other diseases like malaria and cholera because 'it lacked both the "glamour" necessary to sustain political and scientific interest and the economic impact necessary to ensure official intervention'.[8] Although, in recent years, a number of medical historians, for example, Linda Bryder, Barbara Bates, Niels Brimnes, David Barnes, Helen Bynum and many others, have portrayed a larger historical picture of tuberculosis and its interrelationships between state, society and wider contemporary medical sphere.[9]

Throughout the nineteenth century, British imperialism acquired nearly a total 10 million square miles of land and 400 million people to its own colonial holdings. By the end of the century, it had spread almost all over the world and became the strongest and largest empire in Europe. The scope of the current chapter will be limited to the British Empire and of its colonies in the Indian Ocean. The process of British domination in India began after the Battle of Plassey (1757) and by within 1818, large areas of Indian subcontinent (excluding Punjab) came under their jurisdiction. Burma was annexed and brought under the Indian administration. Australia and New Zealand developed rapidly, and huge tracts of west land were added to Britain's Canadian possession. In 1841, Hong Kong too became a part of the British Empire. A large part of Africa was under British control and by the end of 1890 tropical Africa was divided among the major European powers, against the will of the indigenous people living in that region. Dozens of small islands in the Pacific too were seized along with a large portion of Malay Archipelago in Southeast Asia. There were also a number of important regions where Britain dominated the economy, albeit without any formal colonial possession.[10]

MEN, MONEY AND MACHINE: METROPOLITAN EXPERIENCE

In Europe, tuberculosis was rhetorically described as 'Captain of death'. The disease was connoted by different terms such as 'consumption', 'pulmonalis' or 'white plague'. The word tuberculosis is well known today and needs no explanation, and yet it seems to have appeared in print for the first time around 1840, and came into common use only during the next fifty years.

Tuberculosis also known as 'phthisis' or 'romantic disease' greatly influenced the literary world of Europe. For instance, Shakespeare's plays such as *Timon of Athens* (1623), *Much Ado about Nothing* (1599) and *The Tempest* (1610) contain description of the classical symptoms of tuberculosis, such as 'wasting disease', 'rotten lungs' and 'wheezing lungs'. Tuberculosis had never appeared as a terrible or devastating disease in pre-industrial world. Tuberculosis emerged in Europe, as argued by Mark Harrison, largely due to industrialization and later it spread rapidly elsewhere as a result of greater economic changes.[11] Rene and Jean Dubos have argued that the increase of tuberculosis was intimately connected with the rise of industrial and urbanized society.[12] Thanks to the immense greed of British expansionism, diseases like tuberculosis that were previously confined to their own geographical areas began to travel at epidemic and pandemic speed in the wake of industrial revolution followed by imperialism and the establishment of global trading network.[13] To be more specific, as a direct result of imperialism, local market is now connected with global market, and thus the scale and scope of British trade continued to expand throughout the century. Tuberculosis was one of the biggest silent killers in the British colonial cities aggravated by overcrowding, poverty, insanitary conditions and the rapid unhealthy urbanization process. Even in the coal mining areas of Britain tuberculosis was prevalent.[14] Cities and port cities became important and changed dynamically overnight for the interests of the empire's trade and commerce, and large numbers of people flocked from the villages to cities in search of job and other opportunities in the nineteenth and twentieth centuries. Throughout the nineteenth century both European and internal immigration had transformed many villages into major metropolis with increasing numbers of workshop and factories. A new phase of urban history began with the urbanization of the nineteenth century and the expansion of industries. The periphery of cities attracted millions of job seekers from countryside within a few decades. If we look at the British colonial cities, we find more or less similar picture. Even in colonial cities of the Malayan peninsula, especially Singapore, before and after 1940 tuberculosis was a major cause of morbidity and mortality, as shown by Lenore Manderson.[15] The population of British Bengal in 1921 was 44 million and a decade later it had increased to 51million.[16] The growth of Calcutta as an industrial city with its several negative effects helped in further spread of tuberculosis. The smoke which these factories produced had direct impact on the health of the people. David Arnold's research on pollution in modern India revealed that since the end of nineteenth century, dark poisonous smoke from factories, workshops, railway yards or steamships crowded at the port of Hooghly had been continuous source for atmospheric pollution in Bengal.[17] Growing and nurtured in local and international capital, these 'new industries' had tremendous effects on politics as well as in economy, and hence were difficult to control. Interestingly, the opposition to the 'Poisons Act of 1904' did not come from public or the poor, but from the owners of the Calcutta jute mills. Shortly afterwards, in 1915, the city's steamship business organizations similarly opposed an amendment to the 'Bengal Smoke Nuisance Abatement Act' because they saw such act as a curtailment of their business freedom.[18] The Bengali journal *Swasthya Samachar* complained of the volume of smoke emission from the factory chimneys, especially in the Manicktala area in Calcutta. A. C. Chatterjee, director of Public Health of Bengal, wrote in 1939 in *Amrita Bazar Patrika* that more than one-fifth of the total deaths of babies were due to respiratory disease, for which smoke nuisance was primarily responsible.[19] Dr A. Lankester had devoted an entire chapter to the subject of 'Tuberculosis in Cities and Towns' in his influential tuberculosis

Table 14.1 Statement showing the number of deaths from tuberculosis in Calcutta, Bombay and Madras, 1904–1919

	Calcutta		*Bombay*		*Madras*	
Year	*Deaths from TB*	*TB Rate per Mille*	*Deaths from TB*	*TB Rate per Mille*	*Deaths from TB*	*TB Rate per Mille*
1904	1,608	1.8	3,548	4.57	318	0.6
1905	2,052	2.4	3,183	4.10	832	1.6
1906	2,201	2.6	4,052	4.14	736	1.4
1907	2,241	2.6	3,440	3.51	641	1.2
1908	2,101	2.5	3,023	3.09	717	1.4
1909	1,919	2.3	2,862	2.92	774	1.4
1910	1,971	2.3	2,830	2.90	459	0.9
1911	2,060	2.3	2,694	2.75	760	1.5
1912	1,931	2.3	2,794	2.85	672	1.3
1913	2,196	2.5	2,452	2.19	481	0.9
1914	2,137	2.4	1,889	1.92	738	1.4
1915	1,920	2.1	1,710	1.74	759	1.5
1916	1,738	1.9	1,902	1.94	876	1.7
1917	1,539	1.7	2,118	2.16	1,067	2.1
1918	1,826	2.0	2,513	2.56	1,488	2.9
1919	1,889	2.1	2,780	2.83	1,309	2.5

Source: Arthur Lankester, *Tuberculosis in India: Its Prevalence, Causation and Prevention* (Calcutta 1920), 45.

survey report in India. Table 14.1 shows that the mortality from tuberculosis had been generally high in three presidency cities in India.

TUBERCULOSIS IN INDIAN OCEAN WORLD

Tuberculosis was not uncommon in Indian Ocean World[20] (though in Pacific it was completely new) but rapid urbanization in the late nineteenth century took the disease to an alarming level.

The urban scenario had changed. The mass urban migration and epidemic diseases tended to take devastating forms over the time. Urban working and living conditions reflected expanding world of industrialization and the fact that cities were being drawn into the world market. As a result, when Maori began to move in significant numbers to New Zealand cities in the second half of the twentieth century they tended to be crowded into poorer and rapidly became associated with squalor, poverty and most importantly infected with tuberculosis. In Hong Kong, tuberculosis ran at a very high rate for the whole of the 1940 and continued to do so after the Second World War.[21] Similarly in the case of colonial Sri Lanka, Margaret Jones's extensive research has shown that tuberculosis became one of the leading causes of death between 1900 and 1948, along with malaria and dysentery.[22] Randall M.

Packard argued in the context of Southern Africa that tuberculosis has spread rapidly in modern times and basically due to colonization and movement of industrial migrant labours. Since the mines in South Africa required a lot of migrant labour, the problem of tuberculosis was most prevalent there. The commercial importance of Kimberley and Johannesburg, two South African cities rich in gold and diamonds, led to the transformation of ragged, poverty-inflicted mining camps into major metropolitan areas in just a few decades. In the second half of the nineteenth century, workers in various mining areas of South Africa and India had to work in crowded and unhealthy environments, where accidents were common as were fatalities, and miners risked the possibility of contracting respiratory and other diseases. Poor housing and living conditions stimulated the spread of tuberculosis more rapidly among the lower classes. Because of the cost, few factories and even fewer workshops had piped water, sufficient latrines for their workers or waste disposal systems. Workers put in long hours near dangerous machinery and carried heavy loads and had little time to rest. The workers themselves did not realize the importance of breathing clean air, consuming healthy food and bathing. Most of the time they had to spend hours after hours surrounded with factory dust, dirt and industrial poisons. In case of colonial India too, the industrial workers contracted the disease very easily due to their unhealthy working condition. In both Africa and India, the contrast with the 'pre-industrial past' was noticeable. Needless to say, close links between migrant labour, mining and the dissemination of diverse diseases were an important consequence of this pattern (Steere-Williams in this volume).

Migration of people was also responsible for the spread of tuberculosis. Migration did not only occur from villages to cities just within the state. With the abolition of slave economy, plantation owners began to look for alternative sources of labour. Historians have seen the 'massive labour migration' within British Empire, as indenture labour resulted in transformation of many regions into disease zone.[23] From 1830 onwards, labourers were mostly from Asians and between 1879 and 1920 about 60,000 South Asians went under indentured to work in Fiji. By 1838, there were some 25,000 South Asians working on sugar plantations of Mauritius. Some 30,000 South Asians built Kenya's railway in the late 1890s, over a third of whom were killed or seriously injured in the process. Altogether, more than a million South Asians worked under indenture in the British Empire.[24] Tuberculosis mortality rates were high in these plantations.

Insanitary facilities made life miserable, uncomfortable and often short lived. Crowded and unhealthy conditions led to the spread of disease easily among workers and at the same time they acted as prime agents of various unknown diseases including tuberculosis among the local people. For instance, Fiji was a host of virulent epidemics of measles, tuberculosis and influenza in the years of indenture.[25] Moreover, World War I had enhanced the movement of the troops across the globe and helped to spread tuberculosis more widely.[26] Railways and steamships across the British Empire (especially after the construction of Suez Canal in 1860) have connected different regions with wider imperial network and indirectly helped to spread the disease.

UNDERSTANDING TUBERCULOSIS IN 'NATIVE ENVIRONMENT'

How exactly did British imperial medical authorities observe tuberculosis in the wider empire? Who did they blame the disease for? Did race matter at all, and if so, then to what extent? We will try to find the answer to these questions one by one. In many cases, colonial medical authorities considered that climate, environment and above all the indigenous people of the colonies to be the sources of diseases and importance was given on environmental conditions, such as air, water and light for understanding of disease. With the advent of 'Asiatic Cholera' in nineteenth century, the idea that East was unclean and unhealthy became an axiomatic truth among the European people. Thus, Ranald Martin's *Medical Topography*, published in 1837, reveals the superiority of white people:

> The natives have yet to learn, in public and private sense, that the sweet sensations connected with cleanly habits, pure air, are some of the most precious gifts of civilization, and a taste for them tends to give a distaste to degrading and grovelling gratification.[27]

Lord Morley, secretary of state for India, while writing about Indian medical services narrate it as the best in the world, but found only 'two things' bad in India: 'climate' and the 'natives'.

Philip Curtin described India in his book as a home of all dreadful diseases and epidemics where the ruling class migrated only to face death.[28] So the East was continually depicted as dark, while the West was enlightened and civilized. On the other hand, such discourse, as argued by Mark Harrison, 'boosted Europeans' confidence in their ability to rule parts of the globe with climates very different from their own.[29] Imperialism was to them not only the conquest of territory and people but also a civilizing mission. Thus, the conquests of unknown vulnerable diseases from Africa to Asia were a part of their civilizing process.

In the British Empire, especially in the context of India, military medical officers and European-based tuberculosis experts began to discuss the problem of tuberculosis and referred it as a 'social disease' from the beginning of early twentieth century. The medical officers had understood the high incidence of tuberculosis in the colonies due to the socio-economic condition of the people along with their personal cultural habits.[30] So in this 'social' and 'cultural frame', importance was given to indiscriminate spitting, superstitious theories surrounding childbirth, sleeping habits, overcrowding, poverty, marriage customs and above all, the seclusion of women as explanations for tuberculosis.[31] For instance, Arthur Lankester, in his report on the prevalence on tuberculosis among women in India, repeatedly pointed out the various social evils:

> In the whole of my tour through the cities of India no single fact was more constantly brought to my notice by ceaseless reiteration than the direct dependence on consumption upon the system *purdah* seclusion of women.[32]

Similar study was carried out by Margaret Jones, who in her investigation on tuberculosis in Hong Kong referred to Dr J. M. Atkinson (medical director 1900–1911). Atkinson argued in 1911 in his annual report that high mortality rates from tuberculosis in Hong Kong were caused in part by the 'inveterate habit of lower class Chinese of spitting in public buildings, offices, staircases, footpaths and wharves'.[33] In case of New Zealand, Turbot's influential study of tuberculosis among Maoris of Wajapu county emphasized social factors like poverty and more importantly changes in lifestyle.[34]

Ironically, the medical authorities often considered poverty as a secondary cause. In British India, the Government of Bengal identified poverty, malnutrition and overcrowding as chief factor causing tuberculosis while authorities in Bombay located tuberculosis with 'a disease of overcrowding and general insanitary conditions'.[35] In India, anti-tuberculosis campaign in 1930s stressed how the disease could be prevented by human behavioural changes.

VIRGIN SOIL, RACE, TUBERCULOSIS

An interesting argument was put forward by the colonial authorities in this context, that is, the concept of 'Virgin soil'. This concept was well established in Australia and Aborigines were blamed for their movements towards towns and cities abandoning open air lifestyle. However, in case of Colonial Africa, a new approach was taken and the British medical authorities tried to understand tuberculosis in Africa by considering 'race' as a factor for spread of the disease like what was done in Germany and America.[36] It is not possible to write a history of tuberculosis in twentieth century without the discussion of race. Historians have discussed the relationship between tuberculosis and race and spent more time writing about the passage of disease from 'primitive' to 'civilized' peoples than in actually controlling it.[37] Applying the 'virgin soil theory'[38] to Africa, it was acknowledged that the Europeans brought tuberculosis here, but at the same time they also promoted that higher incidence of tuberculosis was predominant in blacks or non-European people in general as they are physiologically weak, backward, ignorant as well as biologically and culturally inferior.[39] Thus, German eugenicists regarded tuberculosis as 'the friend of race' because it ultimately pushes the unfit members of society to the brink of death. In the beginning of twentieth century, white physicians blamed blacks as one of the main sources and spreaders of tubercle bacillus, and thus strong association of tuberculosis with a few specific communities in America, including immigrant polish Jews, black, African American (as opposed to white Americans who were relatively safer), had been firmly established. With the help of various surveys of autopsies and investigation on post-mortem, medical authorities came to the conclusion that lungs of black people lacked the specific ability to produce the fibrous tissue necessary for localizing the disease. We will hear the same story from Lyle Cummins, the leading British authority on the disease in first half of twentieth century, who wrote in 1935 that 'native races' lacked toughness and would only develop resistance to tuberculosis on a historical timescale.[40] The most frightening reflection of tuberculosis and its relation with race was found in Nazi Germany, in which at Neuengamme concentration camp Nazi doctor Kurt Heissmeyer used to infect Jewish children and adults and monitor the development of the germs. Later, in Nazi-occupied Poland and Soviet Union, the *Schutzstaffel* (SS) with the help of mobile X-ray diagnosed more than 100,000 people and all were shot to death.[41]

Responding to Disease: Indian Medical World and Tuberculosis in British India

> 'In the land of the ox-cart, one must not expect the pace of a motor car'. (Resolution, 23 May 1914, Government of India, Department of Education)[42]

By the beginning of the nineteenth century, it was generally believed that India had hardly any tuberculosis occurrence. By the middle of the nineteenth century, tuberculosis was thought to be common particularly among British troops, and in some areas it was thought to be common among natives as well, such as in the districts of Madras. While tuberculosis was not a new disease in India, as a result of colonization along with the urbanization and industrialization the physical and social environment of the country changed. Initially tuberculosis was considered to be widespread in urban areas. However, after 1900, tuberculosis spread to the rural areas through migrant populations.[43] These populations were mostly from labourers who had migrated to the cities and towns in search of work. Those infected had no other option but to return to their rural homes.

In colonial India, probably for the first time, a representative from India, Dr Alexander Crombie, was sent to attend the Congress on Tuberculosis in Berlin, which was held in May 1899.[44] After his return from the Congress, Crombie submitted a report to the Government of India in October 1899 which was the first official documentation on the causes, prevalence and prevention of tuberculosis in India. However, these reports accepted that tubercular disease occurred due to the presence and multiplication of tubercle bacillus, discovered by Dr Robert Koch. Two later reports by Lankester in 1916 and by Cummins in 1932 also adopted a similar view.[45] From 1860, colonial governments directed their attention to the importance of collecting proper statistics for identifying births and deaths. The organization for reporting births and deaths to the authorities was rudimentary. In the rural areas this duty was generally conducted by the village watchman.[46] From 1900, sanitary officials concentrated on the prevalence of tuberculosis among inmates in jails. From 1885, the progressive rise of tuberculosis was noticed among the jail population,[47] with death rates from tuberculosis in Indian jails notably higher than in England and Wales.[48] In 1902, the Government of India gave instruction to all local governments to focus special attention to the problem of tuberculosis. From the official point of view, it was not until 1911 that medical practitioners and sanitary officials believed in the prevalence of tuberculosis in India. For the first time, the acknowledgement came from the medical professionals at the 'First All India Sanitary Conference' held in Bombay in 1911.[49]

Both the indigenous and medical practitioners of Western medicine thought that 'tuberculosis' was an outcome of modern civilization. They critically saw the socio and cultural aspects where moral degeneration occurred as a consequence of the adaption of so-called Western lifestyles. In 1932, Naindra Ranjan Sengupta wrote[50] in the *Journal of Indian Medical Association* that senseless imitations of the Western tinned, bottled, supercooked and universal adaption of tea had neither food value nor vitamins. In the cities, cinema halls and theatres confined people to closed halls, which caused the spread of tuberculosis. The increasing number of rice mills meant that people were eating refined rice instead of pounded rice, causing a loss of vitamin B and other nutrients, which finally resulted in loss of vitality.[51] Contemporary observer criticized the adoption of Western dress like tight trousers, shirts, coats, caps and shoes instead of traditional garments, since they had completely denied the fresh air to the body.[52] Unwise fashion or clothing by the Indians was mentioned by Lankester:

> Of those whose homes are in the cities, and who are dependent upon the Indian tailor for their cloths, are compelled by 'fashion' to wear clothes which tend to contract the chest, preventing to dangerous extent the full expansion of the lungs.[53]

Drinking coffee and tea was seen as causing indigestion and sleeplessness and meat eating, smoking, drinking and chewing tobaccos were viewed as the means through which the germ could spread from affected persons. Thus, the Indian medical practitioners vehemently criticized the cheap imitation of the Western methods and attitudes which according to them undoubtedly helped the spread of disease and its extension and frequency of epidemics. It is interesting to note that in the 1880s at a time when the campaign to expose the tyranny of the plantation worker was at its peak, Sundari Mohan Das (1857–1950), the renowned doctor, and Krishna Kumar Mitra (1852), the nationalist leader, gave up drinking tea for good as a mark of protest.

Kumud Ranjan Mallick (1883–1970), a well-known Bengali poet of the 1930s, described in his poem the fate of tea-addicted Ramsuk Tiwari, who migrated to Bengal for seeking his fortune.[54] It is true that there is no clinical relationship between tuberculosis and tea drinking. Still, these references are useful to project how the changed drinking habits of the Indians were looked upon as a cause of declining health.

There was a rise of prices particularly after the First World War (1914–1918) as a result of which the poor people suffered the most. They were left with no other option and thus many of them were forced to starve as a result of which, one could easily be a victim of tuberculosis. Economic exploitation of India under the British Raj resulted in a series of famines followed by epidemic outbreak. A famine in northern India between 1860 and 1861 killed around 2 million people. More than 6 million people died in famines that spread throughout the country in 1870, and in the late 1890s famine took another 5 million lives. The monsoon failures of 1896 and 1897 in parts of India brought severe famines exacerbated by simultaneous outbreak of plague in 1897. Bengal famine of 1943 led to the spread of smallpox, malaria, cholera, tuberculosis and millions of people died from starvation.[55] Between the two world wars the progress of industrialization in India had been spectacular. Expansion of industrial activities had increased profits and industrialists had accumulated wealth. The working class, on the other hand, had been condemned to a life of poverty and squalor.[56] Industrialization in India started with the establishment of the large number of the jute and cotton textile mills. Indian capitalists had invested their capital in industrial enterprises, when the British founded the textile mills in Bombay and Calcutta after the mid-nineteenth century. In the textile industry, the deliberately hot and humid air, filled with tiny, irritating fibres, sped up the thread as well as spread of the bacteria. According to statistics, the number of factories in British India increased between 1894 and 1914 from about 800 to almost 3,000, while the average daily number of employees rose from 35,000 to 9,50,000.[57] The smoke which these factories produced had direct impact on the health of the people. One can hardly find an exhaust fan in these mills. Housing of the industrial workers had never formed a part of the scheme of industrialization nor had the government introduced any legislative measures to improve the conditions of housing in the industrial areas. The rapid transport facilities, growing industrialization and urbanization transformed tuberculosis into a serious problem. Thus, Lankester remarks:

> 'Most remarkable increase (of tuberculosis) amongst the aboriginal tribes in Chota Nagpur' was due to 'the growing practice for the men to go to work as coollies in Calcutta or in the Bengal coal mines' for five or six months in each year . . . both from towns and village districts in the neighborhood of Calcutta, Bombay, Lahore and other cities, I obtained ample evidence of the spread of the consumption from the central city to parts around, within a considerable radius.[58]

For this very similar reason, Hazaribagh and its surrounding districts, which were famous for the treatment of the disease, were gradually infected with tuberculosis due to the constant influx of the cases from Calcutta and other parts of Bengal.[59] Increasing dust nuisance of the Indian cities on account of increasing number of motor cars and buses had direct repercussions on the incidence of tuberculosis. The particles of carbons had resulted in causation of diseases like tuberculosis. Development of transport and communication system made tuberculosis spread further in the interiors. Increased numbers of motor cars, buses and lorries had been one of the chief sources of poisonous smoke. In 1929, the total numbers of registered motor cars in Calcutta were 25,569, motorcycles 4,334, motor lorries 2,448, taxi cabs 1,861 and motor buses 702.[60] These figures were increasing day by day. People through the columns of the newspaper had expressed their deep grievances against this. Correspondents to newspaper expressed their concerns about this hazard. In 1925, a person named Satya Ghosh wrote a letter to the editor of the *Calcutta Municipal Gazette* complaining of the smoke nuisance from the engine yards in Narkeldanga.

He provided a vivid picture of the health hazards posed by such close proximity to the residential area. In his own words,

> In day time again, the soot deposits caused by winter dew and laid on the roofs and terrace make it impossible for people to get their cloths dried in the sun owing to their getting dirty. The location of the yards was to a certain extent permissible at a time when the surrounding tracts of land beyond the canal were a sort of wilderness. But the time has changed; these suburban places today come to occupy an important place in Calcutta. It is therefore high time for Government to remove these locomotive yards to a suitable distance far from the thickly populated human habitation.[61]

A. C. Chatterjee, the director of Public Health, talked about the dense thick bluish smoke emanating from the exhaust pipes of large vehicles due to bad or defective oil. At times it was so thick that one could not see anything on the road about a hundred yards away.[62] Under the British rule, the Indian population became more mobile within the national boundary. With the advancement of better communication system, movement of people accelerated. Developments in transport systems like railways have facilitated the system of communication but at the same time strengthened and increased the spread of diseases.[63]

CONCLUSION

From 1750 onwards, the impact of disease invasion gradually reached its final stage as territorial empires were established, armies as well as cities grew in size, and most importantly, as a product of imperialism and colonialism, new forms of transport and communication were developed which proliferated the spread of infectious diseases like tuberculosis. European colonialism drastically changed and expanded the geographical boundaries of the diseases and destructed the life of indigenous communities. The picture was pretty much the same from Australia to Africa or from Hazaribagh to Hong Kong. The identification of tuberculosis in the colonies of British Empire and the onset of discussion and discourse centred on it took place a little later than other diseases. The colonial authorities had their own perceptions of tuberculosis, as we saw numerous attempts have been made in the colonies to describe the disease in terms of race or racial theories and sometimes it was identified as simply a social disease, where human activities were blamed. In the case of India we noticed that educated middle class and contemporary medical practitioner severely criticized and attacked the so-called Western modernity and economic exploitation of the rulers. Most importantly, due to the pre-existing presence of tuberculosis in India, the rulers introduced new discourse to understand the aetiology of the disease contrary to colonial Africa.

Let's come to the present situation. What is the status of tuberculosis in the twenty-first century? According to the World Health Organization, someone is infected with tuberculosis germs every second. An estimated 1.6 million people died from tuberculosis in 2005, and in 2006 nearly 9.2 million new cases and 1.7 million deaths were reported due to tuberculosis worldwide, with 90% occurring in low- and middle-income countries. A new strain of tuberculosis began to appear from the 1980s, called multi-drug-resistant TB, resistant to the most powerful tuberculosis drugs, isoniazid and rifampicin. Tuberculosis remains a leading cause of death among patients who are infected with HIV/AIDS, accounting for some 13% of global AIDS deaths. The coronavirus disease (COVID-19) pandemic had a devastating effect on tuberculosis. The most affected areas of COVID-19 have also witnessed the highest tuberculosis burden. Recent investigation by the United Nations express that poverty will increase as much as half billion, mostly among the poor people of Africa, Southeast Asia, Central and South America.[64] The biggest challenge, as to how the nation states will deal with tuberculosis along with poverty and hunger in the coming years, still looms large.

NOTES

1. Ladurie Le Roy, "A Concept: The Unification of the Globe by Disease," in his *Mind and Method of the Historian,* trans. Siân Reynolds and Ben Reynolds (Brighton: Harvester, 1981), 28–83.

2. Alfred W. Crosby, *The Colombian Exchange: The Biological Consequences of 1492* (Westport: Praeger Publication, 1971); N. David, *Born to Die: Disease and New World Conquest, 1492–1650* (Cambridge: Cambridge University Press, 1998); D. Stannard, *American Holocaust: Columbus and the conquest of the New World* (Oxford: Oxford University Press, 1992).

3. However, in areas such as Asia and the East and West Indies diseases represented a primary disadvantage to empire. See Phillip D. Curtin, *Death by Migration: Europe's Encounter with the tropical world in the Nineteenth Century* (Cambridge: Cambridge University Press, 1989).

4. Alfred W. Crosby, *Ecological Imperialism: The Biological Expansion of Europe, 900–1900* (Cambridge: Cambridge University Press, 1986).

5. L. Newson, "Pathogens, Places and Peoples" in *Technology, Disease and Colonial Conquest, Sixteenth to Eighteenth Centuries*, ed. G, Raudzens (Boston: Brill, 2001), 167–210; N. D. Cook, "Disease and Depopulation of Hispaniola, 1492–1518", *Colonial Latin American Review* 2, no. 1–2 (2013), 213–45. Similarly in the case of New Zealand we shall see that as white settler colonialism progressed (1840s onwards) the indigenous Maori populations were marginalized and their numbers decreased significantly, see Alfred W. Crosby, *Ecological Imperialism,* 217–269; Judy Campbell explores the impact of European diseases on aboriginal population of Australia, see Judy Campbell, *Invisible Invaders: Smallpox and Other Diseases in Aboriginal Australia, 1780–1880* (Carlton South: Melbourne University Press, 2002).

6. P. Levine, *Prostitution, Race and Politics: Policing Venereal Disease in the British Empire* (New York: Routledge, 2003); I. J. Catanach, "Plague and the Tensions of Empire: India 1896–1918," in *Imperial Medicine and Indigenous Societies* ed. David Arnold (Manchester: Manchester University Press, 1988), 149–171; M. Espinosa, "The Invincible Generals: Yellow Fever and the Fight for Empire in Cuba, 1868–1898," in *Biomedicine as a Contested Site: Some Revelations in Imperial Contests* ed. Poonam Bala (Lanham, MD: Lexington Books, 2009), 67–79; Mark Harrison, *Medicine in an Age of Commerce and Empire: Britain and its Tropical Colonies 1660–1830* (Oxford: Oxford University Press, 2010); Rohan Deb Roy, *Malarial Subjects: Empire, Medicine and Nonhumans in British India 1820–1909* (Cambridge: Cambridge University Press, 2017); Alison Bashford, *Imperial Hygiene: A Critical*

History of Colonialism, Nationalism and Public Health (Basingstoke: Palgrave Macmillan, 2004).

7. Christian W. McMillen, *Discovering Tuberculosis: A Global History, 1900 to the present* (New Haven: Yale University Press, 2017); Mark Harrison, & Michael Worboys, "A Disease of civilization: Tuberculosis in Britain, Africa and India 1900–39", in *Migrants, Minorities and Health, Historical and Contemporary Studies*, ed. Lara Marks & Michael Worboys (London: Routledge; 1995), 93–124; Michael Worboys, "Tuberculosis and Race in Britain and Its Empire, 1900–50," in *Race, Science and Medicine 1700–1960*, ed. Waltraud Ernst & Bernard Harris (Routledge, 1999), 144–167.

8. Harrison and Worboys, "A Disease of civilization", 116.

9. David S. Barnes, *The Making of a Social Disease: Tuberculosis in 19th Century France* (Oxford: Oxford University Press, 1990); Barbara Bates, *Bargaining for Life: A Social History of Tuberculosis, 1876–1938* (University of Pennsylvania Press, 1992); Niels Brimnes, *Languished Hopes: Tuberculosis, the State and International Assistance in Twentieth-Century India* (New Delhi: Orient Blackswan, 2016); Linda Bryder, *Below the Magic Mountain: A Social History of Tuberculosis, 1876–1938* (Oxford: Oxford University Press. 1992); L. Bryder, F. Condrau, & M. Worboys eds., *Tuberculosis Then and Now: Perspective on the History of an Infectious Disease* (McGill-Queen's University Press, 2010); D. Rene, & J. Dubos, eds., *The White Plague: Tuberculosis, Man and Society* (London: Victor Gollancz, 1953); G. Jones, *Captain of all these Men of Death: The History of Tuberculosis in 19th and 20th Century Ireland* (New York: Rodopi B.V. 2001); Helen Bynum, *Spitting Blood: The History of Tuberculosis* (Oxford: Oxford University Press, 2012).

10. British trade dominated in Argentina and Brazil. They relied heavily on British investors. The policy was successful in so far as Britain was, throughout the century, the main European nation trading in the region. See Willie Thompson, *Global Expansion: Britain and its Empire, 1870–1914* (London: Pluto Press, 1999).

11. Mark Harrison, & Michael Worboys, "A Disease of civilization," 110–111.

12. R. Dubos, & J. Dubos, *The White Plague: Tuberculosis, Man and Society* (New Jersey: Rutgers University Press, 1952, reprint 1987, 1996).

13. David Arnold, "The Indian Ocean as a Disease Zone, 1500–1950," *South Asia: Journal of South Asian Studies* 14 No. 2 (1991), 1–21; also, J. N. Hays, *The Burdens of Disease: Epidemics and Human Response in Western History* (New Brunswick, NJ: Rutgers University Press, 2000); W. Beinart, & L. Hughes, *Environment and Empire* (Oxford: Oxford University Press, 2007).

14. Aurthur Mclvor, Ronald Johnston, and M. Lung, *A History of Dust Disease in British Coal Mining* (Aldershot: Ashgate, 2007).

15. L. Manderson, *Sickness and the State: Health and Illness in Colonial Malaya 1870–1940* (Cambridge: Cambridge University Press, 1996), 120.

16. M. Mann, *South Asia's Modern History: Thematic Perspectives* (Routledge: London, 2015), 283.

17. David Arnold, *Toxic Histories: Poison and Pollution in Modern India* (Cambridge: Cambridge University Press, Cambridge 2016), 192–195.

18. Michael R. Anderson, 'The Conquest of Smoke: Legislation and Pollution in Colonial Calcutta', in *Nature, Culture and Imperialism: Essays on Environmental History of South Asia*, ed. David Arnold & Ramchandra Guha (Delhi: Oxford University Press, 1995), 293–335.

19. I have discussed this in my article, Suvankar Dey, "Captain of Death: Tuberculosis in colonial Bengal", in *Occasional Paper: New Scholarship in Indian Military History*, ed. P, Stanley (Canberra: University of Canberra Press, 2019), 3–9.

20. Monica H. Green & Lori Jones, "The Evolution and Spread of Major Human Disease in the Indian Ocean World", in *Disease Dispersion and Impact in the Indian Ocean World Studies*, ed. Gwyn Campbell & Eva-Maria Knoll (Palgrave Macmillan, 2020), 25–57; Arabinda Samanta, "Living the Shadow of Death: Tubercular Body In Colonial Bengal," in *Contextualizing the body: An Indian Experience*, ed. Sudit Krishna Kumar & Suvobrata Sarkar (New Delhi: Manohar, 2020), 165–177.

21. Margaret Jones, "Tuberculosis, Housing and the Colonial State: Hong Kong, 1900–1950", *Modern Asian Studies* 37, no. 3 (2003): 654.

22. Margaret Jones, *Health Policy in Britain's Model Colony: Ceylon (1900–1948)* (New Delhi: Orient Blackswan, 2018).

23. Ralph Shlomowitz and John McDonald, "Mortality of Indian Labour on Ocean Voyages, 1843–1917", *Studies in History* 6, no. 1 (1990): 35–65.

24. See Madhavi Kale, *Fragments of Empire: Capital, Slaver, and Indian Indentured Labor Migration in the British Caribbean* (Philadelphia: Philadelphia University Press, 1998).

25. Philippa Levine, *The British Empire: Sunset to Sunrise* (Great Britain: Pearson Longman, 2007), 82–103.

26. John F. Murray, "Tuberculosis and World War I," *American Journal of Critical Care Medicine* 192, no. 4 (2015): 411–14.

27. Partho Datta, "Ranald Martin's Medical Topography (1837): The emergence of public health in Calcutta", in *The Social History of Health and Medicine in India,* ed. Biswamoy Pati & Mark Harrison (London: Routledge, 2009), 15–31.

28. Curtin, *Death by Migration,* 1–39.

29. Harrison, *Public Health in British India,* 44.

30. B. Eswara Rao, "From Rajayak s(h)ma (disease of kings) to Blackman's plague: Perception on Prevalence and Aetiology of Tuberculosis in the Madras Presidency, 1882–1947," *Indian Economic and Social History Review* (2006): 457–485. doi: 10.1177%2F001946460604300403

31. Niels Brimnes, *Languished Hopes*, 33–35.

32. Arthur Lankester, *Tuberculosis in India: Its Prevalence, Causation and Prevention* (Kolkata: Butterworth & Co, 1920), 140.

33. Jones, "Tuberculosis, Housing and the Colonial State," 653–682.

34. Crosby, *The Colombian Exchange*; Martin Daunton & Rick Halpern, eds. *Empire and Others: British Encounters with Indigenous Peoples, 1600–1850* (Philadelphia: University of Pennsylvania Press, 1999).

35. Niels Brimnes, *Languished Hopes*, 33.

36. Worboys "Tuberculosis and Race in Britain and Its Empire, 1900–50," 144–167.

37. David McBride, *From TB to AIDS: Epidemics Among Urban Blacks Since 1900* (Albany: State University of New York Press, 1991), 9–30; Katharine Ott, "Race-ing Illness at the Turn of the Century", in *Fevered Lives: Tuberculosis in American Culture Since 1870* (Cambridge: Harvard University Press, 1996), 100–110. For theories on Mexican American susceptibility, see Emily K. Abel, "From Exclusion to Expulsion: Mexicans and Tuberculosis Control in Los Angeles, 1914 –1940", *Bulletin of the History of Medicine* 77, no. 4 (2003): 823–49; and Natalia Molina, *Fit to be Citizens? Public Health and Race in Los Angeles, 187-1939* (Berkeley: University of California Press. 2005), 133–136. For similarities between explanations of the high incidence of tuberculosis among "primitive peoples" in India and Africa, see Harrison and Worboys "A Disease of Civilization," 93–124. For theories on susceptibility in South Africa specifically, see Randall M. Packard, *White Plague, Black Labor: Tuberculosis and the Political Economy of Health and Disease in South Africa* (Berkeley: University of California Press, 1989), 194–210. For theories on racial susceptibility in general, see Warwick Anderson, "Immunities of Empire: Race, Disease, and the New Tropical Medicine, 1900–1920," *Bulletin of the History of Medicine* 70, no. 1 (1996): 94–118.

38. In the early nineteenth century, Western medical practitioners believed in the theory of virgin soil. According to this theory, some races and regions were virgin or less infected with the tubercle bacillus, particularly among African races and tropical regions. For details, see Harrison and Worboys, "A Disease of civilization," 110–111.

39. Packard, *White Plague,* 194–210.

40. L. S. Cummins, "Studies of Tuberculosis Among African Natives", *Tubercle* (1935), 13, cited in Worboys, "Tuberculosis and Race in Britain and its Empire, 1900–50," 144–167.

41. Bynum, *Spitting Blood;* Paul Weindling, *Health, Race, and German Politics between National Unification and Nazism, 1870–1945* (Cambridge: Cambridge University Press, 1989), 548.

42. Quoted by Niels Brimnes, *Languished Hopes*, 23–51.

43. Lankester, *Tuberculosis in India*, 14.

44. The main objects of Congress were "to exchange the information and experience gained throughout the world as to methods available for stamping out this disease. Papers will be read, and clinical and pathological demonstrations will be given . . ." *Proceedings of The Home Department, July, 1901, Objects of Congress*, File No: IOR/P/6115, July 1901, Asian and African Collection, British Library. London.

45. Bikramaditya Kumar Choudhary, "Colonial Policies and Spread of Tuberculosis: An Enquiry in British India", *Journal of Health & Development* 4, no. 1–4 (2008): 65–84.

46. Tuberculosis inquiry by Dr. Ukil 1929, 74/29, Public Health (Sanitary) Branch, National Archives of India, National Archives of India, hereafter NAI.

47. NAI, Home Department, Jail Branch, File No. 38 Jails of 1926.

48. *Annual Report of the Public Health Commissioner with the Government of India, 1899*, File no: IOR/V/24/3652, Asian and African Collection, British Library. London.

49. *The Proceedings of the first All India Sanitary Conference* held at Bombay on 13 and 14 November 1911, 2.

50. Dr. N. Sengupta, (M.D), "Points in the Prophylaxis and Treatment of Tuberculosis", *Journal of Indian Medical Association* 1, no. 7 (1932): 278–281.

51. P. Basu, *The Middleclass People in Calcutta: Being a Study of the Economic Conditions of the Middleclass People in Calcutta, and Their Effects upon the Health and Morals of the Rising Generation* (Kolkata: Chuckervertty Chatterjee & Co. Ltd, 1925).

52. R. M. Packard argued in the context of South Africa that newly Westernized Africans may have been particularly susceptible to TB. Thus, early Christian converts who adopted Western dress as a mark of their new enlightened status were among the first to feel the vice of poverty and suffered high rates of TB. See Packard, *White Plague,* 49.

53. Lankester, *Tuberculosis in India,* 162.

54. He says that because of Ramsuk's addiction of tea he began to suffer from dyspepsia and lost weight considerably:

"অবশেশে অসুশের সংবাদ পাইয়া
দদে দেশে দেশয় এশ া দদেয়াল ভাইয়া
শের লদশ া প্রেশেই চা োওয়াটা বন্ধ দব ভাোয় বশ দসলে দে ন্দে"।

(Ultimately, his brother received the news of his illness and came to his place from the countryside. the brother stopped his consumption of tea forcibly and began to rebuke him in own dialect) (translation mine). See Gautama Bhadra, *From an Imperial Product to a National Drink: The Culture of Tea Consumption in Modern India* (Centre for studies in Social Sciences, Kolkata, 2005), 3.

55. Rajarshi Mitra, "The famine in British India: Quantification Rhetoric and Colonial Disaster Management," *Journal of Creative Communications* 7, no. 1–2 (2012): 153–174.

56. S. Upadhyay, "Indian Working Class Housing: Survey and Suggestion," *The Calcutta Municipal Gazette, 1949, May 14th* (1949): 53.

57. Michael Mann, *South Asia's Modern History: Thematic Perspective* (London: Routledge, 2015), 283.

58. Lankester, *Tuberculosis in India*, 13.

59. Suvankar Dey, "The Silent Killer: Tracing the Trajectory of Tubercular Deaths in Colonial Bengal", *Indian Journal of History of Science* 55, no. 2 (2020).

60. *List of Motor Vehicles Registered in Calcutta (Corrected up to 1st July 1929),* (Kolkata: Bengal Secretariat Book Depot, 1929), 508–681.

61. Letter to the editor of Calcutta Municipal Gazette, 30th January, 1925.

62. A. C. Chatterji, "The Smoke Demon of Calcutta" *Amrita Bazar Patrika,* (1939, Feb 5), 25.

63. Arabinda Samanta discussed the connection of railway embankments with malaria, see Arabinda Samanta, *Living with Epidemics in Colonial Bengal 1818–1945* (New Delhi: Manhohar, 2017).

64. Matthew J. Saunders and Carlton A. Evans, "COVID-19: Tuberculosis and Poverty: Preventing a Perfect Storm," *European Respiratory Journal,* 56 (2020): 2001348.

BIBLIOGRAPHY

Abel, Emily K. "From Exclusion to Expulsion: Mexicans and Tuberculosis Control in Los Angeles, 1914–1940." *Bulletin of the History of Medicine* 77 no. 4 (2003): 823–49.

Anderson, Warwick. "Immunities of Empire: Race, Disease, and the New Tropical Medicine, 1900–1920." *Bulletin of the History of Medicine* 70, no. 1 (1996): 94–118.

Annual Report of the Public Health Commissioner with the Government of India, 1899.

Arnold, David. "The Indian Ocean as a Disease Zone, 1500–1950." *South Asia: Journal of South Asian Studies* 14, no. 2 (1991): 1–21.

Barnes, David S. *The Making of a Social Disease: Tuberculosis in 19th Century France.* Oxford: Oxford University Press, 1990.

Bashford, Alison. *Imperial Hygiene: A Critical History of Colonialism, Nationalism and Public Health.* Basinstoke: Palgrave Macmillan, 2004.

Basu, P. *The Middleclass People in Calcutta: Being a Study of the Economic Conditions of the Middleclass People in Calcutta, and Their Effects upon the Health and Morals of the Rising Generation.* Kolkata: Chuckervertty Chatterjee & Co. Ltd, 1925.

Bates, Barbara. *Bargaining for Life: A Social History of Tuberculosis, 1876–1938.* University of Pennsylvania Press, 1992.

Beinart, W., and L. Hughes. *Environment and Empire.* Oxford: Oxford University Press, 2007.

Bhadra, Gautama. *From an Imperial Product to a National Drink: The Culture of Tea Consumption in Modern India.* Kolkata: Centre for studies in Social Sciences, 2005.

Brimnes, Niels. *Languished Hopes: Tuberculosis, the State and International Assistance in Twentieth-Century India.* New Delhi: Orient Blackswan, 2016.

Bryder, Linda. *Below the Magic Mountain: A Social History of Tuberculosis, 1876–1938.* Oxford: Oxford University Press. 1992.

Bryder, Linda., F. Condrau, and Michael Worboys, eds. *Tuberculosis Then and Now: Perspective on the History of an Infectious Disease.* McGill-Queen's University Press, 2010.

Bynum, Helen. *Spitting Blood: The History of Tuberculosis.* Oxford: Oxford University Press, 2012.

Calcutta Municipal Gazette, 30 January, 1925.

Campbell, Judy. *Invisible Invaders: Smallpox and Other Diseases in Aboriginal Australia, 1780–1880.* Carlton South: Melbourne University Press, 2002.

Catanach, I. J. "Plague and the Tensions of Empire: India 1896–1918." In *Imperial Medicine and Indigenous Societies,* edited by David Arnold, 149–171. Manchester: Manchester University Press, 1988.

Chatterji, A. C. "The Smoke Demon of Calcutta" *Amrita Bazar Patrika,* February 5, 1939.

Choudhary, Bikramaditya Kumar. "Colonial Policies and Spread of Tuberculosis: An Enquiry in British India." *Journal of Health & Development* 4, no. 1–4 (2008): 65–84.

Cook, N. D. "Disease and Depopulation of Hispaniola, 1492–1518." *Colonial Latin American Review* 2, no. 1–2 (2013): 213–45.

Crosby, Alfred W. *Ecological Imperialism: The Biological Expansion of Europe, 900–1900.* Cambridge: Cambridge University Press. 1986.

Crosby, Alfred W. *The Colombian Exchange: The Biological Consequences of 1492.* Westport: Praeger Publication, 1971.

Curtin, Phillip D. *Death by Migration: Europe's Encounter with the Tropical World in the Nineteenth Century.* Cambridge: Cambridge University Press, 1989.

Datta, Partho. "Ranald Martin's Medical Topography (1837): The Emergence of Public Health in Calcutta." In *The Social History of Health and Medicine in India*, edited by Biswamoy Pati and Mark Harrison, 15–31. London: Routledge, 2009.

Daunton, Martin, and Rick Halpern, eds. *Empire and Others: British Encounters with Indigenous Peoples, 1600–1850.* Philadelphia: University of Pennsylvania Press, 1999.

David, N. *Born to Die: disease and New World conquest, 1492–1650.* Cambridge: Cambridge University Press, 1998.

Dey, Suvankar. "Captain of Death: Tuberculosis in colonial Bengal." In *Occasional Paper: New Scholarship in Indian Military History*, edited by Peter Stanley, 3–9. Canberra: University of Canberra Press, 2019.

Dey, Suvankar. "The Silent Killer: Tracing the Trajectory of Tubercular Deaths in Colonial Bengal." *Indian Journal of History of Science* 55, no. 2 (2020).

Dubos, R., and J. Dubos. *The White Plague: Tuberculosis, Man and Society.* New Jersey: Rutgers University Press, 1952, reprint 1987, 1996.

Espinosa, Maria. "The Invincible Generals: Yellow Fever and the Fight for Empire in Cuba, 1868–1898." In *Biomedicine as a Contested Site: Some Revelations in Imperial Contests,* edited by Poonam Bala, 67–79. Lanham, MD: Lexington Books, 2009.

Green, Monica H., and Lori Jones. "The Evolution and Spread of Major Human Disease in the Indian Ocean World." In *Disease Dispersion and Impact in the Indian Ocean World Studies*, edited by Gwyn Campbell & Eva-Maria Knoll, 25–57. Palgrave Macmillan, 2020.

Harrison, Mark. *Medicine in an Age of Commerce and Empire: Britain and Its Tropical Colonies 1660–1830.* Oxford: Oxford University Press, 2010.

Harrison, Mark, and Michael Worboys. "A Disease of Civilization: Tuberculosis in Britain, Africa and India 1900–39." In *Migrants, Minorities and Health, Historical and Contemporary Studies*, edited by Lara Marks and Michael Worboys, 93–124. London: Routledge; 1995.

Hays, J. N. *The Burdens of Disease: Epidemics and Human Response in Western History.* New Brunswick, NJ: Rutgers University Press, 2000.

Jones, G. *Captain of all these Men of Death: The history of Tuberculosis in 19th and 20th century Ireland.* New York: Rodopi B.V. 2001.

Jones, Margaret. *Health Policy in Britain's Model Colony: Ceylon (1900–1948)*. New Delhi: Orient Blackswan, 2018.

Jones, Margaret. "Tuberculosis, Housing and the Colonial State: Hong Kong, 1900–1950." *Modern Asian Studies* 37, no. 3 (2003): 654.

Kale, Madhavi. *Fragments of Empire: Capital, Slaver, and Indian Indentured Labor Migration in the British Caribbean.* Philadelphia: Philadelphia University Press, 1998.

Lankester, Arthur. *Tuberculosis in India: Its Prevalence, Causation and Prevention.* Kolkata: Butterworth & Co, 1920.

Levine, P. *Prostitution, Race and Politics: Policing Venereal Disease in the British Empire*. New York: Routledge, 2003.

Levine, Philippa. *The British Empire: Sunset to sunrise.* Great Britain: Pearson Longman, 2007.

List of Motor Vehicles Registered in Calcutta (Corrected up to 1st July 1929).

Manderson, L. *Sickness and the State: Health and Illness in Colonial Malaya 1870–1940.* Cambridge: Cambridge University Press, 1996.

Mann, M. *South Asia's Modern History: Thematic Perspectives.* Routledge: London, 2015.

Mann, Michael. *South Asia's Modern History: Thematic Perspective.* London: Routledge, 2015.

McBride, David. *From TB to AIDS: Epidemics Among Urban Blacks Since 1900.* Albany: State University of New York Press, 1991.

Mclvor, Aurthur, Ronald Johnston, and M. Lung. *A History of Dust Disease in British Coal Mining.* Aldershot: Ashgate, 2007.

McMillen, Christian W. *Discovering Tuberculosis: A Global History, 1900 to the present.* New Haven: Yale University Press, 2017.

Mitra, Rajarshi. "The famine in British India: Quantification rhetoric and Colonial disaster management." *Journal of Creative Communications* 7, no. 1–2 (2012): 153–174.

Molina, Natalia. *Fit to be Citizens? Public Health and Race in Los Angeles, 1879–1939.* Berkeley: University of California Press. 2005.

Murray, John F. "Tuberculosis and World War I." *American Journal of Critical Care Medicine* 192, no. 4 (2015): 411–14.

Newson, L. "Pathogens, Places and Peoples." In *Technology, Disease and Colonial Conquest, Sixteenth to Eighteenth Centuries,* edited by G Raudzens,167–210. Boston: Brill, 2001.

Ott, Katharine. *Fevered Lives: Tuberculosis in American Culture Since 1870.* Cambridge: Harvard University Press, 1996.

Packard, Randall M. *White Plague, Black Labor: Tuberculosis and the Political Economy of Health and Disease in South Africa.* Berkeley: University of California Press, 1989. *Proceedings of the Home Department, July, 1901*

Rao, B. Eswara. "From Rajayak s(h)ma (disease of kings) to Blackman's Plague: Perception on Prevalence and Aetiology of Tuberculosis in the Madras Presidency, 1882–1947." *Indian Economic and Social History Review* (2006): 457–485. https://doi.org/10.1177%2F001946460604300403

Rene, D., and J. Dubos, eds., *The White Plague: Tuberculosis, Man and Society*. London: Victor Gollancz, 1953.

Roy, Ladurie Le. *Mind and Method of the Historian,* trans. Siân Reynolds and Ben Reynolds. Brighton: Harvester, 1981, 28–83.

Roy, Rohan Deb. *Malarial Subjects: Empire, Medicine and Nonhumans in British India 1820–1909.* Cambridge: Cambridge University Press, 2017.

Samanta, Arabinda. "Living the Shadow of Death: Tubercular Body in Colonial Bengal." In *Contextualizing the Body: An Indian Experience* edited by Sudit Krishna Kumar and Suvobrata Sarkar, 165–177. New Delhi: Manohar, 2020.

Samanta, Arabinda. *Living with Epidemics in Colonial Bengal 1818–1945.* New Delhi: Manohar, 2017.

Saunders, Matthew J., and Carlton A. Evans. "COVID-19: Tuberculosis and Poverty: Preventing a Perfect Storm." *European Respiratory Journal* 56 (2020): 2001348.

Sengupta, N. "Points in the Prophylaxis and Treatment of Tuberculosis." *Journal of Indian Medical Association* 1, no. 7 (1932): 278–281.

Shlomowitz, Ralph, and John McDonald. "Mortality of Indian Labour on Ocean voyages, 1843–1917." *Studies in History* 6, no. 1 (1990): 35–65.

Stannard, D. *American Holocaust: Columbus and the Conquest of the New World.* Oxford: Oxford University Press, 1992.

The Proceedings of the first All India Sanitary Conference

Thompson, Willie. *Global Expansion: Britain and Its Empire, 1870–1914.* London: Pluto Press, 1999.

Ukil, Dr. A. C. 1929, 74/29, Public Health (Sanitary) Branch, National Archives of India, National Archives of India.

Upadhyay, S. "Indian Working Class Housing: Survey and Suggestion." *The Calcutta Municipal Gazette*, 1949, May 14th (1949): 53.

Weindling, Paul. *Health, Race, and German Politics between National Unification and Nazism, 1870–1945.* Cambridge: Cambridge University Press, 1989.

Worboys, Michael. "Tuberculosis and Race in Britain and Its Empire, 1900–50." In *Race, Science and Medicine 1700–1960*, edited by Waltraud Ernst and Bernard Harris, 144–167. Routledge, 1999.

Index

About the Contributors

Sahara Ahmed is professor of history, Rabindra Bharati University, West Bengal, India. Her publications focus on management and policies, forest management and development among others. Her select publications include "Conflicting Claims: The Colonial State Forests and Forest Dwellers in the Jalpaiguri District, 1869–1947", in Ranjan Chakrabarti (ed.), *Situating Environmental History* besides other publications, including "Flood Mayhem and the Colonial Government Disaster Management and Policy Implementation in the District of Jalpaiguri, c. 1880–1950", in *Calcutta Historical Journal*; "A legacy of Participation: Forest Management and Development, Jalpaiguri, c. 1880–1980", in *Itihas Probondhamala*; and Essay on "Andal" in *Dictionary of Historical Places, Bengal, 1757–1947*, ed. Ranjan Chakraborti, 1st edition (2013, Primus Books), among others.

Poonam Bala is a visiting scholar at Cleveland State University (USA) and Professor Extraordinarius in history at the University of South Africa (UNISA), South Africa. She has published extensively on medicine, policies and colonial empires as well as on disease and new biotechnologies, cancer and poverty in a social context. Her select publications include *Imperialism and Medicine in Bengal: A Socio-Historical Perspective* (Sage); ed. *Medicine and Colonialism: Historical Perspectives in India and South Africa* (Routledge); ed. *Learning from Empire: Medicine, Knowledge and Transfers under Portuguese Rule* (Cambridge Scholars), with a recent publication including, *"Ayurveda (re-)invented: Engagements with Science and Religion in Colonial India"* in Dorothea Lüddeckens, Philipp Hetmanczyk et al (eds.), *The Routledge Handbook of Religion, Medicine and Health* (Routledge), 421–34.

Mark F. Briskey is senior lecturer of criminology and coordinator of the Criminology Internships programme at Murdoch University, Australia. Prior to his academic career, he was employed by the Australian Government where he served in Australia and on several long-term overseas postings in Indonesia, Bangladesh, Sri Lanka and Pakistan. Mark was also formerly the head of the Australian Graduate School of Policing. His most recent publication is a chapter comparing Australian right-wing extremism between the 1930s and the current day within, *Back to the '30s? Recurring Crises of Capitalism, Liberalism, and Democracy* (Palgrave Macmillan), 24 September 2020, and a chapter contribution in the next edition of the *Cambridge Handbook of Forensic Psychology.*

Apalak Das is assistant professor of history, Rani Birla Girls' College, University of Calcutta, West Bengal, India. His publications include "Institutionalization of Leprosy Researches in Calcutta School of Tropical Medicine (CSTM) and other Programmes from 1920s to 1950s", *Indian Journal of History of Science*; "Transforming the Space: The 'Tribal Mind' through the Survey of Bengali Literature", in ed. Mahua Sarkar, *A Collage of Environmental History* and "Colonial Health Care in India", in the *Palgrave Encyclopedia of Health Humanities*, Springer Nature (forthcoming).

Sohini Das is a researcher at Jadavpur University, West Bengal, India with research interests focussed primarily on environmental history. Her select publications include *"Comparative study between Political thought of Phule and Ambedkar"* in ed. *Chittabrata Palit, Dalit Movements in Bengal*; *"The Early Strikes: An enquiry into the 1737 Cyclone and 1864 Cyclone"* in (ed.) *Chittabrata Palit, Natural Calamities in Colonial Bengal (Institute of Historical studies)*, and *"Medicine at the Margins: A Study of Indigenous Medical Knowledge in Western India"* in (ed.) *Aparajita Dhar, Pondering the Past: A Collection of Essays on Polity, Economy and Institutions.*

Suvankar Dey is assistant professor of history, Sidho Kanho Birsha University, Purulia, West Bengal, India. His publications include *Health has a history: Revisiting Bengal* (forthcoming); "King's Disease: Tuberculosis in colonial Calcutta (1900–1947)" in Debashis Bandyopadhyay and Pritha Kundu (eds.), *Imperial Maladies: Literatures on Healthcare and psychoanalysis in India*, besides other book chapters and research articles. His recent publication is an edited volume, *Health has a History: Revisiting Bengal*, 2021.

Matthew E. Franco is adjunct professor of history, Goucher College, Baltimore, Maryland, USA. His research focuses on the function of geographic science in the Bourbon Reforms, the history of cartography and the early modern Spanish world. He has also taught at the Johns Hopkins University, the University of Maryland, Baltimore County and Mount St Mary's University. His select publications include "Markings on the Map and Pillars in the Land: The Legacy of Spanish Imperial Geography", *Journal of Iberian and Latin American Studies* (invited contribution for a special issue, *New Directions in the Political History of the Ibero-Atlantic World c. 1750–1850*); "'The sooner they become American, the better': Spanish Imperial Geography and the Early Republic in the Age of Jefferson" (in press with American Philosophical Society Publication Department for special issue of the *Proceedings*); "Books, Bodies, and Messages in Bottles: Mapping Spanish Sovereignty in the Straits of Magellan" (accepted in *Endeavour*).

Amina Ameir Issa has been working as a historian at the Stone Town Conservation and Development Authority, a World Heritage City in Zanzibar, Tanzania; formerly, lecturer in history, State University of Zanzibar; and director of Museums and Antiquities and deputy principal secretary in the Ministry of Tourism and Heritage of Zanzibar. Her areas of interest include history of Zanzibar Stone Town and cultural history of Zanzibar Island, history of Western Medicine, public health and disease in colonial Zanzibar. Her select publications include 'Dhows and Epidemics in the Indian Ocean Ports'; 'Wedding Ceremonies and Cultural Exchange in an Indian Ocean port city: the Case of Zanzibar Town', and others published in *Social Dynamics* and *Journal of Culture and African Women Studies*. 'Women, Kanga and Political Movements in Zanzibar, 1958–1964'.

Saurav Kumar Rai is senior research assistant, Research and Publication Division, Nehru Memorial Museum and Library, Teen Murti House, New Delhi, India. His publications include "Invoking 'Hindu' Ayurveda: Communalisation of the Late Colonial Ayurvedic Discourse", *Indian Economic and Social History Review* (pp. 411–426); "Brahmanizing Ayurveda: Caste and Class Dimensions of Late Colonial Ayurveda Movement in Upper India" in *Summerhill: IIAS Review*, Vol. XXV/No. 2/Winter 2019, pp. 4–9; "Characterization of Medical Practitioners in Premchand's Writings" in *Shodhak*, Vol. 49/Pt. B/May–Aug 2019, pp. 166–173, besides others published in *History and Sociology of South Asia* and *Proceedings of the Indian History Congress*. He is also author of an undergraduate history textbook, *Debating Modern Indian History* (New Delhi: Manak Publications, 2021).

Jeff Ramsay is chairman, Livingstone Kolobeng College, Gaborone, Botswana. His select publications include (with Barry Morton), *Historical Dictionary of Botswana*, Fifth Edition; Khama-Real Leadership for Real

Delivery 2008–2013, Leapfrog, Gaborone, Contributor, *Historical Dictionary of Botswana*, Fourth Edition, co-author with Fred Morton and Themba Mgadla, "Batswana in African Pioneer Corps (1942–46)" in *Shield of the Nation: The Story of the Botswana Defence Force*, and *Comrad Fish, Memoirs of a Freedom Fighter in the Botswana Underground* (compiled with Barry Morton).

Arabinda Samanta is former professor of history at the University of Burdwan, West Bengal, India. A prolific writer on the social history of epidemics and medicine in colonial India, he is the author of *Malarial Fever in Colonial Bengal: Social History of an Epidemic* (2002), *Living with Epidemics in Colonial Bengal, 1818–1945* (2017) and co-editor of *The Revolt of 1857: Memory, Identity, History* (2009), *Life and Culture in Bengal: Colonial and Post-Colonial Experiences* (2011), *Praakrik Biparjay O Manush* (2003), *Saahityer Itihaas Kimba Itihaaser Sahitya* (2002), *Rog, Rogi O Raastra* (2004). He has been a visiting fellow at Zakir Husain Centre for Educational Studies, Jawaharlal Nehru University, New Delhi, at the Wellcome Trust Centre for the History of Medicine at University College, London (UK) and at the Rockefeller Archive Center, New York, USA.

Jacob Steere-Williams is associate professor of history, College of Charleston, South Carolina, USA. His publications include *The Filth Disease: Typhoid Fever and the Practices of British Epidemiology* (University of Rochester Press, Studies in Medical History along with several Public History Essays and Media Appearances including "What can we learn from past pandemics", UNESCO Webinar 23 July 2020, Interview appearance, Charleston, WCBD News, Mt. Pleasant; "History's Ears are Ringing", Royal College of Physicians of London, Wiley Publishing, and Library Journal Webinar; Interview appearance, Charleston Fox News 24; 'Charleston learned the Hard Way What Happens When You End a Quarantine Too Soon' *Post and Courier* besides several other publications.

Elizabeth van Heyningen is an honorary research associate in history at the University of Stellenbosch, South Africa, University of Stellenbosch, South Africa. Her research interests include the history of Cape Town, the history of colonial women and the social history of medicine. Her publications include *Cape Town: The Making of a City* and *Cape Town in the Twentieth Century* both with N. Worden and V. Bickford-Smith, and several research articles including a chapter in a book on the siege of Mafeking, on women in the siege. Her book *The Concentration Camps of the South African War. A Social History* (2013) was shortlisted for the *Sunday Times* Alan Paton prize in 2014. In 2017, she was a joint editor of *Selections from the Letters* *of President M.T. Steyn, 1904–1910*. Her recent project is papers of the three white women associated with the Industrial and Commercial Workers Union (I.C.U.), with a recent chapter for new history of the I.C.U.

Russel Viljoen is professor of history at the University of South Africa (UNISA), South Africa, with expertise that relates to indigenous Khoikhoi Studies. He has published extensively on the indigenous Khoikhoi, including the social history of disease and medicine in colonial contexts and its impact on indigenous communities in colonial South Africa. His select publications include a monograph, *Jan Paerl: A Khoikhoi Cape Colonial Society, 1761–1851* (Brill, 2006), "Moravian Missionaries, Khoisan Labour and the Overberg Colonists at the end of the VOC era, 1792–1795", in Bredekamp, H.C. and Ross, R. (eds), *Missions and Christianity in South African History*; "'Disease, Doctors and De Beers Capitalists': Smallpox and Scandal in Colonial Kimberley, South Africa, during the Mineral Revolution and British Imperialism, 1882–1883", in Bala, P, (ed.) *Biomedicine as a Contested Site: Some Revelations in Imperial Contexts*, besides others. His forthcoming book is titled, *Khoikhoi, Microhistory and Colonial Characters at the Cape of Good Hope* (Lexington, 2023).